CONTEMPORARY HEALTH PSYCHOLOGY

This radical new textbook provides readers with a balanced, research-focused, critical understanding of health psychology through an inclusive lens, addressing issues relating to diversity, inclusion and decolonisation of the curriculum. In so doing, it offers a new understanding on established topics in the field of health psychology to create a more comprehensive and nuanced understanding of health and illness that reflects the diversity of human experience.

The book explores the importance of biopsychosocial processes in health and illness, through an exploration of socio-cultural factors beyond the restrictive Western-centric models of health to include Indigenous populations and marginalised groups. Within this book, readers are introduced to the negative health impacts of direct and transgenerational colonialism, racism, restrictions on cultural practices, freedoms and institutionalisation. This includes recognising the impact of systemic oppression on health outcomes and advocating for policies that address health disparities of diverse populations in order to tailor interventions to meet their specific needs. Research studies present examples of how sexual orientation, gender identity, ethnicity, culture and disabilities intersect with health outcomes in the exploration and the perpetuation of health disparities.

Primarily written for undergraduates, the book also provides a firm foundation for graduate students, teachers and practitioners in psychology, nursing and the allied health professions.

Dr Lynn Dunwoody is a Lecturer in Health Psychology in the School of Psychology, Ulster University, United Kingdom. She has been engaged in teaching, training and research of health psychology for over 30 years, has been involved in curriculum development for British Psychological Society (BPS) stage 1 and 2 training in health psychology since 2007 and is the Head of Assessment for the Stage 2 Qualification in Health Psychology. She is a Health and Care Professions Council (HCPC)-registered Health Psychologist and a Chartered Psychologist with the BPS. Lynn's research is health psychology focused on the areas of adversarial growth, Cognitive Behaviour Therapy (CBT) and quality of life in relation to cancer; physical activity and cancer rehabilitation, palliative care, psychosocial interventions and physical activity in community-dwelling adults, along with the psychological and physical benefits of walking and being a volunteer community walk leader.

BPS Core Textbooks Series

Series editor: Simon Goodson

Routledge in partnership with British Psychological Society are pleased to present their flagship textbook program, the *BPS Core Textbooks Series*. Aimed at a global undergraduate readership, these volumes are designed to be core texts for course adoption, covering all key subject areas in Psychology.

Diversity, equity and inclusion are at the heart of the series. Each book includes a strong focus on all aspects of diversity, including decolonising the curriculum and an understanding of the value of multiple perspectives. There is also a spotlight on employability, to explain why a grounding in basic theoretical areas is necessary for careers in Psychology. There is also a focus on real-world applications and life skills, to help students explore the use of psychological theory to answer real-world questions. These full colour books include a range of pedagogical features, illustrations and figures, with content to emphasise critical thinking and study skills and the unpicking of pseudoscience.

Books are available in traditional print format, as well as our innovative enhanced eBook format. This includes integrative features such as popup keyword definitions, hypertext links to web-based resources, short-answer/open-ended questions, multiple-choice and true/false quizzes and video clips. There is a series website hosting additional digital resources for both students and instructors to tie in with learning objectives.

The books in the *BPS Core Textbooks Series* are essential reading in the core areas in any Psychology honours degree or conversion-level course. They are also relevant as secondary reading in related disciplines.

Titles in the series:

Cognitive Psychology in a Changing World
Linden Ball, Laurie Butler, Sue Sherman & Helen St Clair-Thompson

An Introduction to Cyberpsychology, 2nd edition
Edited by Gráinne Kirwan, Irene Connolly, Hannah Barton, Marion Palmer

Contemporary Health Psychology
Edited by Lynn Dunwoody

For more information about this series, please visit: www.routledge.com/our-products/book-series/BPSCT

CONTEMPORARY HEALTH PSYCHOLOGY

An Inclusive and Culturally-Responsive Approach

LYNN DUNWOODY

Routledge
Taylor & Francis Group
LONDON AND NEW YORK

Designed cover image: Getty © SolStock

First published 2026
by Routledge
4 Park Square, Milton Park, Abingdon, Oxon OX14 4RN

and by Routledge
605 Third Avenue, New York, NY 10158

Routledge is an imprint of the Taylor & Francis Group, an informa business

British Library Cataloguing-in-Publication Data
A catalogue record for this book is available from the British Library

ISBN: 9781032729442 (hbk)
ISBN: 9781032707433 (pbk)
ISBN: 9781003423157 (ebk)
ISBN: 9781003774488 (ebk+)

DOI: 10.4324/9781003423157

Typeset in Stone Serif
by KnowledgeWorks Global Ltd.

Access the Instructor and Student Resources: https://routledgelearning.com/bpscoretextbooks/

The BPS Core Textbooks Series is committed to creating an inclusive environment for all our readers. We acknowledge that language use is constantly evolving and best endeavours have been made to ensure that our language guidelines are up to date at the time of publication. Further, in some cases, the terminology exists within original records and has been retained to inform users on viewpoints at the time. Therefore, textbooks may contain references to potentially challenging terminology relating to protected characteristics which could be considered offensive. It in no way reflects the attitudes of the authors, the British Psychological Society or Routledge.

Disclaimer: Working within your competence

The British Psychological Society acknowledge that delivering services to a necessary professional standard requires specialist knowledge, skills, training and experience. Students should be aware of the importance of working within the recognised limitations of their competence and expertise to ensure ethical and effective practice, seeking supervision or guidance when necessary. This is stated in the BPS Code of Ethics and Conduct.

Contents

1 Health psychology context setting

Careers, cultures and diversity

Chapter contents

- A brief introduction to health psychology.
- Health psychology careers.
- Culture and diversity in healthcare contexts.
- An introduction to decolonisation and intersectionality.

Chapter objectives

After reading this chapter, you should be able to answer the following questions:

- What health contexts do health psychologists work in?
- What psychological information do health psychologists draw on in their practice?
- Why is it important for health psychologists to understand the impacts of decolonisation on health and healthcare?
- Outline the difference between sex, gender, sexual orientation and gender identity.
- Describe and provide examples of what is meant by minoritised groups and intersectionality.

Brief introduction to health psychology

We know that living with a **physical health condition**, for example, heart disease, diabetes or cancer, can influence people's thoughts, emotions and behaviours. Depression and anxiety can result in people engaging in lifestyle behaviours that are detrimental to physical health (Marks et al., 2000). That said, **health psychology** is mainly concerned with physical health rather than mental health conditions; it involves the interrelationship of how biomedical, psychological, social and cultural factors influence people's physical health. Improvements in sanitation, clean drinking water, better nutrition and medication have helped to reduce the burden of **infectious diseases**. People are living longer, but they are having to cope with **chronic diseases** and/or disability caused by

DOI: 10.4324/9781003423157-1

heart problems, stroke, diabetes, cancer, lung problems and obesity (see Chapters 2, 5 and 9). The challenges of living with and trying to prevent these long-term conditions that are influenced by lifestyle behaviours (e.g. smoking, diet and being sedentary) led the way for the development of health psychology. However, lifestyle factors are subject to wider influences, which include income, educational level and **ethnicity**; the geographical location that a person lives in; having a disability, gender identity and sexual orientation; and being from an **Indigenous** population.

Health psychology careers

The contexts in which health psychologists work

Health psychologists play a vital role in improving health outcomes by applying psychological theory, research and evidence to real-world physical health challenges. They train and supervise other healthcare professionals and psychologists. Health psychologists deliver educational materials about health psychology theories and specific types of therapies; they design, develop and evaluate **health interventions** to prevent disease and to improve and manage physical health conditions. Teaching and research are also part of a health psychologist's remit; this includes topics, such as research and research methods, statistics, research ethics, how to conduct **audits** and **service evaluations**. Team working, leadership and **patient and public involvement** help shape health research, services and policies. Health psychologists support other healthcare professionals, patients, families, communities and workplaces in the delivery of behaviour change interventions and skills.

Health promotion

Working within **health promotion**, health psychologists help people to take control of and to improve health habits using education, support and healthy lifestyle initiatives. For example, this includes behaviours related to smoking, overeating, eating sugary or high-fat foods, reducing sedentary lifestyles and avoiding risky sexual practices, all of which can be harmful to health. Health psychologists also contribute to disease prevention by devising strategies that help reduce barriers to the uptake of **screening** to detect diseases such as breast, bowel and cervical cancers at an asymptomatic stage and through the uptake of various vaccinations that are targeted at specific populations and age groups. With a globally ageing population who are living with chronic diseases, health psychologists assist people to cope with disease symptoms, to adhere to medical advice/treatments and to cope with the side effects of treatments.

Working with teams

Health psychologists have an important role to play in a range of healthcare settings and contexts, one particular focus is in chronic health conditions. This can range from working at an individual level with patients to working with families, carers and other healthcare professionals. Work can include being part of a **multidisciplinary team (MDT)**, managing teams and/or advising on strategies to improve health. An MDT consists of healthcare professionals from different disciplines working together to provide integrated patient care. Each member of the MDT will have expertise in a certain area of patient care, team members may include anaesthetists, clinical physiologists, dieticians, doctors, nurses, occupational therapists, pharmacists, physiotherapists, health psychologists, radiologists, social workers and surgeons. The exact makeup of the team will depend on the nature of the disease being treated. These healthcare professionals will have their own specialist knowledge and they will share information and assessments to ensure that all treatment options are considered to provide patients with the best possible treatment outcomes. A patient may not see every one of these healthcare professionals, but each of them may have had some input into the patient's care.

Working in chronic disease contexts

Working within MDTs and patients across a range of diseases, health psychologists help improve patient outcomes. For example, assisting patients to prepare for medical procedures by putting in place strategies to help a patient to lose weight prior to surgery, or supporting a patient and their family to prepare for transplant surgery by offering support and guidance on post-transplant adjustments, such as adhering to lifelong medications. When people have chronic pain, health psychologists can provide education about chronic pain, the role of stress, emotions and pain perceptions. This may help patients identify triggers that make their pain worse and strategies may be devised to manage flare-ups in pain. To help patients cope with chronic pain, a health psychologist may explore and challenge negative thoughts about pain, ways to reduce pain-related anxiety and depression, encouraging physical activity, relaxation and improving sleep. Over 50% of patients living with and beyond cancer **experience cancer-related fatigue** (CRF), which is a pervasive type of fatigue thought to be related to cancer treatments, such as surgery, chemotherapy and radiation. Health psychologists help people engage in lifestyle management including individually tailored progressive physical activity, relaxation and/or **mindfulness**. Health psychologists can help patients to manage unhelpful thoughts and devise strategies to target sleep problems, create collaborative goals to maintain everyday activities and conserve energy. These are just a few examples of how health psychologists work with patients who have chronic diseases.

Strategic working

At a more strategic level, health psychologists devise interventions based on psychological theories that can be used to train other staff to deliver and evaluate them. This may include interventions that have tangible effects on the health service and patient transition through the healthcare system. Between diagnosis and receipt of treatment, health psychologists can help prepare patients for coming into hospital through the design and delivery of **prehabilitation** programmes, with a focus on getting patients nutritionally, emotionally and physically fit for treatment. For example, promoting healthy eating, reducing alcohol consumption, supporting smoking cessation and encouraging physical activity. Depending on the type of treatment or procedure, psychological preparation may also be required to deal with treatment-related anxiety and post-treatment barriers to successful **rehabilitation** to help the patient recover from treatment or illness. Prehabilitation programmes help speed up patient recovery, reduce the length of hospital stay and the likelihood of readmission. Shorter hospital stays mean patients are at lower risk of developing hospital-acquired infections, help to free up beds for other patients and reduce treatment waiting lists.

What knowledge do health psychologists use?

Health psychologists draw on knowledge from a range of different areas of psychology, such as biopsychology, to understand the structure and function of the brain, nervous system, immune and endocrine systems (see Chapter 4). Knowing about an individual's health perceptions, emotions, thoughts and how they interact when making sense of disease symptoms (see Chapter 5), along with the impact of stress and coping mechanisms, is important for health outcomes (see Chapter 8). Social psychology is of use to health psychologists in the assessment and understanding of health behaviours, which may be influenced by **social norms** and the role of significant others, such as role models and media influencers (see Chapter 7). With a focus on health and disease during an individual's lifespan, health psychology also draws on knowledge, research and practice in **palliative care** and **end-of-life care** (see Chapter 11). Health psychologists are interested in the intersections of **culture**, disability, gender identity and sexual orientation educational level, socioeconomic status (SES) and ethnicity that may result in unequal or unfair care due to **discrimination** and **stigma** associated with marginalised identities. The impacts of dominant countries taking over control of land and dominating Indigenous Peoples by subjugating their culture, values, language, knowledge and ways of life during **colonisation** have also had negative impacts on health and contributed to long-term health problems (see Chapter 9). Knowledge and understanding of research methods and different types of analyses are essential areas of interest for health psychologists, so that they can conduct well-designed research, evaluate psychological interventions and make use of questionnaires and other outcome measures (see Chapter 3). Psychological insights into personality can offer explanations of individual differences in health behaviours and links to the experience of stress (Chapter 8). Patients' understanding of health information can impact adherence to medical advice and medication (see Chapter 6), support successful pain management (see Chapter 10) and influence factors associated with the development of chronic diseases (see Chapter 9). Finally, viewing health psychology through a critical lens helps health psychologists understand **social injustices** experienced by some marginalised groups within society who are not afforded the same rights to healthcare as others. This may be due to the dominant culture holding more influence and access to resources due to **power imbalances** that exist on a global, societal, organisational and personal level (Prilleltensky & Prilleltensky, 2003), with an emphasis on respecting equity, equality (see Box 1.1), diversity and inclusion. This is not an exhaustive account of the role of various aspects of psychology that can be applied to health and disease but should serve as an indication of some of the ways in which health psychologists draw on psychological theory and knowledge within their practice.

BOX 1.1
EQUITY AND EQUALITY IN HEALTH, WHAT IS THE DIFFERENCE?

The terms equity and equality sound similar, but they have important differences. **Health equity** is about providing everyone with the specific support they need to live as healthy a life as possible. It is concerned with allocating healthcare resources based on need. **Health equality** involves equal access to healthcare support, e.g. access to appointments with a doctor, getting treatment at emergency departments and access to prescribed medication. This sounds good in theory, but in practice it may not work due to health inequities, which are consistent, preventable and unjust differences in healthcare access and outcomes between groups (McCartney et al., 2019). For example, people may have equal access to scheduling a medical appointment, but due to financial penalties, an individual may not be able to take time off work to attend the appointment, may not have access to transport or may be unable to afford the costs of prescribed medication. People with physical disabilities often experience inequities in accessing healthcare and have unmet needs (Umucu et al., 2025). For example, to discuss problems with healthcare professionals, an individual who is deaf or has difficulty hearing may require someone to help with sign language, but interpreters are not always available, especially at short notice when health emergencies occur (James et al., 2022). In addition, patients who do not speak the language of the dominant culture may be exposed to communication errors of up to 22% when they use informal bilingual family members. Heath et al. (2023) found a 12% error rate for professionally translated information, which has the potential to impact patient safety. Health inequities occur when culturally appropriate care is not provided for people from ethnic minorities (Joo & Liu, 2021), Indigenous Peoples (Statistics Canada, 2024) and sexual and gender minority populations (Lamba et al., 2023).

Where do health psychologists work?

Health psychologists practice in a diverse range of contexts and services, which include private practice, universities, the National Health Service (NHS), government, charities, community organisations, schools, prisons and private organisations. Health psychologists may address issues identified by health-related organisations, including NHS trusts, health authorities and public health bodies. Those who use the services of health psychologists include individuals, families, groups, communities, large organisations and health professionals who work at a population level. Health psychologists treat, advise and conduct research with a range of people, including those who are healthy, patients, families, carers and other healthcare professionals. They work across the lifespan from pre-natal and post-natal phases of pregnancy, through childhood and teenage years, to young adults, adults and older people. Their work may be focused on specific health problems and on health promotion and disease prevention, which can include the design, delivery and evaluation of health interventions.

Outside of the healthcare service, health psychologists may work in independent practice and in higher education institutions (HEIs), such as universities.

Health psychologists have a role in educating the next generation through teaching and supervising trainees on postgraduate training courses and teaching psychology to undergraduate students. Research is also an important aspect of a health psychologist's work; this involves not just designing and conducting research but also working with and leading teams to apply for funding to conduct research. Once completed, research needs to be disseminated; health psychologists publish and share the outputs of research in academic journals; at conferences; in policy documents, at public information sessions, in public and healthcare professional facing documents, podcasts, videos and web pages. Research involves working in teams that may be within and across HEIs, in partnership with healthcare organisations and through regional, national and international collaborations. Conducting and planning research requires collaboration with external organisations, such as charities, governmental bodies, voluntary and community groups, the health service, the public, patients, families and carers.

UK training to become a health psychologist

Becoming a health psychologist in the UK involves completion of an undergraduate degree in psychology (or equivalent), followed by specialist postgraduate training. While it is possible to apply health psychology knowledge to various work settings without being a health psychologist, within the UK, health psychologists must, by law, be registered with the Health and Care Professions Council (HCPC), which is the statutory regulator for all practitioner psychologists. It is a criminal offence to call yourself a health psychologist if you are not on the HCPC register. Most health psychologists are also chartered members of the British Psychological Society (BPS), which is the professional body for psychologists in the UK.

At the current time, to train as a health psychologist in the UK, you must have completed a BPS-accredited undergraduate degree in psychology or a conversion course that confers Graduate Basis for Chartered Membership (GBC). If you have a non-UK undergraduate qualification, you can apply to the BPS to have this assessed for eligibility for GBC. Once GBC has been achieved, you need to complete stage 1 of training, which involves successful completion of an accredited MSc in Health Psychology; this covers the knowledge and core skills necessary to progress to stage 2 of training, which is at doctoral level. The latter involves at least two years of full-time supervised practice within health psychology settings, covering professional skills, psychological interventions, research, working as an expert in a **consultancy** capacity to provide expert health psychology advice and guidance to clients. The final aspect of a stage 2 qualification is delivery of teaching and training. Stage 2 training can be completed through a university-based professional doctorate in health psychology, a PhD plus a portfolio of practice in health psychology or through the BPS-independent route, called the Qualification in Health Psychology (QHP). Regardless of the route taken, successful completion confers eligibility to apply to the HCPC for entry onto the register as a practitioner health psychologist. You may also apply to become a chartered psychologist with the BPS and to join the BPS Division of Health Psychology as a full member. If your health psychology postgraduate training (including the practice component) has been completed outside the UK, it is possible to apply to the HCPC to have your education, training and experience assessed against the standards of proficiency for health psychologists.

Culture and diversity in healthcare contexts

As we will see in Chapter 2, the **biopsychosocial approach** to health and disease moves beyond the narrow focus of the **biomedical model** that views the causes of disease as genetics, viruses, bacteria, chemical imbalances and trauma. Rather than viewing people as helpless victims of disease, the biopsychosocial approach recognises the importance of biomedical, psychological and social factors in health and disease. For example, in conditions such as heart, lung diseases and cancer, an individual's knowledge about health and their health behaviours can influence both risk and recovery. Social factors, such as family relationships, occupation, ethnicity and income, also shape patterns of health and disease. Through a biopsychosocial lens, individuals are seen as having some responsibility for their own health, as they can promote health by engaging in health-related behaviours, such as eating a balanced diet, getting enough rest and being physically active. However, the opposite is also true, as individuals may engage in behaviours that can be compromising to health, such as smoking, drinking excessively, overeating or eating an unhealthy diet. At first glance, the biopsychosocial model appears to offer a comprehensive approach to explaining differences in people's health and disease, yet it does not always account for broader issues such as health inequities. People from different genders, sexual orientations, ethnic minority backgrounds, Indigenous communities or those living with disabilities may face systemic barriers that limit their ability to make healthy choices. For this reason, many health psychologists argue that an ecological view of health and disease is more appropriate (see Chapter 2). This perspective emphasises the interrelationships of interpersonal, organisational, community and policy factors (McLeroy et al., 1988), along with the role of different social identities, such as gender, ethnicity and socioeconomic status (SES), which may intersect to shape health experiences and outcomes.

An introduction to decolonisation and intersectionality

The importance of decolonisation

Historically, many countries across the globe were dominated by invading nations, mainly from the West, who removed Indigenous Peoples from their lands, imposed colonialist ideologies, religions and education. This resulted in subjugation of Indigenous culture, ways of living, languages and healthcare practices. It created a hierarchy of power that exploited and abused Indigenous Peoples. Colonialisation imposed Western ideals and thinking, which have been referred to as 'dominant Western worldview' and this was deemed by colonisers as superior to Indigenous knowledge. Within this textbook, Western refers to thinking and ways of understanding that are based on mainly European and/or North American culture and scientific knowledge. Over the past number of years, there has been renewed interest in decolonising the higher education curriculum, but it is important to note the process of **decolonisation** has a longer history (Jan & Osterhammed, 2017). The United Nations Declaration on the Rights of Indigenous Peoples (UNDRIP) (2007) protected Indigenous Peoples' rights to make decisions about their own healthcare and it emphasised respect for culture, the use of traditional healing practices and medicines. It stipulated that Indigenous Peoples should have the same access to high-quality healthcare as non-Indigenous populations and that holistic health, which includes connections to the land, language, family and community, was to be respected. This was meant to include processes to eliminate the enduring effects of colonisation, typified by discriminatory attitudes, assumptions, institutional structures and **paternalistic power relations** in formerly colonised societies, but as we will see throughout this textbook, colonisation continues to shape and contribute to health inequities.

Decolonisation of the curriculum

Decolonisation of knowledge has a long history within postcolonial societies; however, it came to prominence within universities in 2015 at the University of Cape Town and spread to the UK. This created a groundswell of thinking about the need for educators to reflect on historical injustices, conscious and unconscious biases, especially those that continue to persist in healthcare teaching, research and practice today (Carleton-Boylan et al., 2024). Higher educational institutions (HEIs) in the UK have, due to student pressure, started to examine their historical links to benefactors involved in the slave trade and colonialism. This has led to the removal of some commemorative statues from campuses and the renaming of buildings by several institutions. While this acknowledges some of the injustices of the past, it is necessary to go further by updating the curriculum, so that students are afforded the opportunity to learn about the impact of colonialism, exploitation and injustices that continue to impact health practices of today. This is especially true in situations where healthcare knowledge and techniques were developed through nonconsensual experimentation on Indigenous People, ethnic minorities and people with disabilities (Carleton-Boylan et al., 2024). Thus, for decolonisation to be meaningful, it is important to go beyond the perfunctory action of adding non-White European authors to reading lists, it is essential that we all understand and reflect on the impact that colonialisation has had on Indigenous Peoples, ethnic minority populations and the negative consequences on health and healthcare for these groups. In so doing, there is a need to educate students and healthcare professionals about diversity in health outcomes, access to healthcare, along with the needs and experiences of minority groups. We need to learn about respecting non-Western perspectives and practices of health and healthcare that are often ignored in health professional teaching and subjugated by the past and present colonialist attitudes that 'West is best'.

According to Sherwood and Edwards (2006), decolonisation is a process, which requires researchers and practitioners to critically reflect on their own values, beliefs and assumptions to appreciate and accept that alternative world views, knowledge systems and ways of working are equally valid. It is common to find that reading lists, research examples and societal exemplars used in healthcare teaching, research and research funding are biased towards White American and **Eurocentric** populations, with scant attention to the impact of colonialisation and/or minority voices. Even when minority voices are considered, it is usually to paternalistically apply **Western conceptualisations** of health, illness and healthcare. This typically interprets higher rates of disease in minority groups, as being due to deficiencies that rest within these individuals who require 'fixing' by adhering to Western health practices. This perpetuates oppression and discrimination and ignores the strengths of collectivist-based health practices and Indigenous knowledge.

Where possible throughout this textbook, the author has sought to draw on examples of the impacts of colonialism and Western knowledge on health, disease, healthcare practices and how health outcomes and interventions need to consider axes of **intersectionality**. Drawing on a quotation from Morreira et al. (2020, p. 2) serves to highlight that this health psychology-focused textbook will be a starting point for many learners, as "there is no one single way of implementing decolonial [and intersectional] thought and practice in the classroom, and that this may well be recognised as a strength rather than a limitation".

It is important to note that when talking about decolonising the curriculum, it is a process that adds to knowledge, it is not a mechanism for erasing Western-centric knowledge, research and ideas. Decolonisation helps to give voice to non-White, non-European people and encourage diversity. While it is not within the scope of this book to 'decolonise' health psychology, it is hoped that the content will help students, researchers and healthcare professionals to consider their conscious and unconscious colonialist assumptions, knowledges and biases that have been gained through education. Moreover, it is necessary to consider these factors when reading scholarly literature on health psychology, interacting with and developing health interventions for people from minority groups and other cultural backgrounds. There are many excellent textbooks on health psychology that cover a much broader range of topics and in much greater depth than this text, but they do not consider the Indigenous ways of knowing and traditional knowledge about health and healthcare practices that have been subjugated to facilitate the 'superiority' of Western medicine. The aim of this textbook is to consider mainstream health psychology knowledge and give equal consideration (where possible) to Indigenous Peoples, ethnic, sexual and gender minorities and people with disabilities.

Indigenous Peoples

It is recognised that there are over 476 million Indigenous Peoples around the globe, spanning almost 100 countries (United Nations, n.d.). Their cultures, languages, lands and human rights have been and continue to be subjugated by colonialism, which has resulted in **intergenerational trauma**. When writing about Indigenous Peoples, there can be political tensions, with some countries denying indignation and referring only to ethnic minorities (Kozlov et al., 2007). India, China and the Siberian area of Russia have large populations of Indigenous Peoples, but there is very little information on their health or research with these groups (Coates, 2004). For pragmatic reasons, this textbook will focus on the Indigenous Peoples within Canada, Australia, New Zealand and the US, as most of the literature, health-related polices and changes in health practices have taken place in these counties. That is not to deny or negate the colonial subjugation of other Indigenous populations around the globe who are still living and coping with the many traumas inflicted by non-Indigenous settlers on their lands.

Indigenous Peoples around the world are diverse in their culture, language and traditions, even within the same country, making it difficult to provide an all-encompassing definition of Indigenous Peoples. That said, self-identification as Indigenous has been recognised by the United Nations (2007) and Martínez Cobo (1981) highlighted that Indigenous Peoples have continuous links to the land that predate colonisation, they identify as being distinct from the non-Indigenous population and are committed to protecting their ancestral lands for the next generation.

Use of the term 'Indigenous Peoples' has been viewed as being problematic due to its broad application to diverse groups who have distinct languages, cultures, lands, spiritual beliefs and traditions. While acknowledging the problem of terminology, the use of more specific identifiers, such as First Nations, Inuit and Métis to describe the Indigenous Peoples of Canada, Native Americans and Alsakan Natives in the US, Aboriginal and Torres Strait Islanders of Australia and Māori in New Zealand, allows for clear distinctions between Indigenous groups. However, researchers do not always specify the particular Indigenous communities that have been studied. Where specific Indigenous groups have been named, they will be reported within this textbook, otherwise research will be discussed using the term Indigenous Peoples. While there is diversity among Indigenous Peoples both within- and between countries, they all share a common history of colonialisation.

Colonialisation has deprived Indigenous Peoples of their land, rights, wealth, sovereignty and wellbeing (Durie, 2004). Their voices have often been silenced, especially in health-related research, which has been based on practices that ignore Indigenous viewpoints (Sherwood & Edwards, 2006). For Aboriginal, Torres Strait Islanders, Māori, First Nations, Inuit, Métis, Native American and Alaskan Native Peoples, land has meaning that goes beyond property ownership or monetary wealth, it has spiritual meaning and cultural significance for the community. Being dispossessed of land and Indigenous knowledge systems impacts health and health improvement of these Peoples. Western approaches to health emphasise the role of individual behaviours and the medicalisation of health and illness. While there may be some recognition of Indigenous conceptions of health, it seems that Western policies and practices predominate and separate health from Indigenous People's lives, traditions and knowledge that have been handed down through community Elders, all of which are central to the development of their holistic health (Sherwood & Edwards, 2006). These authors point to the continued application of Western world views on health, which contributes to health inequities in Aboriginal and Torres Strait Islanders of Australia.

Minority ethnic groups

A minority ethnic group refers to a group of people who have a shared and distinct culture, history, language and/or traditions that are different from those of the majority who live in a country. BAME is often used to refer to people who are from Black, Asian and Minority Ethnic backgrounds and cultures. However, the author wishes to acknowledge that BAME is not an inclusive term, as it implies that people from various ethnic groups are homogenous, in addition, the acronym emphasises one group over another. There are variations in the power and inequities experienced by people from different cultural backgrounds and using BAME excludes other mixed-ethnicity groups. For example, saying someone is of an Asian ethnicity is a broad descriptor, as it does not delineate between someone who is Indian, Pakistani, Chinese, Vietnamese or who may describe themselves as British Asian. Within this textbook when exploring previous research, the acronym BAME will be reported when it is used by researchers within their publications. However, terminology is an important consideration when writing and talking about communities that have been marginalised due to culture, beliefs and identities. To avoid treating distinctly diverse groups as if they were one and the same, where possible, the specific ethnic group will be reported or the term minority ethnic group will be used (Lokugamage et al., 2022).

In the UK, the colonial legacy that permeated all society is still prevalent within the healthcare system today. This includes paternalistic attitudes, unequal power dynamics and the value placed on White Eurocentric perspectives in health education and practice. This may have negative consequences on the health needs of ethnic minority communities, as cultural sensitivities may not be factored into healthcare provision. This may contribute to a clash of cultural health practices and a lack of understanding from both the healthcare professional and the patient viewpoints. In addition, language barriers can have negative impacts on healthcare utilisation and communication between health professional staff and patients. Across England and Wales, 8.9% of the population do not speak English (or Welsh in Wales), that means around 5.1 million people (Office for National Statistics, 2022) may have difficulty in accessing healthcare information and services. Moreover, the needs of patients who have multiple marginalised identities, such as ethnicity, gender orientation, sexual orientation and disabilities, must be addressed, as they have all been linked to poorer health outcomes (Marmot et al., 2020).

One way to try and overcome such inequities is to engage in targeted interventions; however, research shows that not all interventions are impactful and can fail due to cultural insensitivity or lack of responsiveness to the needs of the diverse communities they were designed to help. To enhance the experiences of patients from ethnic minority communities, it is essential that healthcare staff are upskilled in relation to the health beliefs, culture and traditions associated with the populations they work with. Embedding **cultural competence** training into the curriculum for healthcare professional students and trainees can lead to **cultural sensitivity** and improved health outcomes for ethnic minority communities. Furthermore, the legacy of paternalistic delivery of healthcare needs to be disbanded by listening to the voices of patient representatives and community groups. This may help empower minority groups to engage in a partnership way of working to improve health outcomes. Taking such an approach will facilitate the sharing of cultural practices and beliefs, embedding patient choice in decision-making and hopefully promoting patient-centred care.

Sex and gender terminology

To ensure the usage of correct terminology, it is important to know the difference between the terms such as sex and gender. Sex describes the physiological and anatomical differences between males and females, which are based on their reproductive organs, chromosomes and hormones. Typically, males will have XY and females XX chromosomes and these will help to determine if the individual develops male or female reproductive organs and associated hormones. The American Psychological Association (APA, 2020) defines gender as a socially and culturally defined construct that is characterised by certain behaviours, attitudes, feelings, activities and expectations related to the 'psychological sense' of a person's sex. How a person sees themselves in terms of gender is their gender identity, which can be different to their biological sex. An individual can change their gender identity, which means it may not align with their ascribed sex at birth. There are a range of gender identities, for example, girl or a woman, boy or a man, transgender, gender-neutral, non-binary and gender-queer, but this is not an exhaustive list. A person whose sex at birth and gender identity corresponds, for example born female and identifies as a woman, may self-designate as a cisgender woman, whereas someone born as a male and self-identifies as a man may refer to themselves as a cisgender male. Being transgender means an individual's gender identity or their gender expression differs from their sex assigned at birth. Transgender individuals may self-identify as being a transgender man or a transgender woman and people who avoid binary terms may prefer to self-identify as non-binary, gender fluid or gender-queer.

It is important to note that gender identity is independent of sexual orientation, the latter is concerned with who a person is physically and emotionally attracted to. For example, a person who self-identifies as being a woman (gender) and has a relationship attraction to men would be described as heterosexual (sexual orientation). A man who is attracted to men and women may refer to themselves as being bisexual. An individual, who self-describes as a woman (gender identity) who is attracted to other women (sexual orientation), may refer to themselves as lesbian and a man (gender identity), who is attracted to other men (sexual orientation), may refer to themselves as gay. It should be noted that the terminology used for sexual orientation here may not be all-encompassing and might not reflect everyone's perspectives or experiences. The American Psychological Association (2020) recommended that we should report the gender identity and sexual orientation of people as specifically as possible and not assume that people fit into discrete gendered categories due to their appearance.

Various acronyms are used to embrace gender identities and sexual orientations. The majority of the population are heterosexual and cisgender, and people who do not identify with these two descriptors are commonly referred to in research studies as sexual and gender minorities (SGMs). In addition, various acronyms are used in the literature when referring to people who are not cisgender or heterosexual, and these include LGB (lesbian, gay and bisexual), LGBT (with the addition of transgender), LGBTQI (with the addition of queer or questioning and intersex) and LGBTQI+ (the use of plus to indicate other gender and sexual identities not already listed). Indigenous populations in the US use the term 'two-spirit' as a widely accepted term to describe non-binary genders, but this term can also reflect a specific role in traditional ceremonies. The acronyms LGBTQI+ and variants of this are peppered through the research literature. It is acknowledged that people from these groups do share some commonalities regarding inequities in healthcare provision and experience of stigma and discrimination. However, it should be noted that the individual communities within these collective descriptors may have specific and unique healthcare needs.

Two other descriptors used in research are sexual minorities and gender minorities, in the former, individuals are identified in terms of their sexual orientation (e.g. lesbian, gay, bisexual), whereas the latter is concerned with gender identity (e.g. transgender, gender diverse, gender fluid). An IPSOS (2021) survey across 27 countries indicated that 80% of people self-identified as heterosexual, 4% as bisexual, around 3% as gay, lesbian or homosexual and 1% as pansexual, omnisexual, asexual or 'other', with the remainder being uncertain or even declined to reply to the question. In terms of gender identity, 1% identified as transgender, non-binary, nonconforming or gender fluid. Researchers may also refer to people from LGBTQI+ communities as belonging to gender and sexual minority groups (GSMs), but it is important to note that many people from LGBTQI+ groups may reject the notion of being referred to as minority, as it can be associated with stigma and discrimination. Thus, the terminology used within this book will vary according to the population that has been included in specific research studies and where possible, care has been taken to ensure that language used is as inclusive as possible.

LGBTQI+ communities, discrimination and stigma

Individuals from LGBTQI+ communities often experience stigma and discrimination due to prejudices that are engrained by religious and/or cultural beliefs. These are then perpetuated by social norms and stereotypic ideas of the binary gender identities that are associated with biological sex i.e. being male or female. In terms of sexual orientation, within the UK, decriminalisation of same-sex acts between men occurred in 1967 in England and Wales, but not until 1980 in Scotland and 1982 in Northern Ireland. In Canada, decriminalisation occurred in 1969, in Australia and China in the late 1990s and statewide in the US in 2003. However, there are still 64 countries across the globe spread out in Africa, the Middle East, Pacific Islands and the Caribbean that criminalise same-sex acts. Iran, Saudi Arabia, Yemen, Mauritania, Nigeria, Uganda and Brunei retain the death penalty, while in other countries long prison sentences and corporal punishment are the norm (The International Lesbian, Gay, Bisexual, Transexual and Intersex Association, n.d.).

The AIDS (acquired immunodeficiency syndrome) epidemic in the early 1980s caused by HIV (human immunodeficiency virus) had far-reaching consequences on the health of LGBTQI+ communities. HIV can be transmitted from an infected person to a non-infected person through bodily fluids in semen, vaginal fluids through unprotected sex, unscreened blood products used in hospitals, shared hypodermic needles in people who inject themselves with drugs and from mothers to babies during pregnancy, childbirth and breastfeeding. People diagnosed with AIDS/HIV experienced stigma that included negative attitudes, behaviours, lack of understanding, misinformation about the disease and assumptions that those who had a diagnosis of AIDS/HIV were either gay men, sex workers or intravenous drug users. Hence, people with AIDS/HIV faced multiple challenges in dealing with the medical aspects of the disease. They experienced stigma from the public and the healthcare professionals who were treating them, along with discrimination in the form of verbal and/or physical abuse and social isolation, even from their own family members. The negative experiences and associations of an AIDS/HIV diagnosis have contributed to past and present minority stress in LGBTQI+ communities, which has had negative consequences on their physical and mental health (Frost et al., 2015). Such experiences have contributed to health inequities, which we will explore throughout this textbook.

Intersectionality

People have multiple identities that are associated with age, ethnic group, religion, sexual orientation, gender identity, disability and/or chronic illness, which interact with and contribute to privilege and oppression. When two or more of these identities intersect, people may experience multiple and heightened levels of stigma, discrimination, oppression and marginalisation. People may not only experience privilege based on their ethnicity (White, British) and gender (man, woman), but may also be discriminated against due to their sexuality (gay). Intersectionality also interacts with societal systems and power to create subjugation and privilege and people who have two or more minority identities may experience greater discrimination. For example, a White American, lesbian women with a disability may experience discrimination on the basis of sexual orientation and disability; however, a Black African American, transgender women with a disability may experience a greater degree of discrimination, as they have multiple minority identities, which may all intersect and contribute to inequities in accessing and receiving healthcare that is appropriate to meet their needs.

Colonisation, education, economic, governmental, historical, social and legal factors may be associated with various types of oppression and discrimination that are directed towards individuals or groups, resulting in various types of inequities. Such relationships can be quite complex and have been summarised by Simpson (2009) in an intersectionality wheel diagram (see Figure 1.1). This illustrates the complexities of intersectionality that include aspects of identity that may be positively or negatively influenced by income, housing, education, occupation, etc., various types of discrimination and stigma that can impact others and self-perceptions, availability and access to and/or use of healthcare services. The outer circle provides examples of historical and current influences and systems that perpetuate inequities. Health interventions or policies that fail to take into account intersectional identities may be doomed to fail, as they will not consider the impact of co-experienced stigmas (Turan et al., 2019).

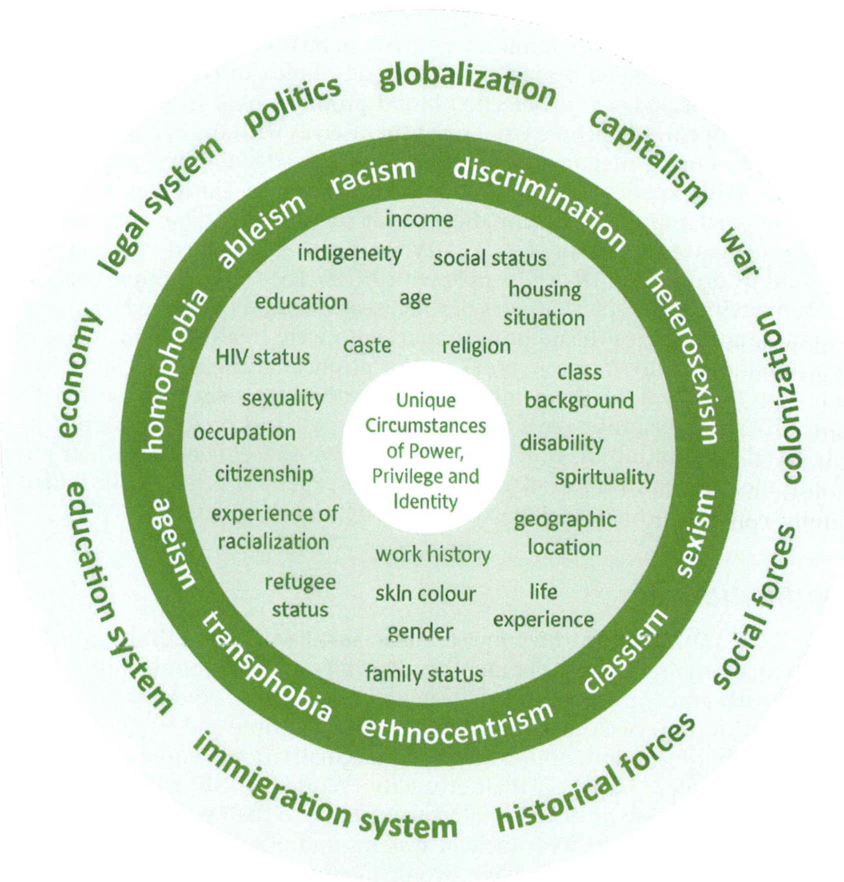

https://www.criaw-icref.ca/publications/everyone-belongs-a-toolkit-for-applying-intersectionality/

Figure 1.1
Intersectionality displayed in a wheel diagram

Source: Simpson (2009) reproduced with kind permission from the Canadian Research Institute for the Advancement of Women (CRIAW)

Chapter summary

In what health contexts do health psychologists work?

Health psychologists help individuals, families, groups, communities and populations to improve their health, by working with patients, the public, members of MDTs, other psychologists and researchers in health promotion, research and chronic disease. They work in a variety of health settings including hospitals, communities, workplace settings and strategic levels across the lifespan.

What psychological information do health psychologists use in their practice?

Health psychologists draw on a range of psychological evidence, research and research methods from biopsychology, personality, information about health perceptions, emotions, thoughts and how they interact when making sense of disease symptoms. Stress, coping and adherence may be influenced by own and other's beliefs and health behaviours. Social psychology is of use in exploring values, beliefs and social norms associated with gender identity, sexual orientation, ethnicity and culture, social injustice, power, stigma and discrimination.

Why is it important for health psychologists to understand the impacts of colonisation on health and healthcare?

Colonisation has had detrimental impacts on the health of Indigenous Peoples, their knowledge, ways of living and traditional healthcare practices have been subjugated by Western knowledge. Health psychologists and other healthcare professionals need to acknowledge the negative impacts of colonisation and ensure that their practice is culturally competent and sensitive to Indigenous holistic health, which includes respect for connections to the land, language, family, community and traditional health practices.

Outline the differences between biological sex and gender, sexual orientation and gender identity

Biological sex refers to physiological and anatomical differences between males and females, which are based on their reproductive organs, chromosomes and hormones. Gender is a social and cultural construct that reflects certain behaviours, attitudes, feelings, activities and expectations. Gender identity is the 'individual's internal sense of being a man, woman or another non-binary gender and can be different to the sex that was ascribed at birth'. Sexual orientation is concerned with who a person is physically and emotionally attracted to.

Describe and provide examples of what is meant by minoritised groups and intersectionality

Minoritised groups are those that are disadvantaged in some way, which may be due to paternalistic power relationships associated with colonisation, belonging to an ethnic, LGBTQI+ group, having a disability, low educational level, low income or living in a deprived area. Intersectionality is concerned with the overlap of these minoritised identities that can result in discrimination, stigma and health inequities.

Keywords

Physical health condition: One that affects the physical body, for example, heart disease, diabetes or cancer can influence people's thoughts, emotions and behaviours.

Health psychology: The interrelationship between how biological, psychological, social and cultural factors influence people's physical health.

Infectious diseases: These are diseases caused by bacteria, viruses, fungi and parasites.

Chronic diseases: Long-term conditions lasting more than six months, which can be managed, but not fully cured.

Ethnicity: Refers to shared common cultural values, customs and language, which may also have shared histories and traditions.

Indigenous: These people are the original inhabitants of a region or country, who have distinct languages, cultural, social and historical traditions that are closely tied to their ancestral lands and share a common history of having been dominated by non-Indigenous settlers.

Health interventions: Programmes or strategies to prevent disease, improve and manage physical health conditions.

Audits: Evaluations of health services or interventions to see if they meet a predetermined standard.

Service evaluation: Used to explore and assess what a service has achieved in terms of health outcomes.

Patient and public involvement: The active participation of patients and the public to help shape health research, services and policies.

Health promotion: Helps people to take control of and to improve health habits.

Screening: To detect diseases at an asymptomatic stage.

Multidisciplinary team: Healthcare professionals from different disciplines working together to provide integrated patient care.

Cancer-related fatigue: Persistent overwhelming tiredness that is not helped by sleep or rest and can persist for years.

Mindfulness: Bringing attention to present-moment thoughts, feelings, bodily sensations and the immediate environment, without judgement.

Prehabilitation: Getting patients nutritionally, emotionally and physically fit for treatment.

Rehabilitation: Helps the patient recover from treatment or illness.

Social norms: The shared rules or expectations for behaviour of a group or society.

Palliative care: The assessment and treatment of physical, psychological and spiritual wellbeing in serious illness.

End-of-life care: Comfort, dignity and quality of life in the final stages of a terminal illness.

Culture: The shared beliefs, values, customs, behaviours and traditions of a group or society.

Discrimination: The impact of unequal or unfair care.

Stigma: Negative attitudes or prejudice associated with marginalised identities.

Colonisation: The impacts of dominant countries taking over the control of land, dominating Indigenous Peoples by subjugating their culture, values, language, knowledge and ways of life.

Social injustices: Some groups within society who are not afforded the same rights to healthcare as others or are treated differently due to marginalised identities.

Power imbalances: Groups, such as the dominant culture, holding more influence and access to resources, which leads to inequality and inequity.

Health equity: Providing everyone with the specific support they require to lead as healthy a life as possible.

Health equality: Providing equal access to healthcare support.

Consultancy: The provision of expert health psychology advice and guidance to clients.

Biopsychosocial approach: Recognises that biomedical, psychological and social factors can influence health and disease.

Biomedical model: Views disease as being due to genetics, viruses, bacteria, chemical imbalances and trauma.

Decolonisation: This is a process that involves colonised countries or Peoples gaining independence, control of their land, culture and the right to self-determination. It also includes challenging knowledge and practices based on Western-dominated perspectives related to healthcare and psychology.

Paternalistic power relations: These are unequal power relations, in which the dominant group or person makes decisions for and imposes their authority without consulting those who will be affected.

Eurocentric: Viewing European culture, values and knowledge as being the acceptable standard or the standard that other cultures should aspire to, while devaluing other cultures and their knowledge.

Western conceptualisations: Involves thinking and ways of understanding that are based on mainly European and/or North American culture and scientific knowledge.

Intersectionality: This is the concept of an individual or group having multiple identities, such as gender identity, sexual orientation, ethnicity, low educational attainment and low socioeconomic status.

Intergenerational trauma: This refers to trauma that is passed down from one generation to another that has psychological and physical health implications, even when descendants did not have any direct exposure to the original traumatic events.

Cultural competence: Knowledge of the impact that social and cultural factors have on patients from the non-dominant culture and the importance of being sensitive to such factors when communicating with patients and delivering care.

Cultural sensitivity: Involves being aware of cultural values, beliefs, traditions and knowledge of others' culture and being respectful of them when interacting with or treating patients.

Key Readings

González, R., Carvacho, H., & Jiménez-Moya, G. (2022). Psychology and indigenous people. *Annual Review of Psychology, 73*, 431–459. https://doi.org/10.1146/annurev-psych-012921-045304

Heard, E., Fitzgerald, L., Wigginton, B., & Mutch, A. (2020). Applying intersectionality theory in health promotion research and practice. *Health Promotion International, 35*(4), 866–876. https://doi.org/10.1093/heapro/daz080

Lawrence, W., & Barker, M. (2016). Improving the health of the public: What is the role of health psychologists? *Journal of Health Psychology, 21*(2), 135–137. https://doi.org/10.1177/1359105314528013

Reflective Questions

1 Is there an area of physical health that would make you want to pursue a career in health psychology? Would you prefer to work with children, teenagers, adults or the elderly and why?
2 Do you think decolonising health psychology is important, if so, why?
3 Do you think overlapping identities like ethnicity, gender identity, sexual orientation and socioeconomic status can affect someone's healthcare experiences? Can you give an example?

References

American Psychological Association. (2020). *Publication manual of the American Psychological Association: The official guide to APA style* (7th ed.). American Psychological Association. https://apastyle.apa.org/products/publication-manual-7th-edition

Carleton-Boylan, G., Crossley, S., Siebert, P., Ajanaku, N., Iqbal, A., John, A., Sandhu, S., Williams, C., Leach., Patel, R., Buchanan, H., Taggar, J., Leonardi-Bee, J., Morling, J., Qureshi, I., Hubber, L., Bethea, J., & Wilson, E. E. (2024). Inclusivity and decolonisation of the post-graduate public health curriculum: Reflections from a student-led approach. *Public Health in Practice, 7,* 100507. https://doi.org/10.1016/j.puhip.2024.100507

Coates, K. S. (2004). *A global history of Indigenous Peoples: Struggle and survival.* Macmillan.

Durie, M. (2004). Understanding health and illness: Research at the interface between science and indigenous knowledge. *International Journal of Epidemiology, 33,* 138–143. https://doi.org/10.1093/ije/dyh250

Frost, D. M., Lehavot, K., & Meyer, I. H. (2015). Minority stress and physical health among sexual minority individuals. *Journal of Behavioral Medicine, 38,* 1–8. https://doi.org/10.1007/s10865-013-9523-8

Heath, M., Hvass, A. M. F., & Wejse, C. M. (2023). Interpreter services and effect on healthcare: A systematic review of the impact of different types of interpreters on patient outcome. *Journal of Migration and Health, 7,* 100162. https://doi.org/10.1016/j.jmh.2023.100162

IPSOS (2021). *LGBT+ Pride 2021 global survey*. Retrieved October 10, 2024, from https://www.ipsos.com/en/ipsos-lgbt-pride-2021-global-survey

James, T. G., Coady, K. A., Stacciarini, J. R., McKee, M. M., Phillips, D. G., Maruca, D., & Cheong, J. (2022). They're not willing to accommodate deaf patients: Communication experiences of deaf American sign language users in the emergency department. *Qualitative Health Research, 32*(1), 48–63. https://doi.org/10.1177/10497323211046238

Jan, J. C., & Osterhammed, J. (2017). *Decolonization: A short history*. Princeton University Press.

Joo, J. Y., & Liu, M. F. (2021). Culturally tailored interventions for ethnic minorities: A scoping review. *Nursing Open, 8*(5), 2078–2090. https://doi.org/10.1002/nop2.733

Kozlov, A., Vershubsky, G., & Kozlova, M. (2007). Indigenous peoples of Northern Russia: Anthropology and health. *International Journal of Circumpolar Health, 66*(1), 1–184. https://doi.org/10.1080/22423982.2007.11864603

Lamba, S., Obedin-Maliver, J., Mayo, J., Flentje, A., Lubensky, M. E., Dastur, Z., & Lunn, M. R. (2023). Self-reported barriers to care among sexual and gender minority people with disabilities: Findings from the PRIDE study, 2019-2020. *American Journal of Public Health, 113*, 1009–1018. https://doi.org/10.2105/AJPH.2023.307333

Lokugamage, A. U., Robinson, N., Pathberiya, S. D. C., Wong, S., & Douglass, C. (2022). Respectful maternity care in the UK using a decolonial lens. *Springer Nature Social Sciences, 2*, 267, 1–32. https://doi.org/10.1007/s43545-022-00576-5

Marks, D. F., Murray, M., Evans, B., & Willig, C. (2000). *Health psychology: Theory, research and practice* (2nd ed.). Sage Publications.

Marmot, M., Allen, J., Boyce, T., Goldblatt, P., & Morrison, J. (2020). *Health equity in England: The Marmot review 10 years on*. Institute of Health Equity. Retrieved September 30, 2025, from https://www.instituteofhealthequity.org/resources-reports/marmot-review-10-years-on/the-marmot-review-10-years-on-full-report.pdf

Martínez Cobo, J. R. (1981). *Study of the problem of discrimination against Indigenous populations*. United Nations. Retrieved September 30, 2025, from https://www.un.org/development/desa/indigenouspeoples/publications/2014/09/martinez-cobo-study/

McCartney, G., Popham, F., McMaster, R., & Cumbers, A. (2019). Defining health and health inequalities. *Public Health, 172*, 22–30. https://doi.org/10.1016/j.puhe.2019.03.023

McLeroy, K. R., Bibeau, D., Steckler, A., & Glanz, K. (1988). An ecological perspective on health promotion programs. *Health Education Quarterly, 15*(4), 351–377. https://doi.org/10.1177/109019818801500401

Morreira, S., Luckett, K., Kumalo, S. H., & Ramgotra, M. (2020). Confronting the complexities of decolonising curricula and pedagogy in higher education. *Third World Thematics, 5*(1–2), 1–18. https://doi.org/10.1080/23802014.2020.1798278

Office for National Statistics (2022). *Language, England and Wales census* 2021. Retrieved September 30, 2025, from https://www.ons.gov.uk/peoplepopulationandcommunity/culturalidentity/language/bulletins/languageenglandandwales/census2021

Prilleltensky, I., & Prilleltensky, O. (2003). Towards a critical health psychology practice. *Journal of Health Psychology, 8*(2), 197–210. https://doi.org/10.1177/1359105303008002659

Sherwood, J., & Edwards, T. (2006). Decolonisation: A critical step for improving Aboriginal health. *Contemporary Nurse, 22*(2), 178–190. https://doi.org/10.5172/conu.2006.22.2.178

Simpson, J. (2009). *Everyone belongs: A toolkit for applying intersectionality*. Canadian Research Institute for the Advancement of Women (CRIAW). Retrieved April 14, 2025, from https://www.criaw-icref.ca/publications/everyone-belongs-a-toolkit-for-applying-intersectionality/

Statistics Canada (2024). *Health care access and experiences among Indigenous people, 2024*. Retrieved May 21, 2025, from https://www150.statcan.gc.ca/n1/daily-quotidien/241104/dq241104a-eng.htm

The International Lesbian, Gay, Bisexual, Transexual and intersex Association (n.d). *Legal frameworks, criminalisation of consensual same-sex sexual acts*. Retrieved October 9, 2024, from https://database.ilga.org/criminalisation-consensual-same-sex-sexual-acts

Turan, J. M., Elafros, M. A., Logie, C. H., Banik, S., Turan, B., Crockett, K. B., Pescosolido, B., & Murray, S. M. (2019). Challenges and opportunities in examining and addressing intersectional stigma and health. *BMC Medicine, 17*(1), 7. https://doi.org/10.1186/s12916-018-1246-9

United Nations (2007). *The United Nations Declaration of the Rights of Indigenous Peoples.* Retrieved October 28, 2024, from https://www.un.org/development/desa/indigenouspeoples/wp-content/uploads/sites/19/2018/11/UNDRIP_E_web.pdf

United Nations (n.d.) *Indigenous Peoples: Respect NOT dehumanization.* Retrieved February 20, 2025, from https://www.un.org/en/fight-racism/vulnerable-groups/indigenous-peoples

Umucu, E., Vernon, A. A., Pan, D., Qin, S., Solis, G., Campa, R., & Lee, B. (2025). Health inequities among persons with disabilities: A global scoping review. *Frontiers in Public Health, 13,* 1538519. https://doi.org/10.3389/fpubh.2025.1538519

Video Resources

Holman, D., Salway, S., & Bell, A. (n.d). *Intersectionality and health explained.* Sociological Studies, University of Sheffield. [Video]. http://youtube.com/watch?v=rwqnC1fy_zc

University College London (n.d.). *Why is my curriculum White* [Video]. https://www.youtube.com/watch?v=Dscx4h2l-Pk

2 Historical and cross-cultural views of health and the development of health psychology

Chapter contents

- Early views on health and disease.
- Scientific advances and the changing nature of disease.
- The role of psychological, social and cultural factors on health and disease.
- 'West is best', the ethnocentrism of healthcare practices and beliefs.
- Indigenous models of health.
- Cultural appropriation of Indigenous healing practices.
- Culture and health.
- Cultural awareness, competence and safety.

Chapter objectives

After reading this chapter, you should be able to answer the following questions:

- Explain how early views about health and disease have changed over time.
- Identify factors that have influenced the changing nature of disease.
- Compare and contrast the contributions that the biomedical, biopsychosocial and ecological models have made to understanding health and disease.
- Outline what is meant by ethnocentrism in health and why this reflects biased thinking.
- How do Western and Indigenous models of health differ?
- Outline the difference between cultural awareness, sensitivity and safety.

Early views on health and disease

In some non-Western cultures, health and disease have been linked to spirituality, community wellbeing and harmony. The Indigenous Peoples of Australia, Canada, New Zealand and US view health and disease as intertwined with

DOI: 10.4324/9781003423157-2

spiritual, environmental, cultural and social factors; they also stress the importance of harmony with nature (WHO, n.d.). The idea of harmony between the body, mind and spirit is of vital importance in the Ayurvedic medical system in India. Disease prevention and the restoration of health within Traditional Chinese Medicine (TCM) highlights the balance between two energy forces called Yin and Yang. These examples, which go back thousands of years, emphasise the holistic nature of health, along with the importance of the mind-body link. During the time of the Greek physician Hippocrates (c. 460–377 BCE), who is seen as the founding Father of Western medicine, the **mind-body link** was also acknowledged and as we shall see in this chapter, the importance of the mind-body link in health and disease has fluctuated over time.

Hippocrates

Hippocrates proposed the 'humoral theory' to explain disease, which was based on four bodily humours (also known as bodily fluids), these are blood, phlegm, black bile and yellow bile. An imbalance in these bodily humours could also have negative impacts on an individual's psychological state. Imbalances in blood were associated with fever and inflammation; an abundance of black bile could cause digestive problems and depression; and an excess of phlegm was linked with fatigue and respiratory problems, whereas too much yellow bile was associated with liver problems. To maintain the balance between these bodily humours, bleeding, taking medicines, the avoidance of excesses, eating special diets and taking exercise were prescribed. This 'humoral theory' also described personality temperaments; people with a predominance of blood were cheerful and happy; too much black bile was associated with being sad and melancholic; an excess of phlegm with lethargy and calmness; and an excess of yellow bile with anger and irrationality. Later (2nd century AD), the Roman physician Galen's dissection of animals led to discoveries about anatomy, physiology and the difference between arteries and veins. This helped to advance Western thinking about disease and Hippocrates' theory was extended to include humoral imbalances within bodily organs.

The role of the Church

The humoral theory prevailed into the Middle Ages, but spiritual and religious explanations for disease were prevalent in Western Europe; churches and religion assumed a leading role in healing people who were sick. At this time, disease was regarded as a punishment from God, plagues were attributed to God's anger and people with mental illnesses were seen as being possessed by demons. The Church controlled medical practices, which were administered by priests or monks who engaged in ritualistic activities to 'cleanse' the body of disease. Monasteries, convents and churches were places where the sick could come for treatments that consisted of prayers, fasting, the laying on of hands and the use of holy water (Wells, 2022). During this period, the body was viewed as containing the immortal 'soul', which was created by God, thus no dissection was permitted, and that development halted scientific advancements in physical medicine until the 1600s.

The Renaissance

Theories about the causes of disease changed in the 17th century when the French philosopher Descartes proposed that the mind (also referred to as the 'soul') was non-physical, while the body was the physical part of a person. Descartes viewed the mind and the body as separate, but knew they could interact, this became known as Cartesian Dualism. According to Descartes, when a person died their 'soul' left their body, this mind-body separation placated Church concerns about the soul being immortal and helped to defend religious beliefs about life after death. It paved the way for human dissection to recommence, leading to advances in knowledge about physiological and anatomical aspects of the body. The invention of the microscope and the role of microorganisms in disease led to the humoral theory being disregarded, previous beliefs about disease and plagues being a punishment from God reduced and in the 1800s, surgery became less of a risk due to the use of antiseptics and anaesthesia.

Scientific advances and the changing nature of disease

During the 18th–19th centuries, most deaths in Western nations were caused by acute (short-duration) infectious diseases, such as influenza, pneumonia, tuberculosis, smallpox, diphtheria, whooping cough, typhoid, cholera and measles. In the early 1990s, the global life expectancy was only 32 years (Dattani et al., 2023); however, the introduction of public health measures to improve sanitation, provision of clean drinking water and improvements in diet within Western countries helped reduce deaths. These factors also helped to lay the foundations for the biomedical model, in which disease could be explained by infections, biochemical imbalances, genetics or trauma. The separation between the mind and the body became the dominant thinking in Western medicine, individuals were seen as helpless victims, unable to do anything to prevent or cure disease, with diagnosis and treatment being the sole remit of doctors.

Later, vaccines and antibiotics also assisted in the control of infectious diseases, death rates decreased and there was an expectation that these advances would lead to the eradication of disease, people would become healthier and live longer. In 2023, the average global life expectancy (see Box 2.1) had increased to just over 73 years (see Figure 2.1); however, this trend was not experienced equally across the world. In the 1950s, countries categorised as being of high income (based on the World Bank Income criteria, see Box 2.2), had a life expectancy of 61.8 years, which was twice that of low-income countries at 31.2 years and in 2023, people living in countries with the lowest incomes still had the poorest life expectancy (see Figure 2.2).

BOX 2.1
LIFE EXPECTANCY

Life expectancy is an approximation of the age that an individual is expected to live to based on their biological sex and age, compared to age- and sex-specific death rates. It can be calculated for individual countries, regions and globally, but not every country registers deaths, especially in Africa (Karlinsky, 2024).

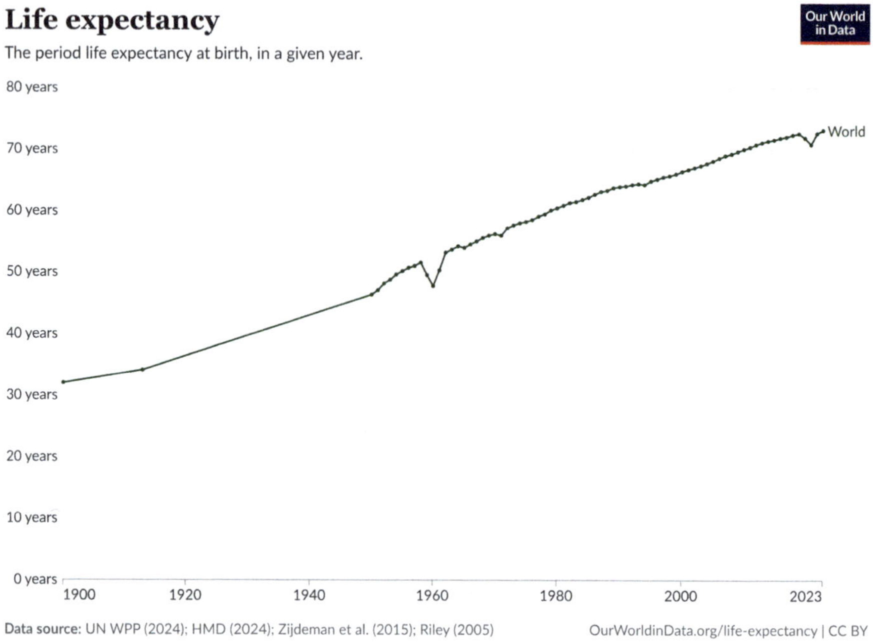

Figure 2.1
Global life expectancy 1900–2023

Source: https://ourworldindata.org/life-expectancy

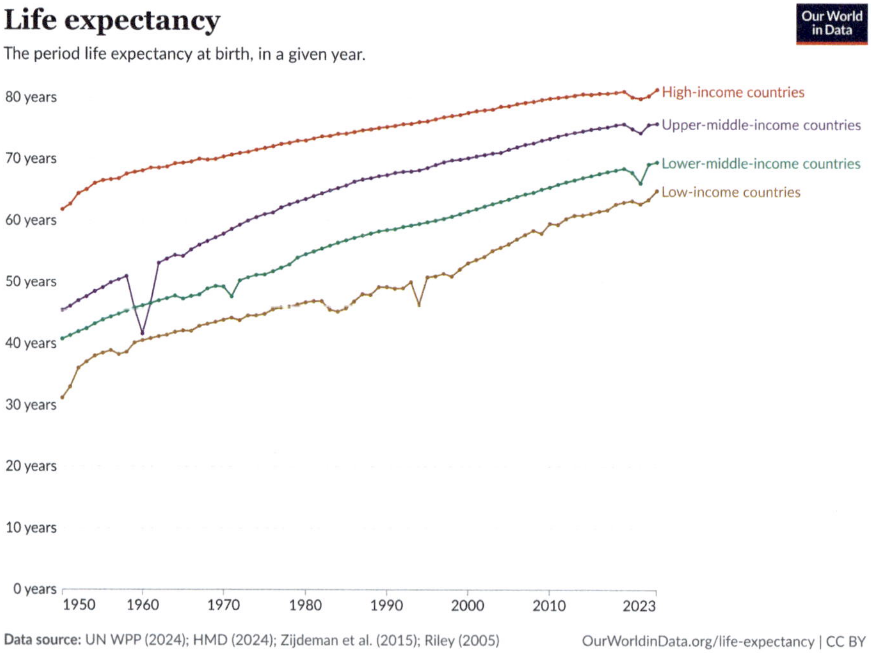

Figure 2.2
Life expectancy across World Bank Income countries 1950–2023

Source: https://ourworldindata.org/life-expectancy

BOX 2.2
WORLD BANK INCOME CRITERIA

The World Bank classifies countries into four groups (low, lower-middle, upper-middle and high) based on their Gross National Income (GNI). This is the total money earned by people and businesses in a country in one year plus any money earned abroad (e.g. through investments or sent home to their country by migrant workers). GNI is used as a 'proxy' measure of health, as higher-income countries tend to have higher healthcare spending, better health infrastructure, technologies, access to medications, higher life expectancy, more disease prevention initiatives, better nutrition, more input into managing long-term conditions and lower levels of infectious diseases in comparison to lower income countries.

Life expectancy also varies within countries, for example, men live nine years longer and women eight years longer than their Indigenous counterparts in Australia (Australian Institute of Health and Welfare, 2024). Similar findings are reported in New Zealand with around seven years higher life expectancy for non-Indigenous men and women compared to Māori (Stats New Zealand, 2021), and likewise for the Indigenous Peoples of Canada (Native Women's Association of Canada, 2025). However, a more marked differential is found for American Indian and Alaskan Native men in the US whose life expectancy is around 15 years lower than their non-Indigenous counterparts and almost eight years lower for women (Fleck, 2023). There are various reasons for this, which will be explored in subsequent chapters.

The move from acute to chronic diseases

In addition to life expectancy, other metrics used to measure the success of Western medicine have included reductions in deaths due to acute diseases, reductions in hospital admissions, quicker recovery from acute diseases and shorter durations of stay in hospital. In terms of life expectancy, the World Health Organization (2024) estimates that by 2030 approximately one out of every six people across the globe will be over the age of 60 years and with changing patterns of disease, the need for healthcare will only grow. Compared to previous generations in Europe, the United Kingdom (UK) and the US, more people are being diagnosed and living longer with chronic diseases, such as heart problems, cancer, lung diseases, type 2 diabetes (T2DM) and dementia (WHO, 2024). Chronic diseases are linked to disability and poorer overall health, which can have negative impacts on quality of life (QoL) (Gimeno et al., 2024; see Box 2.3) and they cannot be fully explained by biomedical factors alone (Donaldson, 2000). In high-income countries, more people are becoming overweight or obese and less physically active, which increases their risk of developing heart disease, T2DM and stroke compared to their more active and normal or lower body weight counterparts. Researchers have started to explore the possible link between chronic diseases, stress, lifestyle, psychosocial and environmental factors (see Chapters 8 and 9).

BOX 2.3
QUALITY OF LIFE (QoL) AND HEALTH-RELATED QUALITY OF LIFE (HRQoL)

QoL is a broad concept that is multidimensional in nature, while there is no one universally accepted definition, it is conceptualised as being subjective, culturally and values based and concerned with life satisfaction. The WHO (1998, p. 1570) defined QoL as, "an individual's perception of their position in life in the context of the culture and value systems in which they live and in relation to their goals, expectations, standards and concerns".

Health-related quality of life (HRQoL) is a subdomain of overall QoL and it focuses on the effects of health and healthcare on an individual's quality of life, which includes the impact of disease, treatments and disability on physical and mental functioning. Within health psychology, HRQoL is an important construct to measure, as it permits healthcare professionals and researchers to evaluate the impact that diseases, treatments and interventions have on individuals. For example, two medications for pain may have similar outcomes in terms of the degree of pain relief they provide, both cost the same amount of money, but which one is the best? In clinical trials of medication, symptom control will be measured, along with medication side effects, which often includes a measure of HRQoL. Pain medications may have unwanted side effects, such as nausea, constipation and make people sleepy, but some patients may find that they can cope with these side effects and taking these factors into consideration along with the reduced pain, they may experience improved HRQoL. Usually, the medication that has the least detrimental impact on HRQoL is the best for the patient. HRQoL is measured using questionnaires, which can assess overall HRQoL, or they can be disease specific.

In 1948, the Framingham Heart Study (FHS) was the first major longitudinal study (a research method that measures the same factors in the same individuals or groups of individuals at different time points over a period of time that can range from months to years) to scientifically explore the causes of heart disease. The study provided evidence that being assigned male at birth, sedentary, a smoker and having a poor diet contributed to high cholesterol (a fatty substance in the blood), high blood pressure and the chances of developing heart disease (Dawber et al., 1957). Researchers also started to examine specific aspects of diet and disease and found that having higher levels of a certain type of blood cholesterol and the consumption of a diet high in saturated fats (fats that solidify at room temperature) were linked with an elevated risk of heart disease (Keys, 1953). Smoking cigarettes was associated with the development of respiratory diseases and lung cancer (Doll & Hill, 1950) and variations in the health of specific occupational groups were linked with stress and physical inactivity. Bus drivers who were sedentary most of their working day had higher rates of heart disease than physically active bus conductors who walked up and down the bus stairs to collect fares (Morris et al., 1953). A growing wealth of evidence showed that while the biomedical model was of great utility in helping to explain, to treat acute diseases and to save lives, it was insufficient to deal with the disability and detrimental impacts of chronic disease on quality of life. It was apparent that a more holistic approach to health was required, one that considered more than just the biomedical aspects of disease. In 1973, the American Psychological Society (APA) Task Force on Health Research was established to help deal with the increase in chronic diseases, which were seen as preventable (APA, 1976) and a year later, Engel (1977) introduced the biopsychosocial model of health. The APA established the Division of Health Psychology along with training for psychologists that focused on physical health and wellbeing. Health psychology became a formally recognised profession within the US in 1978, the European Health Psychology Society (EHPS) was established in 1986 and health psychology became a BPS Division within the UK in 1997 (Quinn et al., 2020).

The role of psychological, social and cultural factors on health and disease

The biopsychosocial model

Engel (1977) realised that the biomedical model was dehumanising, it supported the idea of the mind and body being separate, and it focused on disease, while ignoring psychological and social complexities associated with health. Engel proposed the need to view health and disease as an interplay between the biological, psychological and social factors in people's lives. The bio part of the model still acknowledged the impact of biomedical factors (viruses, bacteria, genetics and trauma), along with the role of biomedical diagnostic tests, medicine, surgery and other treatments, such as radiotherapy. However, the link with psychological (perceptions, beliefs, emotions, **health literacy**, stress and habitual behaviours) and social (family, peers and others, social supports, education, socioeconomic status (SES)) and occupational factors highlighted that individuals and others also had a role to play in the prevention, development and treatment of disease (see Figure 2.3).

Even though Engel did not write about the biopsychosocial model until 1977, the definition of health provided by the World Health Organization in 1948 had already acknowledged that health was more than being free from disease, it was

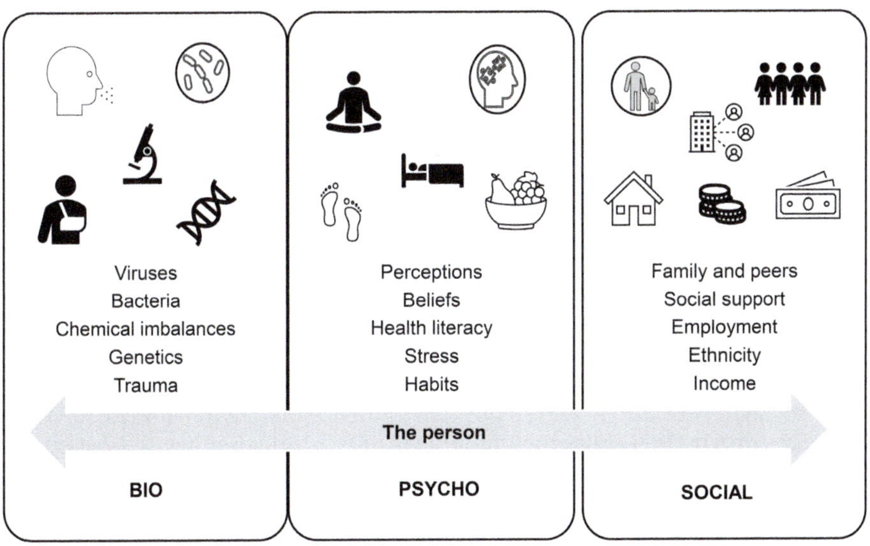

Figure 2.3
The biopsychosocial model
Source: Author, based on Engel (1977)

"a state of complete physical, mental and social well-being". However, this definition ignored the fact that health resources are not freely accessible for all, the enduring impacts of colonisation, along with health discrimination and stigma experienced by ethnic, sexual and gender minorities, those with disabilities and intersectionality. The WHO definition and the original conception of biopsychosocial model have also been criticised for largely ignoring culture. While Engel (1977) did refer to culture acting as a filter through which individuals interpret bodily experiences and make decisions about health, this discussion was based within the dominance of Western medical science. In the broadest sense, culture includes the beliefs, shared traditions, social norms and behaviours of a group of people, which are of central importance to health outcomes (Hatala, 2013). Western-based healthcare practices have often ignored the needs of ethnic, gender and/or sexual minority groups, as well as those living with disabilities and Indigenous populations (Dune et al., 2021). However, it must be remembered that Engel was writing almost 50 years ago, at a time when the evidence base about the impact of psychosocial and cultural considerations was less well known. We now know that non-medical-related inequities, such as low educational attainment and income, high unemployment, inadequate housing and lack of access to adequate healthcare provision (Paradies, 2016) and colonisation have adverse consequences for **morbidity** and life expectancy (Australian Bureau of Statistics, 2018). Thus, a more comprehensive model is required, which includes the multilevel and intersectional factors that exert an influence on health outcomes.

The ecological model of health

McLeroy et al. (1988) developed an ecological model of health that was built on the work of Bronfenbrenner (1979) who highlighted that multiple levels of influence, such as the home environment, school, neighbourhood, external environment, social and cultural factors influenced children's development.

The ecological model of health helps to explain how interconnected factors exert multiple levels of influence on health, which includes individual, interpersonal, organisational, community and policy (see Figure 2.4). McLeory's model was later extended by Simons-Morton et al. (2012) to include physical space and culture. This conceptualisation contains two common principles, namely that behaviour can be impacted by various layers of influence and that these layers of influence interact with each other to have enhancing or detrimental impacts on health (Ding et al., 2011)

This model acknowledges that an individual's health behaviour can be impacted by biomedical factors, individual knowledge, beliefs and personal choices about the worth of engaging in health-related behaviours. For example, an individual may give up smoking, switch to a healthier diet and/or engage in regular physical activity because they have knowledge about health enhancing or health compromising behaviours.

Next, at an interpersonal level, relationships between family, friends, peers and other social networks may exert a positive influence on health behaviours. A parent teaches their child about the importance of brushing their teeth for good oral health. Peers may help an individual engage in regular physical activity by going out running in a group or encouraging healthy eating through meal planning. Friends and family may encourage an individual to seek medical advice for specific disease-related symptoms and discourage health compromising behaviours, such as smoking or excessive consumption of alcohol. Peers and people in the media who consume alcohol to excess, take illegal or non-prescribed drugs, can

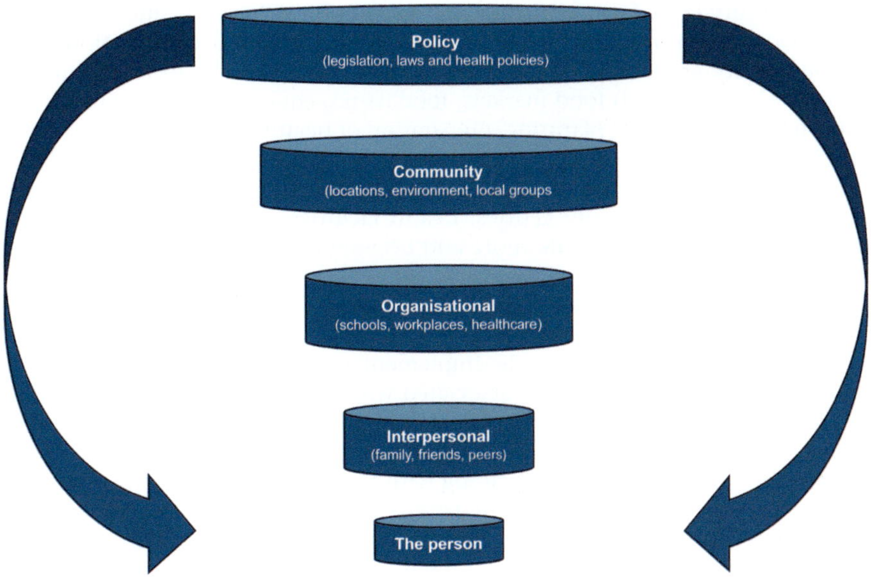

Figure 2.4
The ecological model of health

Source: The author based on McLeroy et al. (1988)

also exert negative influences over an individual's health, as the individual may model their own behaviour on that of others (see Chapter 7).

The organisational level involves schools, workplaces and/or healthcare providers. Workplaces may have health-related strategies that encourage cycle to work schemes, offer relaxation sessions, conduct health checks, offer gym memberships or engage in walking activities at lunchtime. Schools may provide health education, nutritious meals at lunchtime and encourage children to become more physically active by engaging in whole school-based activity sessions, such as the 'Daily Mile' (see Box 2.4).

BOX 2.4
THE DAILY MILE

The Daily Mile was started in Scotland (UK) in 2012 by a primary school teacher who wanted to increase the physical activity of pupils to foster fitness, improve concentration and mental wellbeing. It involves children running, walking or wheeling (in a wheelchair) for 15 minutes (to cover around 1 mile or 1.6 kilometres), usually within the school playground or locality close to their school. The Daily Mile is part of the school day, which requires no specialist equipment or clothing, and children can take part, regardless of their age or ability. Since its inception, the Daily Mile has been adopted in 98 countries around the world.

More information on the Daily Mile is available at: https://thedailymile.co.uk/

Video: An introduction to The Daily Mile from founder, Elaine Wyllie

Website: https://www.youtube.com/watch?v=ai8TD_v6hvU

Community-level factors include the geographical location and the neighbourhood or environment that an individual lives in, local organisations and/or community groups that may impact health. For example, local community initiatives, such as fresh food markets, food banks, education and advice for parents on budgeting, meal planning, preparation of healthy meals and group-based physical activities, offer comprehensive community-level participation. Within neighbourhoods, lighting, physical layout of spaces, along with proximity to shops, libraries, community centres, health facilities and recreational grounds, may encourage people to walk more and become involved in supportive health activities.

At the policy level, legislation, policies and laws may be used to create systemic change to improve health outcomes. For example, a ban on smoking in public spaces and at school gates may be implemented to discourage smoking and to prevent health risks to children associated with **passive smoking**. Health policies may be applied at a population level or targeted at specific groups, including ethnic, gender, sexual minorities and people with disabilities.

The WHO definition of health along with the biopsychosocial and ecological models has moved Western thinking from a purely biomedical approach to one that is more holistic in trying to prevent and treat disease at an individual level. However, the WHO definition of health has been criticised as being too idealistic, because for most people, 'complete physical, mental and social well-being' is a state they are unlikely to attain. Moreover, the biopsychosocial and ecological models lack generalisability for Indigenous populations, as they ignore the impacts of colonisation, intergenerational trauma, connection to the land, ancestry, traditional knowledge and Indigenous world views that emphasise the importance of community over individual health.

BOX 2.1
CRITICAL THINKING

The views of health have changed over time, from Hippocrates' holistic view of balance between bodily humours to today's biopsychosocial and ecological models.

What are the strengths and limitations of the biomedical model?
How does the biopsychosocial model expand on this view?
What extra perspective does the ecological model add?
Think? Are we moving towards a more holistic view of health or redefining health in new ways?

'West is best', the ethnocentrism of healthcare practices and beliefs

With colonisation came Western medicine with its emphasis on the biomedical model and it became the legitimised knowledgebase from which to manage all healthcare initiatives and diseases (Wright, 2007). Indigenous Peoples across the globe have poorer health outcomes than their non-Indigenous counterparts.

Instead of examining how colonisation harmed health through the suppression of holistic cultural practices, ways of life and traditional healing, Oetzel et al. (2021) argued that too much attention has been placed on the 'deficits-based approach', which tends to blame Indigenous populations for their health problems. This **ethnocentric view** is based on Western notions of what is meant by health, with a tendency to think and interpret other cultures and their healthcare practices as inferior (Betancourt et al., 2002). The imposition of Western ethnocentric views that negate the importance of spirituality, links to the land and ancestors, have had negative consequences for Indigenous health outcomes (Moss, 2016).

Indigenous Peoples all view health as being holistic, involving a balance between physical, emotional, mental and spiritual wellbeing. Earlier in this chapter, we learned about the WHO's (1948) all-encompassing definition of health referring to physical, mental and social wellbeing. However, the WHO Global Plan of Action for Indigenous Peoples (WHO, n.d.) has gone even further to propose a more nuanced view of health that recognises Indigenous People's health as "an equilibrium of spirituality, traditional medicine, biodiversity and the interconnectedness of all that exists". Western-based healthcare practices and models of health behaviour (see Chapter 7) emphasise individual responsibility for health (see Chapter 5), while Indigenous Peoples stress the importance of community knowledge, shared values, beliefs and health decision-making, the land and the **spirit world** (Boot & Lovell, 2019; Wilson, 2003). Hence, Indigenous conceptions of health and disease are not based on biomedical or biopsychosocial viewpoints, rather they need to be considered in a more ecological way that includes how relationships, culture and broader social systems interact to influence health and disease. For Indigenous Peoples, healing not only includes offerings to the spirit world, gatherings and community ceremonies that involve traditional healers, but intergenerational trauma associated with colonisation must also be addressed.

The move to 'decolonise' global health, with a focus on challenging issues such as the dominance of Western views of health and knowledge, is included within Article 24 of the United Nations Charter on the Rights of Indigenous Peoples (2007), which affirmed the right of these Peoples to use their own traditional healthcare practices. Within Australia, Canada, New Zealand and the US, there has been some recognition of cultural, spiritual wellbeing, the key role of the land and community needs of Indigenous Peoples. However, Dune et al. (2021) point out that all too often, the continued effects of colonialism persist and contribute to **health disparities**. The imposition of Western ways of thinking about health and disease continues to take precedence over Indigenous models of health. While it is beyond the scope of this book to outline all Indigenous models of health here, two examples explain how the holistic nature of Indigenous health goes beyond Western conceptions.

Indigenous models of health

Te Whare Tapa Whā Model of Māori health

The Māori (the Indigenous Peoples of Aotearoa New Zealand) believe that Western-based healthcare services that are situated within the biomedical model focus on physical health, ignoring Māori spiritual, emotional and cultural health (Rochford, 2004). In attempting to conceive a holistic model of health for Māori communities, Durie (1985) proposed the Te Whare Tapa Whā, which represents Māori cultural values, beliefs and ways of understanding the world and this is conceptualised as four walls of a meeting house. The walls symbolise the four aspects of health, physical, mental and emotional, spiritual, family and social health. Physical health (Taha Tinana) includes bodily sensations, movement, diet, sleep and physical activity. Mental and emotional health (Taha Hinengaro) is about wellbeing related to thoughts and feelings, relaxation, expressions of gratitude, talking to people and that the mind and body cannot be separated. Spiritual health (Taha Wairua) involves heritage, faith, beliefs, values, traditions and connecting with nature by spending time outdoors. Family and social health (Taha Whānau) incorporates the extended family, friends, caring, the community, creation of new friendships and quality of relationships. The 'walls' of the house are of equal size and importance. If the walls of the meeting house are secure and strong, the person will be in good health, damage or change to anyone of these 'walls' will affect balance and harmony, resulting in negative impacts on overall health. In 2000, Fielden et al. reported that the Te Whare Tapa Whā model was expanded to include the fifth aspect that represented the foundations of the house (Taha Whenua), which is associated with culture and belonging, connecting the Māori to the land. The New Zealand Ministry of Health (n.d.) recognise and propose three Māori health models, the first is Te Whare Tapa Whā, as described above. The second is Te Wheke, which is a model based on the eight tentacles of an octopus, the head represents the extended family (whānau) and the eyes indicate general health (waiora). Each of the tentacles are associated with specific holistic aspects of health (Pere, 1991). The third model is the Te Pae Māhutonga (Durie, 1999), it is based on the four stars of the Southern Cross constellation, which signify aspects of health promotion (cultural roots, surroundings, healthy habits and community involvement), grounded in community leadership and autonomy, represented by the two pointer stars of the constellation.

The Medicine Wheel

Many Indigenous Peoples of North America make use of the Medicine Wheel, which has been used in teaching and healing. It comprises four quadrants of a circle (see Figure 2.5), which are interconnected, symbolising the cycle of life and nature, along with harmony and balance. The four differently coloured quadrants can be used to represent the cardinal directions, states of self, seasons, times of the day, stages of life and sacred plant medicines. This is just one example of the Medicine Wheel, as each Indigenous tribal community has their own culture, history and teachings, which are reflected in variations in the colour of quadrants and information that is presented in each quadrant. Balance and harmony are important aspects of health for Indigenous Peoples and we will explore the Medicine Wheel more fully in Chapter 7.

Cultural appropriation of Indigenous healing practices

Indigenous and healing practices, such as Traditional Chinese Medicine (TCM), Ayurveda, yoga and mindfulness, have beneficial outcomes for the mind, body and spirit. Western medicine views these healing practices with scepticism, as

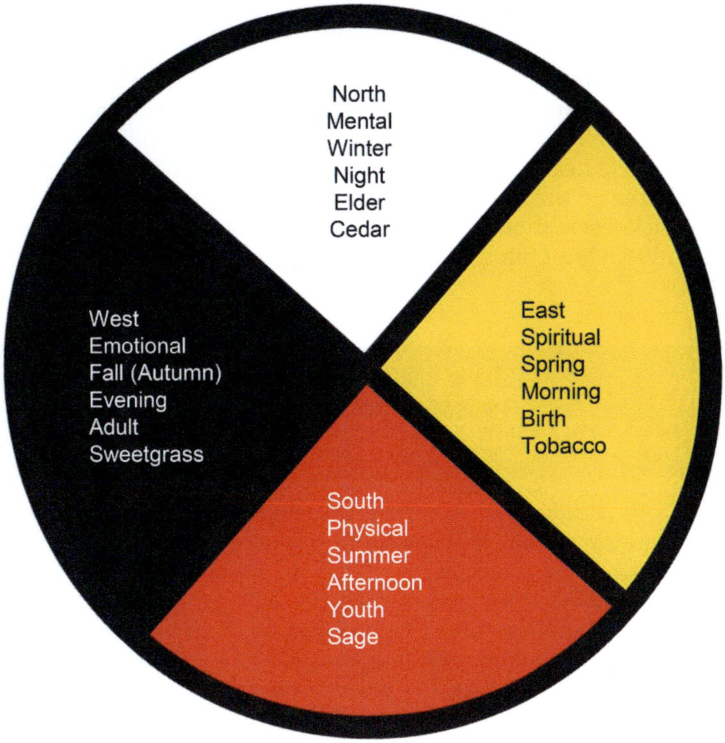

Figure 2.5
The Medicine Wheel

Source: Author based on Greer and Lemacks (2024)

efficacy and worth of a therapy or treatment requires evidence, which is usually based on randomised controlled trials (RCTs) (see Box 2.5). Such an approach is commendable when drug A is being evaluated against drug B or a placebo, but Indigenous and Eastern healing practices do not lend themselves to such an approach (Lokugamage et al., 2020), as treatments are tailored to meet individual patient needs, rather than the same treatment or intervention being prescribed for everyone with the same disease or symptoms. This makes replication problematic, in addition, Indigenous and Eastern healing outcomes address multiple aspects of health that do not lend themselves to quantification, such as spiritual wellbeing, harmony and balance. Despite rejecting the worth of Indigenous and Eastern holistic therapies, such as acupuncture, Ayurveda, yoga and mindfulness, Western medicine, practitioners and researchers have **culturally appropriated** (where the historically dominant culture takes over elements of a colonised culture, without understanding, respect or permission) and rebranded them as **complementary and alternative medicines** ([CAMs]; Lokugamage et al., 2020). Non-Indigenous practitioners mainly use CAMs to complement dominant Western healthcare practices but give little recognition to the colonised societies from which they originated (Ramcharan & Sinjela, 2005). Some attempts have been made to combine Western medicine alongside CAMs, which has become known as integrative medicine (Hollenberg & Muzzin, 2010); for example, mindfulness, which has its basis in Buddhism, has been researched within a Western medical framework as a method for dealing with stress, managing anxiety and depression in people living with and beyond cancer (Carlson et al., 2023). However, it seems that 'integration' means certain aspects of Indigenous and Eastern healing practices have been 'cherry picked' and assimilated into Western medicine, with holistic healing knowledge being suppressed or tokenised. For example, the branding of 'medical' acupuncture to promote pain relief and alleviation of morning sickness without any attempt at understanding or acknowledging the history or underlying philosophy in TCM that emphasises holistic health (Bell et al., 2002).

BOX 2.5
RANDOMISED CONTROLLED TRIALS

A randomised controlled trial (RCT) is a type of experimental design that involves randomisation of participants into two separate groups, one receives the drug or intervention (the experimental group) and the other (the control group) receives no treatment, usual treatment or a placebo (an inert drug or intervention). Randomisation is a way of allocating people to groups by chance (see Chapter 3) to preclude any systematic between group differences that could have an impact on the outcomes of a study. Specific outcome measures (e.g. symptom severity, QoL, depression and/or biomedical tests) are collected prior to the receipt of the intervention/drug and after the end of the study. The outcomes between the two groups are compared to determine if any changes have occurred over time.

Traditional Chinese Medicine

Traditional Chinese Medicine (TCM) was originally used as a method of illness prevention, with an emphasis on balance and harmony in all aspects of life. Health and disease are conceptualised by the balance of Yin and Yang and Qi (vital or life force). Patients, irrespective of how they are feeling, attend their acupuncturist every season to check the balance of Yin, Yang and Qi, and receive treatment to try and ward off disease even before it appears. Fine needles are used to stimulate specific acupuncture points to influence the balance of Qi. These points are situated along the 14 meridians, which connect the surface of the body to the internal organs to regulate the flow of Yin and Yang. The holism of TCM also considers the impact of external aspects of the person's environment that can impact on Qi; this includes climate and weather in the form of heat, cold, wind, moisture and dryness, along with internal factors that contribute to disease, such as emotions, but the latter are not conceptualised in the same way as Western thinking. In TCM, emotions are said to interrupt the flow of Qi, creating an imbalance between Yin and Yang, which is manifested in various symptoms that can contribute to disease. The liver is associated with the emotion of anger, which may cause headaches and dizziness. The heart is linked with joy, worry or overthinking, which may result in palpitations and insomnia. A problem with the spleen may be characterised by indigestion and fatigue, whereas sadness and grief can be injurious to the lungs, resulting in respiratory issues. Finally, fear can be detrimental to the kidneys, which may manifest as low back problems and frequent urination. The flow of Qi can also be influenced by external factors, such as injuries, stress, poor health habits relating to diet, too much or too little sleep, activity or work.

When coming to a diagnosis, the TCM practitioner observes the patient's eyes, nails, skin, and lips, looks at the colour and texture of each. Observation includes the patient's tone of voice, their posture and bodily odours. The patient is asked questions about their symptoms, appetite, thirst and bodily excretions. After this, the practitioner engages in pulse diagnosis and tongue diagnosis, the latter is said to reflect the status of the internal organs and the energy within each meridian. Pulse diagnosis involves palpation of the six deep (Yin) and six superficial (Yang) pulses on lateral (outside) aspect of the wrists, providing information on the overall strength and quality of Qi, relative to each organ. Treatment includes acupuncture, herbs and cupping (a container, usually glass) is placed on the skin and heated, which creates suction and draws Qi into the skin). Moxibustion may be used and this involves the placement of small amounts of burning herbs on acupuncture needles to draw heat into the meridian. The Western use of TCM strips it of the holistic context, complexity and cultural roots, as Yin, Yang, Qi, meridians and acupuncture do not align with Western anatomy, physiology or ways of knowing and positive effects of TCM treatment have often been explained as a mere placebo effect.

Ayurveda

Like TCM, Ayurveda is a holistic approach concerned with the prediction and prevention of disease. It is based on ancient medical practices that originated in India and there is an emphasis on the concept of people having different body types that require differing treatments (Morandi et al., 2011). Unlike Western medicine, Ayurveda states that men and women will have differential responses to treatment, likewise between adults and children (Arnold, 2023). The physiology of the body is considered in terms of five elements, the sky, air, fire, water and earth and five senses (hearing, touch, sight, taste and smell), which are linked with three bodily humours or doshas (Vata, Pitta and Kapha). Optimal health involves a balance between the doshas, whereas disease involves an imbalance (Mantle, 2002). Vata is concerned with the physiological functions of the nervous system, breathing, the heart, blood flow and the motility of the digestive system. Pitta is concerned with appetite, digestion of food, metabolism and the flow of blood and oxygen around the body. Bone, muscle and joint lubrication are associated with Kapha. The doshas are found in nature; hence, they can be disrupted by natural external factors such as the weather, food and seasons, as well as pathogens, such as viruses and bacteria (Postmonitor & Teitelbaum, 2009); they are also subject to internal factors such as emotions (Sharma et al., 2007). The uniqueness of each individual means that when there is an imbalance within their doshas, one individual may exhibit a different disease and series of symptoms, hence there is a need for personalised treatments.

Like TCM, the Ayurvedic practitioner observes the patient and engages in pulse diagnosis. Digestion is a central tenet of Ayurvedic health and there is a belief that all diseases start in the digestive system (Arnold, 2023), hence food and drink are very important factors in health, disease and treatment. Ayurveda emphasises the mind-body connection, along with the impact that significant others may exert on emotions, thus psychosocial aspects of a person's environment can impact health. Treatments may involve massage, diet, yoga, meditation, sound (Lynch et al., 2018), colour therapy (Kurt & Osueke, 2014) and herbal remedies. The individualistic nature of Ayurveda means that like TCM, it does not lend itself to Western scientific efficacy testing through randomised controlled trials (RCTs). Yet, aspects of Ayurveda are being colonised by Western medicine, which disregards the holistic patient assessment, along with treatments that involve a combination of herbal medicines that are used in synergy with yoga and meditation.

When India was colonised, the practice of Ayurveda was supplanted by Western medicine, but after independence in the 1950s, Ayurveda was reintroduced and there are many such clinics and hospitals in India today. However, the herbs and dietary aspects of healing used within Ayurveda for thousands of years have become a focal point for the Western drug industry. Attempts have been made to isolate and identify the chemical components of curcumin (used to help with inflammation) and ashwagandha (used to control stress, improve the immune response and lower blood pressure) to develop new synthetic versions that can be capitalised on by pharmaceutical companies (Arnold, 2023). It is difficult to find any recent statistics, but Posey (1990) pointed out that the commercialisation of certain aspects of Indigenous healing and traditional remedies had a total market value of around US$43 billion (around £32.75 billion), with less than .001% returned to Indigenous Peoples.

Yoga

Yoga has its basis in the Hindu philosophy and has also undergone cultural appropriation. Traditional Indigenous yoga is a holistic practice that involves spiritual development, ethical living, nonviolence and truthfulness (Yama), being content and disciplined (Niyama), movement-based bodily poses (Asana), controlled breathing (Pranayama), detaching oneself from sensory distractions (Pratyahara), concentration (Dhyana) and self-realisation (Samadhi). These aspects are complemented by the yoga of selfless action (Karma), devotion (Bhakti) and knowledge (Jnana). In addition, yoga involves the movement of energy through the chakras (energy centres) to assist healing and achieve spiritual awakening. If the energy with a chakra is weak or becomes blocked, it may cause physical or emotional disease. The use of yoga in Western contexts is often trimmed down to physical postures (Asana), sometimes accompanied by relaxation. This contrasts with the Indigenous conception of yoga in which physical postures are used to prepare the mind for deeper spiritual practices that are targeted on the cultivation of inner balance, health, mental discipline and being 'at one' with the universe and linked to the rhythms of the earth and the sun.

Mindfulness

Mindfulness includes the core practice of meditation in which the individual pays attention, without judgement to the present movement. It also involves loving-kindness (metta), the cultivation of love and compassion (karuna) to self and others to enhance mental and physical health by trying to reduce negative emotions and increase positive ones. Mindfulness is just one aspect of Buddhism that has been selected for its usefulness to complement Western healthcare practices, again without acknowledgement to the philosophy and way of living on which it was based. Buddhism involves the Four Nobel Truths, which relate to suffering, its existence (Dukkha), causes (Samudaya), overcoming suffering (Nirodha) and cessation of suffering (Magga), leading into the Noble Eightfold Path. The latter is a guide for ethical and mental development related to wisdom, ethical conduct and mental discipline. Included in Buddhism is the law of karma, which is about the moral consequences of one's actions, good actions equal good karma or good outcomes and the reverse being true for negative actions. For the Buddhist, the ultimate goal is to reach Nirvana, which is a state of liberation from suffering. Ethical living through the Five Precepts in which the individual consciously tries to avoid harming anything that is living, avoidance of sexual misconduct, stealing, lying and becoming intoxicated. Diet is a central aspect of Buddhism that includes eating a vegetarian diet, but these aspects are selectively missing in most Western applications of mindfulness.

From the examples provided, it is evident that despite intentions from Western healthcare systems to engage in decolonisation, dominance and cultural appropriation of Indigenous and Eastern healthcare practices still persist today. Particular aspects have been 'foraged' as useful adjuncts to Western ethnocentric medicine. Western cultures heralded the biopsychosocial approach to health as a great 'breakthrough' in upholding the WHO (1948) definition of health but seem to have ignored the fact that many Indigenous populations have been using the principles of the biopsychosocial model in healing and in the prevention of disease for centuries, if not for thousands of years. While there are variations in traditions and cultures across and within Indigenous populations, they share a commonality in that their healthcare practices are truly holistic. While biopsychosocial, ecological and Indigenous views about health and wellbeing have different cultural and philosophical underpinnings but they all agree that health is multidimensional and involves some degree of personalisation. However, Western notions about health tend to assume universality in how health is conceptualised, how diseases are treated and how success is measured. Such an approach ignores collectivist dimensions of wellbeing, self-determination, negative consequences of colonisation and cultural appropriation.

BOX 2.2
CRITICAL THINKING

Ethnocentrism in health means judging other cultures' health practices, values and concepts from our viewpoint, which can lead to bias in healthcare, research and practice.

How has health psychology been shaped by Western ideas?
Consider how health professionals may ignore culture beliefs about illness and healing?
How can we make healthcare more culturally respectful and inclusive?
Can you think of an example where cultural misunderstandings affected health outcomes?

Culture and health

Definitions of culture have changed over time, from focusing on geographical belonging, ethnicity, shared identity, customs, habits, beliefs and language to also include gender identity, sexual orientation, socioeconomic status, educational status, religious and spiritual beliefs, age and disability. Culture influences people's perceptions of health and disease; hence, there will be fundamental differences in the approaches to and beliefs about healthcare practices, ways of making diagnoses and treatments. Western healthcare places the onus on the individual to assume responsibility for their own health, which contrasts with Indigenous health practices that are community concerns. This means that Western practices and associated models of health that try to predict and control an individual's behaviour may have less relevance to Indigenous societies, which is something that healthcare professionals and researchers do not always understand or may choose to remain ignorant of (Prilleltensky & Prilleltensky, 2003).

Indigenous Peoples across the globe are still living with the enduring effects of colonisation, such as poorer health, poverty, lower life expectancy and lower access to third-level education compared to their non-Indigenous counterparts. Indigenous health involves interrelated aspects of culture, community, the land, physical, psychological, mental and spiritual health, which cannot and should not be viewed in isolation (Boot & Lovell, 2019). For health partnerships to flourish, Western trained healthcare professionals need to take a bicultural approach to healthcare. They need to have respect for traditional healing beliefs and practices, while recognising diversity in relation to language, culture, ancestral heritage and social relationships among Indigenous and other minoritised groups, even within the same country.

Within England, the 2021 census showed that almost a fifth of the population self-identified as belonging to a non-White ethnic minority group (Office for National Statistics, 2023). While the National Health Service (NHS) in the UK provides free access to healthcare, NHS surveys have indicated that some ethnic minority groups can experience less positive healthcare experiences compared to their White British counterparts (Raleigh, 2023). Similar to Indigenous populations, people from ethnic minorities may have cultural beliefs and needs that are underserved by healthcare providers. The most fundamental and main barrier to accessing care in England is language (Ajayi Sotubo, 2021). The NHS does provide professional interpreters, but to increase patient trust and prevent culture misunderstandings, it is essential that interpreters are sensitive to the cultural contexts of patients and the specific terminology in the healthcare services and departments they are requested to work in (Lehane & Campion, 2018).

Ethnicity is only one non-medical factor that can impact health; gender and sexual orientation, disability, socioeconomic status, educational level and living in deprived neighbourhoods can impact access to healthcare, treatment and health outcomes. However, the intersections of these factors can overlap to create even greater experiences of privilege and oppression (Routen et al., 2023). For example, a recent audit of maternal deaths within the UK, between 2020 and 2022, found that the mortality risk for Black women was three times higher in the year immediately following the birth of their babies compared to White women, whereas Asian women were twice as likely to die. The audit reportedly noted that between 6 weeks and 12 months after giving birth, almost a third of all maternal deaths were caused by suicide or substance abuse. In addition, Black and Asian women experienced delayed birthing interventions and received inadequate pain relief. The audit reported insufficient interpreter services for women who did not speak English as their first language, which hindered informed decision-making and consent. Women from Black and Asian groups were more likely to have lived in deprived areas, characterised by higher unemployment, inadequate housing and diet, all factors that have been linked to poorer health outcomes. The authors of the report stated that fear of stigma and lack of culturally sensitive services for those with mental health conditions were barriers to women seeking help. They also went on to highlight the need for cultural competency training for healthcare professionals to ensure that cultural needs and values are addressed (Felker et al., 2024). From this, it is clear that multiple intersecting factors played a role in the differential treatment and experiences of these women. These findings echo earlier research of there being an association between intersecting identities and **health inequities** (Lokugamage et al., 2020). To reduce misunderstandings, patient dissatisfaction and detrimental health outcomes, there is a need for health professional training that highlights the role of power, privilege and intersectionality on healthcare experiences.

Cultural awareness, competence and safety

Increasing cultural diversity and ethnicity within the US in the 1960s meant that healthcare practitioners and researchers lacked the ability to engage with patients whose culture, values and beliefs were different to those of the White non-Hispanic population. To be able to engage with East Asian refugees, African American and Hispanic populations, healthcare practitioners required training in **cultural awareness**. At that time, training consisted of learning general facts about the lives, behaviours and beliefs of cultural groups. There was an acknowledgement that this superficial approach ignored historical injustices, discrimination, stigma and unconscious bias and was later replaced with training in **cultural competence**. The latter emphasised the importance of health professionals' understanding the impact of social and cultural factors on patients from the non-dominant culture and being sensitive to such factors when communicating with patients and delivering care. However, this approach seemed to be task orientated, in that it helped individual healthcare professionals to acquire knowledge, skills and attitudes about other cultures and once training had been completed, cultural competency was obtained (Kumagai & Lypson, 2009). However, Furlong and Wight (2011) have questioned if training in cultural competence has been reduced to a tick-box exercise, as it assumes that individuals from the dominant culture can assess the cultural competence of colleagues without having the actual lived experience of being from a minority culture. Training in cultural competency has moved on and expanded beyond training individual healthcare professionals, it has become embedded within healthcare organisational approaches to patient care. This involves more than gaining knowledge and awareness of the needs of minority groups and includes changes in behaviour, challenging stereotypic views, self-reflection of the dominant culture along with promotion of inclusion. Despite this, inequities in health prevention strategies and healthcare not only persist but are also perpetuated by negative healthcare interactions.

The term **cultural safety** originated in New Zealand and was developed by Māori nurses (Ramsden, 2002). It includes healthcare professional practice that recognises and reflects on power imbalances in society (systemic racism, White privilege and improving the health of minority groups) and during patient encounters. In their critique of who assesses cultural competence, Furlong and Wight (2011) stated that the recipient of the healthcare interactions, service or research should determine if the care being received is culturally safe. In contrast to cultural awareness or competence, cultural safety is not something that is achieved, passed and crossed off a list as being complete, it is an ongoing process, involving self-awareness and self-reflection. Self-awareness involves health professionals recognising and understanding how their own culture, upbringing, beliefs and values have shaped their thoughts and behaviours. Self-reflection is about understanding how our own cultural identity and beliefs impact our interactions with others and healthcare that is delivered (Dune et al., 2021). To reduce health inequities and negative experiences for minority groups, multiple power imbalances, levels of privilege and bias, healthcare systems ought to be considered within an ecological model (McLeroy et al., 1988). Without organisational and policy changes, the dominant Eurocentric view of health and associated power imbalances that maintain disadvantage will persist (Curtis et al., 2019).

BOX 2.3
CRITICAL THINKING

How do colonial histories still affect health and healthcare today?
Why might one health message or treatment not work for everyone?

Chapter summary

Explain how early views about health and disease have changed over time

Hippocrates viewed health as an imbalance between four bodily humours and Galen expanded this theory further to include bodily organs. During the Middle Ages, people turned to religion for healing, with illness being seen as a punishment from God, dissection was banned until the Renaissance when Descartes stipulated that the mind and body were separate and human dissection recommenced.

Identify factors that have influenced the changing nature of disease

The discovery of the microscope, the role of microorganisms in disease, antiseptics and anaesthetics along with clean water supplies and improved sanitation helped reduce the burden of infectious diseases and improve life expectancy. Later, antibiotics and vaccines led to further improvements in health and the biomedical model became established. Deaths due to infectious diseases have reduced, people are living longer, but at the same time they are having to cope with chronic diseases.

Compare and contrast the contributions that the biomedical, biopsychosocial and ecological models have made to understanding health and disease

The biomedical model has helped in the diagnosis and treatment of acute diseases that were caused by viruses, bacteria and trauma, but it was unable to deal with the increasing burden of chronic diseases caused by lifestyle factors. The biopsychosocial model included not only the biomedical aspects of disease, but also psychological and social factors to explain the role that lifestyle could have on the development and progression of chronic disease. The ecological model took this a stage further to consider how organisational, community and policy factors along with an individual's privilege and power imbalances could impact an individual's health and disease.

Outline what is meant by ethnocentrism in health and why this reflects biased thinking

Ethnocentrism is about viewing Western healthcare practices as superior to other people's health care systems, beliefs and practices. Bias lies in the devaluation of other perspectives and cultural differences.

How do Western and Indigenous models of health differ?

The Western and Indigenous models of health differ in their understanding of what it means to be healthy, the causes of disease and the healing methods used. Western models focus on the physical body, biomedical and lifestyle factors as the causes of disease. Biomedical approaches are taken to treat diseases, based on scientific research and that the individual is responsible for their own health. Indigenous models view disease as an imbalance between mental, emotional, spiritual and physical wellbeing, which is influenced by the family community, ancestors and the land. Colonisation has contributed to imbalances. Healing involves traditional practices that are holistic in nature to restore balance. Health and disease are collective responsibilities, shared with the family, the community and ancestors.

Outline the differences between cultural awareness, competence and safety

Cultural awareness involves knowing that differences exist between cultures in terms of beliefs, values and health practices. Cultural competence means people are considerate and respectful of cultural differences. Cultural safety is about creating an environment that people from other cultures feel safe from discriminatory actions, attitudes and judgements, being aware of power relationships and ensuring that patients and their family members are involved in care decisions.

Keywords

Mind-body link: An individual's thoughts and emotions can affect their physical health and physical health, in turn can affect thoughts and emotions.

Humoral theory: An early explanation that imbalances of bodily humours (blood, phlegm, black bile and yellow bile) caused disease.

Cartesian Dualism: Based on the views of Descartes that the mind and the body were separate, people's thoughts and emotions could not affect physical health.

Life expectancy: An approximation of the age that an individual is expected to live to based on their biological sex and age.

Health literacy: Having the skills, knowledge and ability to find, understand and use health information.

Morbidity: Having a disease or being ill.

Passive smoking: Inhaling others' exhaled smoke from tobacco or the side-stream smoke of the tobacco.

Ethnocentric view: Tendency to think and interpret other cultures and health-care practices as inferior to your own.

Spirit world: The belief that everything has a spirit, for example, ancestors, the land, animals and that they are all connected to the individual.

Intergenerational trauma: Trauma and pain that is passed down from previous generations, e.g. colonisation. The trauma that affects those who did not experience the original event.

Health disparities: Differences in health outcomes between groups of people, caused by a range of different factors e.g. poverty, educational level, discrimination and colonisation.

Culturally appropriated: Where the historically dominant culture takes over elements of a colonised culture, without understanding, respect or permission.

Health inequities: Unfair or unavoidable health differences that are caused by a range of factors e.g. poverty, educational level, culture, ethnicity, colonisation, gender, gender identity and sexual orientation.

Cultural awareness: Learning general facts about the lives, behaviours and beliefs of cultural groups that are different to your own.

Cultural competence: Knowledge of the impact that social and cultural factors can have on people from the non-dominant culture and the importance of treating people fairly and with respect.

Cultural safety: The ability to recognise and reflect on power imbalances to ensure that people are safe from discriminatory actions, attitudes and judgements.

Complementary and alternative medicines: Complementary medicines are those that are used alongside Western medicine e.g. the use of acupuncture for pain relief and taking painkilling medications. Alternative medicines or therapies are used instead of Western ones, e.g. taking herbal remedies instead of Western medications.

Key readings

Lokugamage, A. U., Ahillan, T., & Pathberiya, S. D. C. (2020). Decolonising ideas of healing in medical education. *Journal of Medical Ethics*, *46*(4), 265–272. https://doi.org/10.1136/medethics-2019-105866

McLeroy, K. R., Bibeau, D., Steckler, A., & Glanz, K. (1988). An ecological perspective on health promotion programs. *Health Education Quarterly*, *15*(4), 351–377. https://doi.org/10.1177/109019818801500401

Syed, S., Syed, S., & Bhardwaj, K. (2020) The role of the bio-psychosocial model in public health. *The Journal of Medical Research*, *8*(5), 252–252. https://doi.org/10.31254/jmr.2020.6517

Reflective Questions

1 How have ideas about the causes of illness changed over time, and why does this matter in health psychology?
2 In what ways might Western medicine's focus on science and individual treatment overlook the cultural and community-based approaches to health found in Indigenous healthcare practices?
3 What should a health psychologist do to ensure that their care respects beliefs about health across different cultures?

References

Ajayi Sotubo, O. (2021). A perspective on health inequalities in BAME communities and how to improve access to primary care. *Future Healthcare Journal, 8*(1), 36–39. https://doi.org/10.7861/fhj.2020-0217

American Psychological Association (1976). Task force on health research, contributions of psychology to health research: Patterns, problems, and potentials. *American Psychologist, 31*, 263–274. https://doi:10.1037/0003-066X.31.4.263

Arnold, J. T. (2023). Integrating ayurvedic medicine into cancer research programs part 1: Ayurveda background and applications. *Journal of Ayurveda and Integrative Medicine, 14*(2), 100676.

Australian Bureau of Statistics (2018). *Aboriginal and Torres Strait Islander life expectancy lowest in remote and very remote areas*. Retrieved April 11, 2025, from https://www.abs.gov.au/articles/aboriginal-and-torres-strait-islander-life-expectancy-lowest-remote-and-very-remote-areas

Australian Institute of Health and Welfare (2024). *Aboriginal and Torres Strait Islander Health Performance Framework: Summary report*. Australian Government. Retrieved April 8, 2025, from https://www.indigenoushpf.gov.au/

Bell, I. R., Caspi, O., Schwartz, G. E. R., Grant, K. L., Gaudet, T. W., Rychener, D., Maizes, V., & Weil, A. (2002). Integrative medicine and systemic outcomes research. *Archives of Internal Medicine, 162*, 133–140. https://doi.org/10.1001/archinte.162.2.133

Betancourt, J. R., Green, A. R., & Carrillo, J. E. (2002). *Cultural competence in health care: Emerging frameworks and practical approaches* (Field Report No. 576). The Commonwealth Fund. https://www.commonwealthfund.org/publications/fund-reports/2002/oct/cultural-competence-health-care-emerging-frameworks-and practical approaches

Boot, G. R., & Lowell, A. (2019). Acknowledging and promoting Indigenous knowledges, paradigms, and practices within health literacy-related policy and practice documents across Australia, Canada, and New Zealand. *International Indigenous Policy Journal, 10*(3). https://doi.org/10.18584/iipj.2019.10.3.8133

Bronfenbrenner, U. (1979). *The ecology of human development: Experiments by nature and design*. Harvard University Press.

Carlson, L. E., Ismaila, N., Addington, E. L., Asher, G. N., Bradt, J., Mehta, A., & Rowland, J. H. (2023). Integrative oncology care of symptoms of anxiety and depression in adults with cancer: SIO-ASCO guideline summary and Q&A. *Journal of Oncology Practice, 19*(10), 847–851. https://doi.org/10.1200/OP.23.00358

Curtis, E., Jones, R., Tipene-Leach, D., Walker, C., Loring, B., Paine, S. J., & Reid, P. (2019). Why cultural safety rather than cultural competency is required to achieve health equity: A literature review and recommended definition. *International Journal for Equity in Health, 18*(1), 174. https://doi.org/10.1186/s12939-019-1082-3

Dattani, S., Rodés-Guirao, L., Ritchie, H., Ortiz-Ospina, E., & Roser, M. (2023). *Life expectancy*, Published online at OurWorldinData.org. Retrieved October 23, 2024, from https://ourworldindata.org/life-expectancy

Dawber, T. R., Moore, F. E., & Mann, G. V. (1957). Coronary heart disease in the Framingham study. *American Journal of Public Health and the Nation's Health, 47*(2), 4–24. https://doi.org/10.2105/ajph.47.4_pt_2.4

Ding, D., Sallis, J. F., Kerr, J., Lee, S., & Rosenberg, D. E. (2011). Neighborhood environment and physical activity among youth a review. *American Journal of Preventive Medicine, 41*(4), 442–455. https://doi.org/10.1016/j.amepre.2011.06.036

Doll, R., & Hill, A. B. (1950). Smoking and carcinoma of the lung; Preliminary report. *British Medical Journal, 2*(4682), 739–748. https://doi.org/10.1136/bmj.2.4682.739

Donaldson, L. (2000). Disease emergence and health transitions in the last millennium. *Journal of the Royal College of Physicians of London, 34*, 543–548.

Dune, T., McLeod, K., & Williams, R.(Eds.) (2021). *Culture, diversity and health in Australia*. Routledge.

Durie M. H. (1985). A Maori perspective of health. *Social Science & Medicine, 20*(5), 483–486. https://doi.org/10.1016/0277-9536(85)90363-6

Durie, M. (1999). Te Pae Mahutonga: A model for Mäori health promotion. *Health Promotion Forum of New Zealand Newsletter, 49*, 2–5.

Engel, G. L. (1977). The need for a new medical model: A challenge for biomedicine, *Science, 96*, 129–136. https://doi.org/10.1126/science.847460

Felker, A., Patel, R., Kotnis, R., Kenyon, S., & Knight, M. (Eds). On behalf of MBRRACE-UK (2024). Saving lives, improving mothers' care compiled report - Lessons learned to inform maternity care from the UK and Ireland Confidential Enquiries into Maternal Deaths and Morbidity 2020-22. National Perinatal Epidemiology Unit, University of Oxford. Retrieved June 3, 2025, from https://www.npeu.ox.ac.uk/assets/downloads/mbrrace-uk/reports/maternal-report-2024/MBRRACE-UK%20Maternal%20MAIN%20Report%202024%20V2.0%20ONLINE.pdf

Fleck, A. (2023). *Native Americans still face significant life expectancy pap*. Statistica. Retrieved April 8, 2025, from https://www.statista.com/chart/30991/average-life-expectancy-in-the-united-states-by-racial-and-ethnic-groups/

Furlong, M., & Wight, J. (2011). Promoting "critical awareness" and critiquing "cultural competence": Towards disrupting received professional knowledges. *Australian Social Work, 64*(1), 38–54. https://doi.org/10.1080/0312407X.2010.537352

Gimeno, L., Goisis, A., Dowd, J. B., & Ploubidis, G. B. (2024). Cohort differences in physical health and disability in the United States and Europe. *The Journals of Gerontology*, 79(8), gbae113. https://doi.org/10.1093/geronb/gbae113

Greer, T., & Lemacks, J. L. (2024). The Medicine Wheel as a public health approach to lifestyle management interventions for Indigenous populations in North America. *Frontiers in Public Health, 12*, 1392517. https://doi.org/10.3389/fpubh.2024.1392517

Hatala, A. R. (2013). Towards a biopsychosocial–spiritual approach in health psychology: Exploring theoretical orientations and future directions. *Journal of Spirituality in Mental Health, 15*(4), 256–276. https://doi.org/10.1080/19349637.2013.776448

Hollenberg, D., & Muzzin, L. (2010). Epistemological challenges to integrative medicine: An anti-colonial perspective on the combination of complementary/alternative medicine with biomedicine. *Health Sociology Review, 19*(1), 34–56. https://doi.org/10.5172/hesr.2010.19.1.034

Karlinsky, A. (2024). International completeness of death registration. *Demographic Research, 50*, 1151–1170. https://doi.org/10.4054/DemRes.2024.50.38

Keys, A. (1953). Prediction and possible prevention of coronary disease. *American Journal of Public Health and the Nation's Health, 43*(11), 1399–1407. https://doi.org/10.2105/ajph.43.11.1399

Kumagai, A. K., & Lypson, M. L. (2009). Beyond cultural competence: Critical consciousness, social justice, and multicultural education. *Academic Medicine, 84*(6), 782–787. https://doi.org/10.1097/ACM.0b013e3181a42398

Kurt, S., & Osueke, K. K. (2014). The effects of color on the moods of college students. *SAGE Open, 4*(1). https://doi.org/10.1177/2158244014525423

Lehane, D., & Campion, P. (2018). Interpreters: Why should the NHS provide them? *The British Journal of General Practice, 68*(677), 564–565. https://doi.org/10.3399/bjgp18X699905

Lokugamage, A. U., Ahillan, T., & Pathberiya, S. D. C. (2020). Decolonising ideas of healing in medical education. *Journal of Medical Ethics, 46*(4), 265–272. https://doi.org/10.1136/medethics-2019-105866

Lynch, J., Prihodova, L., Dunne, P. J., Carrol, A., Walsh, C., McMahon, G., & White, B. (2018). Mantra meditation for mental health in the general population: A systematic review. *European Journal of Integrative Medicine, 23*, 101–108. https://doi.org/10.1016/j.eujim.2018.09.010

Mantle, F. (2002). The role of alternative medicine in treating postnatal depression. *Complementary Therapies in Nursing & Midwifery, 8*, 197–203. https://doi.org/10.1054/ctnm.2002.0647

McLeroy, K. R., Bibeau, D., Steckler, A., & Glanz, K. (1988). An ecological perspective on health promotion programs. *Health Education Quarterly, 15*(4), 351–377. https://doi.org/10.1177/109019818801500401

Morandi, A., Tosto, C., Roberti di Sarsina, P., & Dalla Libera, D. (2011). Salutogenesis and Ayurveda: Indications for public health management. *The European Association for Predictive Preventive & Personalized Medicine Journal, 2*(4), 459–465. https://doi.org/10.1007/s13167-011-0132-8

Morris, J. N., Heady, J. A., Raffle, P. A., Roberts, C. G., & Parks, J. W. (1953). Coronary heart-disease and physical activity of work. *Lancet, 262*(6795), 1053–1057. https://doi.org/10.1016/s0140-6736(53)90665-5

Moss, P. (Ed.) (2016). *American Indian health and nursing*. Springer.

Native Women's Association of Canada (2025). *Healthy aging report*. Retrieved April 8, 2025, from https://nwac.ca/assets-knowledge-centre/Healthy-Aging-Report.pdf

New Zealand Ministry of Health (n.d.). *Māori health models*. Retrieved May 27, 2025, from https://www.health.govt.nz/maori-health/maori-health-models/te-wheke

Office for National Statistics (2023). *Ethnic group by age and sex, England and Wales: Census 2021*. Retrieved June 2, 2025, from www.ons.gov.uk/releases/ethnicgroupbyageandsexenglandandwalescensus2021

Oetzel, J. G., Ruru, S., Zhang, Y., Simpson, M. L., Nock, S., Meha, P., Holmes, K., Clark, M., Adams, H., Akapita, N., Ngaia, K., Murphy, S., Moses, R., Reddy, R., & Hokowhitu, B. (2021). Enhancing well-being and social connectedness for Māori elders through a peer education (Tuakana-Teina) programme: A cross-sectional baseline study. *Frontiers in Public Health, 9*, 775545. https://doi.org/10.3389/fpubh.2021.775545

Paradies, Y. (2016). Colonisation, racism and indigenous health. *Journal of Population Research, 33*, 83–96. https://doi.org/10.1007/s12546-016-9159-y

Pere, R. (1991). *Te Wheke: A celebration of infinite wisdom*. Ao Ako Global Learning New Zealand.

Posey, D. (1990). Intellectual property rights and just compensation for Indigenous knowledge. *Anthropology Today, 6*(4), 13–16. https://doi.org/10.2307/3032735

Postmontier, B., & Teitelbaum, M. (2009). An Ayurvedic approach to postpartum depression. *Holistic Nursing Practice, 23*(4), 201–216. https://doi.org/10.1097/HNP.0b013e3181aece5a

Prilleltensky, I., & Prilleltensky, O. (2003). Towards a critical health psychology practice. *Journal of Health Psychology, 8*(2), 197–210. https://doi.org/10.1177/1359105303008002659

Quinn, F., Chater, A., & Morrison, V. (2020). An oral history of health psychology in the UK. *British Journal of Health Psychology, 25*(3), 502–518. https://doi.org/10.1111/bjhp.12418

Raleigh, V. (2023). *The health of people from ethnic minority groups in England.* The King's Fund. Retrieved June 6, 2025, from https://www.kingsfund.org.uk/insight-and-analysis/long-reads/health-people-ethnic-minority-groups-england

Ramcharan, R., & Sinjela, M. A. (2005). Protecting traditional knowledge and traditional medicines of Indigenous Peoples through intellectual property rights: Issues, challenges and strategies. *International Journal on Minority and Group Rights, 12,* 1–24. https://doi.org/10.1163/1571811053890399

Ramsden, I. (2002). *Cultural safety and nursing education in Aotearoa and Te Waipounamu* (Doctoral thesis). Victoria University of Wellington. https://www.croakey.org/wp-content/uploads/2017/08/RAMSDEN-I-Cultural-Safety_Full.pdf

Rochford, T. (2004). Whare Tapa Wha: A Māori model of a unified theory of health. *The Journal of Primary Prevention, 25,* 41–57. https://doi.org/10.1023/B:JOPP.0000039938.39574.9e

Routen, A., Lekas, H. M., Harrison, J., & Khunti, K. (2023). Intersectionality in health equity research. *British Medical Journal, 383,* 2953. https://doi.org/10.1136/bmj.p2953

Sharma, H., Chandola, H. M., Singh, G., & Basisht, G. (2007). Utilization of Ayurveda in health care: An approach for prevention, health promotion, and treatment of disease. Part 1 – Ayurveda, the science of life. *Journal of Alternative and Complementary Medicine, 13*(9), 1011–1019. https://doi.org/10.1089/acm.2007.7017-B

Simons-Morton, B., McLeroy, K., & Wendel, M. (2012). *Behavior theory in health promotion practice and research.* Jones & Bartlett Learning.

Stats New Zealand (2021). *Growth in life expectancy slows.* Stats NZ Tatauranga Aotearoa. Retrieved April 8, 2025, from https://www.stats.govt.nz/news/growth-in-life-expectancy-slows/#:~:text=Life%20expectancy%20at%20birth%20was,to%20live%20to%2084.4%20years

United Nations (2007). United Nations declaration on the rights of Indigenous Peoples. Retrieved October 18, 2024, from https://www.un.org/development/desa/indigenouspeoples/wp-content/uploads/sites/19/2018/11/UNDRIP_E_web.pdf

Video. The Medicine Wheel for spiritual wellness and health Website: https://www.youtube.com/watch?v=YKVkJm5hhNM

Wells, J., (2022) *Health and the medieval church.* Wellcome Collection. Retrieved October 15, 2024, from https://wellcomecollection.org/stories/health-and-the-medieval-church

Wilson K. (2003). Therapeutic landscapes and First Nations peoples: An exploration of culture, health and place. *Health & Place, 9*(2), 83–93. https://doi.org/10.1016/s1353-8292(02)00016-3

World Health Organization (1948) *Constitution of the World Health Organisation.* Retrieved October 24, 2024, from https://apps.who.int/gb/bd/PDF/bd47/EN/constitution-en.pdf?ua=1

World Health Organization (1998). *The World Health Organisation Quality of Life Assessment (WHOQOL): Development and general psychometric properties. Social Science & Medicine, 46*(12), 1569–1585. https://doi.org/10.1016/s0277-9536(98)00009-4

World Health Organization (2024). *Ageing and health.* Retrieved October 24, 2024, from https://www.who.int/news-room/fact-sheets/detail/ageing-and-health

World Health Organization (n.d.). *Frequently asked questions on the health and rights of Indigenous Peoples.* Retrieved April 1, 2025, from https://www.who.int/initiatives/global-plan-of-action-for-health-of-indigenous-peoples/frequently-asked-questions-on-the-health-and-rights-of-indigenous-peoples?utm_source

Wright, J. A. (2007). Practice guidelines by specialist societies are surprisingly deficient. *The International Journal of Clinical Practice, 61,* 1076–1077. https://doi.org/10.1111/j.1742-1241.2007.01436.x

3 Methods and issues in research

Chapter contents

- Epidemiology
- Ontology and epistemology
- Quantitative research designs
- Qualitative research data collection
- Mixed methods
- Decolonisation of research
- Ethical aspects of research
- The replication crisis and open science

Chapter objectives

After reading this chapter, you should be able to answer the following questions:

- Define and explain key concepts and purposes of epidemiological data.
- How ontology and epistemology influence how and what data we collect?
- Explain what is meant by the hierarchy of research designs and how this helps our critical understanding of study bias.
- Discuss the importance of standardisation, validity and reliability when selecting questionnaires.
- Outline methods of qualitative data collection and assess the importance of trustworthiness in qualitative data.
- Discuss the value of using mixed methods.
- Explain why decolonisation of research is important.
- Why do we need research ethics?
- Explain why the replication crisis has implications for open science.

Health psychology covers a wide range of topics and uses a variety of research designs, methods of data collection and analyses. This chapter covers a range of concepts and topics relating to research methods, providing an overview, which will help you to understand how researchers and health psychologists use research to answer specific questions about health and illness. In health psychology, research is conducted in response to an identified gap in the existing literature, which is usually based on previous research findings, or due to patient, healthcare provider or service needs.

DOI: 10.4324/9781003423157-3

Epidemiology

Health psychology makes use of data from **epidemiology**, which is concerned with how diseases affect people. Epidemiologists are interested in who gets sick, how often, why and how infectious diseases spread. This information helps explain the causes of disease, how diseases may be prevented and how to control infectious diseases. Epidemiological information was presented in Chapter 2, in relation to global life expectancy, how a country's income can affect life expectancy and the transition from acute to chronic disease. In interpreting data about disease, it is important to know the difference between prevalence and incidence. **Prevalence** refers to the total number of cases of a disease at a given time, while **incidence** is the number of new cases of a disease at a given time. For example, the British Heart Foundation (2025) reported that the number of people across the globe living with cardiovascular disease (CVD) in 2021 was around 640 million (prevalence) and the number of people with a new diagnosis (incidence) is around 67 million per year. Epidemiological statistics are useful to healthcare providers in exploring how well disease prevention messages and interventions (such as screening people who have no CVD symptoms) are working. These data can also help to determine what additional services and information may be required to prevent and manage specific aspects of disease burden.

Ontology and epistemology

When we conduct research on health and disease, it is helpful to understand the underlying philosophical aspects of how we think about the data that are being collected. To do this, we need to learn about ontology and epistemology, as they influence the types of questions that we ask, the methods used to collect data and subsequent analyses. **Ontology** is concerned with what we think is real or what we believe exists and can be studied. **Epistemology** is concerned with how do we know what we know, that is, how do we gain knowledge. Students sometimes get a bit lost at this point because discussion of ontology and epistemology tends to be quite abstract. To keep the explanation of ontology as simple as possible, we will consider the two major contrasting ontological positions, realist (that is the existence of one reality) and relativist (that is the existence of multiple realities).

Researchers, who favour a pure realist ontological position, see the world (or reality), as not being influenced by human interpretations and perceptions, there is one truth, with no room for subjectivity. This position is characterised by experimentation, use of the scientific method and **objective measurements**. The relativist ontology is the opposite of realist. It supports the idea of their being multiple realities; it is interested in **subjectivity** and acknowledges the role of the researcher coming together with participants to construct realities. An example may be useful to explain the difference between the two ontological positions. What is pain? From a realist ontological perspective, pain is a physical reality due to something being wrong with bodily tissues, muscle, bones or biochemistry. A relativist perspective acknowledges that pain is present, that there may be multiple causes, but pain is not just physical, pain has meaning to the individual, which can be influenced by culture, experience and the context in which the pain occurs (see Chapter 10). A realist ontology involves objective measures to ascertain the cause of pain, this may include blood tests, scans, blood pressure and heart rate. The results of these methods are usually numerical and analysed using statistical tests. The relativist takes the view that pain is a subjective experience that is assessed or measured using interviews, focus groups, pictures, participant diaries, open-ended questionnaires and participatory methods. The resulting data are analysed by qualitative techniques, for example, content, thematic analysis and interpretative phenomenological analysis, which we will look at later in this chapter.

Implications for practice and research

A health professional who believes that disease is only influenced by biomedical factors that can be objectively measured (realist ontology) may ignore social (family, friends, caring and work commitments) and psychological factors (stress, depression and anxiety) that can influence the onset, development and recovery from disease. Taking the opposite approach, only focusing on psychosocial factors and ignoring disease-related issues may be insufficient to deal with conditions that require medication, surgery, chemotherapy or radiation treatment.

A variety of methods are used to collect data in health-related research; these include quantitative and qualitative methods and sometimes a combination of both, which is called mixed methods. **Quantitative methods** are based on numbers and statistics and involve hypothesis testing. A **hypothesis** is a specific statement that is testable, it predicts the relationship between two or more variables in a study or examines if there are numerical differences between different groups or within groups (over time, known as repeated measures) on specific variables. It is essential to formulate a hypothesis (or hypotheses, if more than one is being tested) prior to commencement of a study. **Qualitative methods** are mainly based on words or pictures, the meanings of what people say or how they say it. Qualitative studies do not test hypotheses, rather they pose explorative **research questions**.

Quantitative research designs

Healthcare decisions are based on research, so in learning about health psychology, it is important to understand the different types of research designs, along with the strengths and weaknesses of each. The hierarchy of research designs (Greenhalgh, 1997) provides a structured way of ranking different types of research designs from the most rigorous at the top to the least robust at the bottom (see Figure 3.1), based on the inherent degree of potential research bias in each study design. For example, a case report is an in-depth study of one person, this type of design would provide rich data on how an individual is managing and coping with a disease, but it is unlikely that the findings can be generalised to larger populations. Knowing where a type of research design sits within the hierarchy of research designs can help students, researchers and health professionals to understand how generalisable the results from research might be and where inherent biases lie.

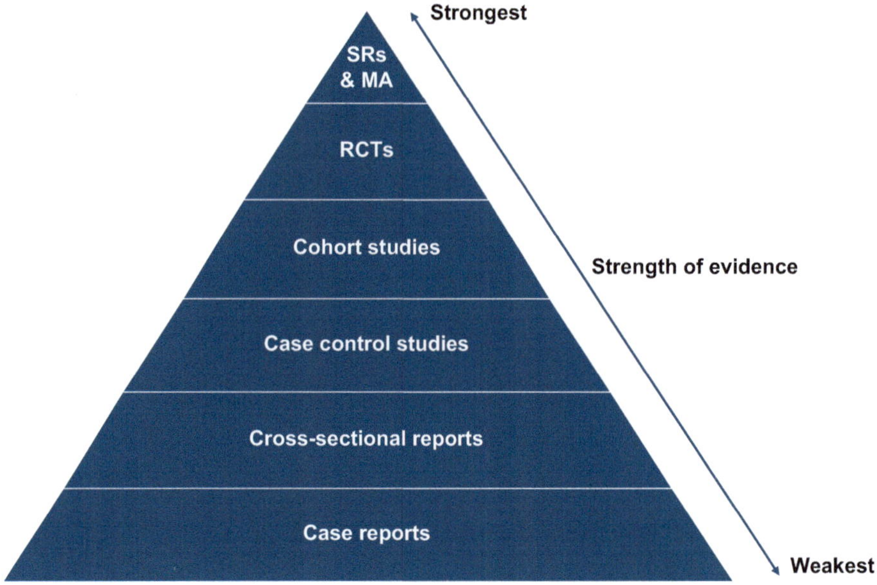

Figure 3.1
Hierarchy of research designs

Source: Author, based on Greenhalgh (1997)

Case reports

A case report is an in-depth study of a single person; the inclusion of multiple case reports is called a case series. There are several journals that are devoted to case reports, and they focus on some unusual aspect of a patient or series of patients. This may include uncommon or new diseases, how to manage them, unique reactions to treatments, adverse side effects of medication or some other finding that has not been previously reported in the literature. Hopkinson et al. (2025) described a patient who was obese (very overweight) who had engaged in lifestyle changes consisting of a diet that included smaller portion sizes, intermittent fasting and following a Mediterranean diet (fruit, vegetables, whole grains, fish, poultry, nuts, seeds, eggs and olive oil) along with exercises (activities that increased the heartrate and breathing, brisk walking, muscle strengthening exercises and yoga). Prior to making these lifestyle changes two years ago, the patient was pain free but developed chronic (lasting more than three months) all over bodily pain within six months of initiating the changes. The patient was diagnosed with fibromyalgia (a long-term condition that features bodily pain and fatigue). The case report highlighted that major changes to physical activity and diet may have been a trigger for fibromyalgia. As this was a previously unreported finding, it suggested that further research into weight loss, exercise and chronic pain is needed. While this is just one patient, this case study may help stimulate discussion and debate about the topic, educate and alert healthcare professionals to be on the lookout for chronic pain in patients who are obese, exercising and following a diet for weight loss. Case reports are descriptive, but as shown in this example, they can provide the first line of evidence for new and slowly emerging healthcare issues and stimulate future research. However, caution is required in generalising the findings of this case report to all patients who are obese and engaging in lifestyle changes, as there may be multiple causes and explanations for chronic pain.

Cross-sectional surveys

Cross-sectional surveys investigate a sample of the population at one time point. The researcher does not intervene in any way to change anything that participants are doing. Participants are usually selected, according to specific inclusion and exclusion criteria related to the research question. At their most basic level, cross-sectional surveys can provide information about how common a disease is or what specific symptoms are present in a population. They can also be used to assess the knowledge, understanding beliefs and attitudes towards a disease or how people manage specific health problems. Such surveys can be descriptive or analytical, while the former may be used to measure the prevalence of certain diseases and symptoms, the latter permits relationships to be tested between variables that have been measured in a survey.

Descriptive cross-sectional surveys

Al Maqbali et al. (2020) conducted a descriptive cross-sectional survey in Oman to assess health professionals' knowledge about cancer-related fatigue. To take part, prospective participants had to be working in a role within the National Oncology Centre that involved interacting with patients who had a diagnosis of cancer. Results indicated that despite participants having a good level of knowledge about cancer-related fatigue, they did not routinely assess patients for this troublesome symptom, which may have been due to not having a questionnaire to measure cancer-related fatigue that was suited to the culture and language in Oman. The authors acknowledged that their findings may not be generalisable to all healthcare professionals due to an over-representation of nurses in the study (75%).

Analytical (or correlational) cross-sectional survey

Hollands et al. (2024) conducted a cross-sectional survey of people who had recovered from a stroke to assess how feeling connected with a stroke support group affected feelings of loneliness and what aspects of the group helped that connection. Survey questions measured loneliness, group identification (e.g. feeling part of the group, sense of belonging, feeling like other group members, having things in common with group members); group resources (receipt of social support from the group) and providing social support for others. Data assessed associations between various aspects of support and loneliness using descriptive and inferential statistics (see Box 3.1). The study showed that people who felt more connected to their support group had lower scores on loneliness. Providing support to others in the group, getting support from others, knowing the purpose of and having collective group goals, along with being with the same group members over time, made members feel more connected to the group. The researchers acknowledged that some of the survey items had not been previously validated (see below) in a stroke population and adaptations had to be made to some survey items to accommodate the needs of people who had language problems due to their stroke. Participants were volunteers, which means that they self-selected to take part in the study. This may have created bias, as people who volunteered for this research may have had opinions or health needs that were not representative of everyone who had experienced a stroke.

BOX 3.1
DESCRIPTIVE AND INFERENTIAL STATISTICS

As the name implies, descriptive statistics involve the description of data and can help to decide what statistical test(s) are appropriate for analysing data. Descriptive statistics are important, as they help summarise data and make it more meaningful. For example, if we just had a list of test scores for 1,000 people, it would not be very meaningful, we need some way of organising and summarising those data, to quantify and describe them. Data can be summarised using measures of **central tendency**. The **standard deviation** provides a measure of how much data deviate from the mean.

As most data analyses in psychology go beyond description, psychologists use statistical techniques to make inferences about data. Based on the results from samples selected from the population, we make inferences about the population, as it would be impossible (due to time and funding) to include everyone in a research study. If we conduct a study to look at quality of life (QoL) in 150 cancer patients and find that quality of life in patients who have stomach cancer declines when they are undergoing treatment compared to their quality of life pre-treatment, this only tells us about those 150 people and not about everyone who has stomach cancer. The results from the sample provide an estimate of quality of life in these patients. By using inferential statistics, we can assess the probability that this estimate reflects quality of life in the wider population who have stomach cancer. We can never be 100% certain about our conclusions, but we can be about 95% confident in the results.

Different types of questionnaires

Throughout this book, reference will be made to self-report outcome measures, which can also be referred to as scales, questionnaires, inventories or measures and cover a range of areas, such as symptoms of a disease, pain, quality of life, stress, coping strategies, to name but a few. Such outcomes may be used to assess individual responses on one occasion, before and after some type of treatment or intervention or on multiple occasions over a prolonged time. Questionnaires can be delivered in paper or online formats, completed by telephone or face to face.

Survey questions can be used to collect information to describe the participants who are taking part in a study, such as age, gender, educational level, income, occupation and where a person lives. These demographic data are used to describe the sample of people who have completed a survey. In addition, demographic information can be used to describe associations between non-medical factors and health. Surveys are usually quick to administer and permit large amounts of data to be gathered within a short timeframe. However, surveys are open to bias, as participants may complete questions in a way that they think the researcher wants them to respond or in a manner that they would like to be viewed. For example, when asked how many fruits and vegetables are eaten per day, an individual might think about the health advice to eat at least five portions. In wanting to appear to have healthy eating habits, they may report eating five or more portions, even if none have been consumed. This is known as social desirability bias, which may be linked to fear of being judged or disapproved of (Miller et al., 2008). There may also be unintentional under or over reporting of health behaviours; Dyrstad et al. (2014) showed that when asked to complete a questionnaire about physical activity, people often overestimated the intensity of physical activity (how hard it was) and underestimated their sedentary behaviour (time sitting or lying down) compared to objective measures recorded on an accelerometer (a small device worn by a person that measures physical activity and sedentary behaviour). Hence, information obtained from surveys may be open to intentional or unintentional errors.

Standardisation, validity and reliability of questionnaires

Standardised questionnaires are designed to measure specific concepts. Each participant receives the same questions, with identical instructions, in the same order for all participants and all questions are scored in the same way for each person. Participants will be presented with specific answers to choose from, e.g. yes/no; strongly agree, agree, neutral, disagree, strongly disagree. Some questionnaires provide the option to indicate that a questionnaire item is 'not applicable', or 'neutral' and others use 'forced responses', meaning that a specific answer is required, e.g. very satisfied, satisfied, dissatisfied, very satisfied. If participants are forced into choosing a response, the answer may not be a true representation of how they think about a topic. Each questionnaire will have a specific method of scoring and usually have 'norms' for specific populations, which permits the researcher to compare the results from their sample to other populations and/or groups. For example, if an individual completes a questionnaire to measure stress and they get a score of 18, to know if this is high, average or low, the score needs to be compared with a population norm, which may include specific values for grouping variables, such as gender, students, ethnic background and disabilities, etc.

For questionnaires to be valid, they need to have face **validity**, which refers to whether test items look as if they measure the intended topic. For example, a stress questionnaire that has items about feeling tense, under pressure, frustrated and sleep problems would have good face validity, as these are the typical aspects of life affected by stress. Conversely, items asking about favourite music and television programmes would indicate poor face validity, because the items have no relevance to stress. Questionnaires need to have content validity, which is concerned with the degree to which the items measure the full concept of what it is designed to measure. We may expect a stress questionnaire to measure emotional responses to stress (e.g. feeling tense and irritable), physical symptoms (headaches, tiredness) and behavioural aspects (eating less, drinking more alcohol). We are also interested in construct validity; this is how well the questionnaire measures the concept of stress. There are a range of ways of doing this, which include assessing the degree to which the questionnaire correlates with a similar measure of stress (convergent validity) and scales that measure something different (divergent validity). Statistical analyses are used to assess whether questionnaire items group together, as predicted by a theory. For example, in a stress questionnaire, items measuring emotions should cluster together. A questionnaire can also be examined for known-groups variability, in this we would expect that people who have very stressful jobs would score more highly on stress compared to those in low stress jobs.

If a stress questionnaire has good test-retest **reliability** and if no major changes have occurred to influence people's stress levels, there should be a moderately high correlation between scores at two different time points (e.g. one or two weeks later). A questionnaire needs to have good internal consistency (also known as

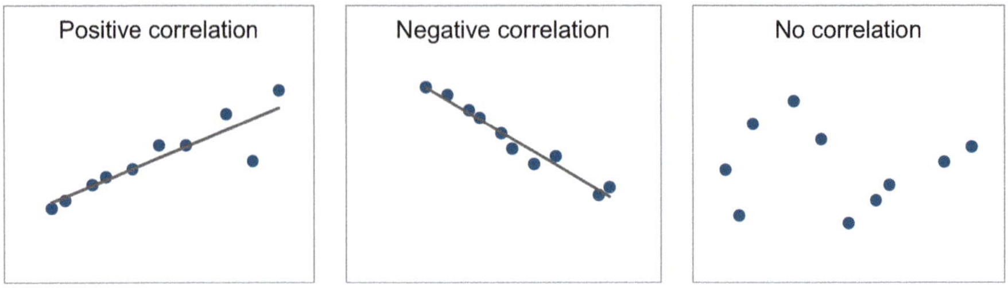

Figure 3.2
Scatterplots of correlations

Source: Author

internal reliability), this shows how well the individual items in the questionnaire group together to measuring similar aspects of stress and the most used statistic to assess it is Cronbach's alpha. An acceptable level of internal consistency is .70 and above.

A correlation is a way of describing the extent of the relationship between two or more variables and it can range from −1 to +1. It is important to remember that when two variables correlate, it does not imply that one variable directly affects the other variable, a correlation just indicates that there is some type of relationship. When both variables increase together, it is described as a positive correlation; when one variable increases and the other decreases, it denotes a negative correlation. If the variables are unrelated, this is referred to as a zero correlation (see Figure 3.2).

Case control studies

Case control studies usually involve a group of people with a disease or a set of symptoms (cases) that is compared to a group who does not have that disease (controls). Case control studies may involve examination of medical records of both groups to try to identify if there is something different about cases that may have contributed to the disease that is not evident in the controls. In some studies, participants in the case group will be matched with those in the control group to try and minimise disease differences that may be influenced by age, biological sex, disability, ethnicity, occupation, etc.

D'Souza et al. (2007) were interested in the link between the human papillomavirus (HPV) and the development of oropharyngeal (in the back of the mouth, flexible muscular part of the roof of the mouth, tonsils, back of the tongue and walls of the throat) cancer. These researchers examined the lifetime sexual histories, oral hygiene, the medical and family histories of cancer, smoking and alcohol intake of people who had a new diagnosis of oropharyngeal cancer compared to controls who had no cancer. The study found that having a higher number of vaginal-sex or oral-sex partners or experience of oral HPV infections increased the risk of developing oropharyngeal cancer. The researchers acknowledged that despite previous research linking smoking and alcohol consumption to the development oropharyngeal cancer, this association was not apparent within the current study. From this, researchers surmised that separate pathways could contribute to the development of oropharyngeal cancer. Case control studies can permit researchers to look at multiple risk factors for disease and data can be extracted directly from medical records or large datasets. However, in research that involves participant recall of diet and physical activity over the past year or lifetime recall of the number of sexual partners, recall bias may a problem, as people may not be able to accurately recall information or they can deliberately over- or underestimate information.

Cohort studies

Cohort studies involve data collection at different time points and follow participants over several years, these are a type of **longitudinal study**. People recruited to cohort studies usually have something in common, such as being born in a certain year, they may be from specific occupational groups or may have been exposed to a certain risk. Cohort studies may involve several 'waves' of data collection. On entry into a study, participants complete the first wave of data, often referred to as baseline, then at the specific times dictated by the research design, subsequent waves of data will be collected using the same outcome measures (questionnaires and/or tests) used at baseline and some additional measures may be included. This permits researchers to track health outcomes over time and can help show how risk factors are associated with disease. One of the most famous cohort studies that we will look at in Chapters 8 and 9 is the Framingham Heart Study (Dawber et al., 1951). It started in 1948 and is still ongoing, having recruited the children and grandchildren of participants who took part in the original study. This study has provided a wealth of information on risk factors associated with the development of CVDs and contributed to the development of disease prevention polices (Tsao & Vasan, 2015). The Nurses' Health Study, which started in 1976, has also been collecting health information on women over several generations. It was initially designed as a longitudinal questionnaire-based survey to examine the impact of oral contraceptive use on cancer. Data collection has been expanded to include physical activity, diet, blood, DNA and tumour samples of women diagnosed with cancer (Bao et al., 2016). The Nurses' Health Survey has shown the impact that lifestyle factors can have on diseases such as type 2 diabetes mellitus, the detrimental health impacts of smoking, the importance of eating a healthy diet, engaging in physical activity and moderating alcohol intake. Findings have also included various risk factors for the development of several cancers and heart disease. All these findings have helped to inform public health policy and health initiatives across the globe (Colditz et al., 2016).

Cohort studies have the benefit of following large groups of people over a long time and usually commence when the study population is relatively disease free, which permits the tracking of lifestyle factors, disease commencement and progression. These types of studies are time and resource intensive, there can be problems keeping track of participants and people drop out. Despite these issues, cohort studies are the mainstay of epidemiological data (Barrett & Noble, 2019).

Randomised controlled trials

Randomised controlled trials (RCTs) are viewed as the 'gold standard' of research designs. They are commonly used in drug trials with participants randomly allocated to the treatment group who receive the drug or the control group who receive a **placebo** (an inert substance such as a tablet that contains no active ingredient). Once participants have consented to take part in the study, baseline measurements are collected. To control for the possibility of there being any known or unknown differences between participants, they are **randomly allocated** to groups, which means everyone has an equal chance of being selected for either group. In double-blind RCTs, participants and researchers do not know who is receiving the drug or placebo and every attempt will be made to make the drug look as similar as possible to the placebo. This is to ensure that researchers do not inadvertently react in different ways when interacting with the two groups and participants' experiences and expectations about the effects of the drug or placebo do not influence the outcomes of the study. Everyone will receive the same instructions, take the drug or placebo at the same time of day, with the same interval between doses and complete the same outcome measures or biomedical tests at the same time points during the study. RCTs do provide very structured and controlled ways of conducting research to minimise bias, but they can be time-consuming and expensive too. They need to have an adequate predetermined sample size and it can sometimes be difficult to recruit enough participants during the lifetime of a study.

Randomised controlled trials are also used to test intervention effectiveness, one group will receive the intervention (intervention group) and the other group will be on the waiting list or in receipt of usual care (control group). Due to the nature of interventions, it is not always possible to blind researchers and participants to group allocation. We could test the hypothesis that healthy, but sedentary adults who are asked to walk 5,000 steps per day for four weeks will report significantly lower levels of perceived stress compared to those who maintain their usual routine (i.e. advised to make no changes to their usual physical activity levels). Our participants need to be over 18 years old who have self-reported moderate stress levels, can walk unaided and do not routinely engage in physical activity (and we would explicitly define what that meant). We randomly allocate participants to the intervention (walking) and control (usual routine) groups and provide everyone with a pedometer to measure their step count. We cannot disguise the fact that one group will be asked to walk and the other will not, hence participants cannot be blinded to the intervention. Stress will be measured prior to the walking intervention and at the end of four weeks, using a standardised, valid and reliable questionnaire. It is possible to blind the researcher who is conducting data analysis to group allocation, as they will only receive the perceived stress scores for group A and B, this is known as a single-blind study. Once the data have been collected, statistical tests will be conducted to assess the primary (main) outcome measure – stress scores between the two groups. However, most interventions of this type will also collect secondary outcome measures; in our example, this is step count. Due to the use of step count data, it will be impossible to blind the researcher conducting the analysis to group allocation, as they will observe the difference in step counts between the groups and be able to guess which is the intervention group.

Systematic reviews and meta-analyses

When commissioners of healthcare services are choosing between different treatments (medications, interventions, surgery, equipment or questionnaires to measure some aspect of patient treatment, experience, symptoms, etc.), they often use high-level evidence from research studies, such as systematic reviews and randomised controlled trials (RCTs), to help them make informed choices. Systematic reviews are a very rigorous way of summarising several research studies that investigate a specific research question. Just because a study has been published in an academic journal does not mean that it is free from bias and systematic reviews assess specific types of bias (see Box 3.2) that may affect interpretation and generalisability of study results. Systematic reviews are conducted in a clearly defined, transparent way and are capable of replication. The starting point for a systematic review is the protocol, which details the very precise research question that will be answered by the review, the types of study designs to be included, the date range, **inclusion criteria** and **exclusion criteria**, the electronic databases used to search for papers, the search terms used to identify papers and details of the critical appraisal tool that will be used to assess aspects of bias inherent within studies.

BOX 3.2
TYPES OF BIAS EXAMINED IN QUANTITATIVE SYSTEMATIC REVIEWS

There are a range of critical appraisal tools that can be used to assess bias. Using a critical appraisal tool means that every study is assessed using the same criteria. Selection bias is concerned with checking if there were any differences in baseline characteristics between the two groups, in how participants were recruited and if they were randomised into groups. Performance bias assesses whether there were any differences in the way the groups were treated (apart from the intervention) and if the study used either single- or double blinding. Detection bias examines if there were any differences between the two groups in terms of the outcome measures used, that the outcomes were standardised and whether the person taking the outcome measures was blinded to group allocation. Attrition bias looks for any differences in the number of participants who dropped out of each group (which may be related to side effects of the treatment or intervention) and how missing data were dealt with. Reporting bias examines if there was any selective reporting of results between the two groups. Taken together, assessment of these types of biases helps researchers come to a conclusion about the quality and credibility of study results.

Systematic reviews can focus on interventions, drugs or treatment effectiveness, the economic costs of a specific type of treatment, the experience of service users (patients) and outcome measures or questionnaires used to assess symptoms and/or quality of life. Universities, colleges and healthcare organisations usually provide access to electronic databases that permit searches for studies that have been published in peer-reviewed journals. Searches can return a lot of studies, which need to be screened against the systematic review's inclusion and exclusion criteria. Mullan et al. (2025) conducted a systematic review to examine the components of interventions to manage head and neck lymphoedema (abnormal levels of swelling in the head, face and neck) associated with treatments for head and neck cancers. These researchers pre-registered the protocol of their systematic review in PROSPERO (The International Prospective Register of Systematic Reviews) (Mullan et al., 2022). Five databases were searched; this identified 2,799 studies, but due to multiple databases being used, 890 duplicates were excluded, a further 1,870 studies were deemed not to meet the inclusion criteria in the first round of screening and 27 in the second, which left 12 studies in the review.

There are two main ways of synthesising and presenting evidence from a systematic review of quantitative studies, and these are **narrative synthesis** and **meta-analysis**. Due to the variety of different outcome tools used to assess lymphoedema, Mullan et al. (2025) found it was impossible to statistically compare the results of intervention outcomes across studies, hence the nature of the review was a narrative synthesis. In assessing the quality of studies, Mullan et al. used the GRADE (Grading of Recommendations Assessment, Development, and Evaluation) tool to assess bias, which showed that the main sources of bias across studies were lack of information surrounding the randomisation process and lack of blinding (Mullan et al., 2025).

In a systematic review with meta-analysis, effect sizes (a statistic that gives an indication of how big the difference is between two groups) from each study are weighted according to the sample size of each study and combined into an overall measure (pooled effect size). This shows the extent and consistency of an intervention, treatment or drug on the **primary outcome measure**. Results of a meta-analysis are usually displayed in a graphical format called a forest plot. McCloy et al. (2022) conducted a systematic review and meta-analysis of the effects of mindfulness-based interventions on fatigue and psychological wellbeing in women with cancer. Their database search identified 1,843 studies, after deduplication and eligibility checks, 20 studies were included in the review. There were variations across studies in terms of the types of cancer, intervention duration and outcome measures. The Cochrane Risk of Bias Tool for randomised trials (Higgins et al., 2019) showed that more than half of the studies were rated as having a high risk of bias, primarily due to a lack of blinding. The latter is common and often unavoidable in mindfulness-based interventions, as participants are actively engaged in meditative practices, hence they cannot be blinded to the intervention. McCloy et al. (2022) concluded that mindfulness led to significant improvements in cancer-related fatigue, depression and anxiety in women with cancer.

Since systematic reviews summarise research findings and provide an indication of the worth of studies and strength of evidence of specific drugs/interventions, they are extremely useful to commissioners of services, researchers and healthcare professionals. They can be used to inform policy, highlight gaps in the literature and make recommendations for future research. For example, McCloy et al. used the results from their 2022 systematic review to design a mindfulness and exercise-based intervention to manage cancer-related fatigue in gynaecological (woman's reproductive organs) cancers (McCloy et al., 2025).

BOX 3.1
CRITICAL THINKING

Bias can be a part of research at many levels from who designs a study, how data are collected, analysed and reported.

What types of biases can you identify in quantitative research designs?
How might researchers guard against bias when using questionnaires?
How do randomised controlled trials try to minimise different types of bias?

Qualitative data collection

Meta-synthesis

A **meta-synthesis** is a bit like a narrative systematic review, instead of combining the statistical results, it combines the findings from individual qualitative studies and uses qualitative critical appraisal tools to assess methodological quality. Selection bias in qualitative studies is concerned with how participants were recruited, if **purposeful sampling** was used (recruiting participants because they are particularly knowledgeable about the topic being investigated) and whether the inclusion and exclusion criteria were appropriate to the aims of the study. Researcher or reflexivity bias is an important consideration, as the researcher's own knowledge, beliefs and assumptions can have an impact on design, data collection, interpretation and reporting. This can be mitigated by reflexivity statements. Interpretation bias may involve misrepresentation or oversimplification of findings, which can reduce the validity of conclusions.

A meta-synthesis starts with a specific research question and follows the same process of specifying participants, types of studies, search terms, etc., as described previously in relation to systematic reviews. Instead of reporting statistical outcomes, a meta-synthesis identifies patterns in themes and/or contradictions across studies. Themes are interpreted to provide an in-depth analysis of findings, going beyond what each study on its own can show, which can reveal new perspectives on an area of interest. Biring et al. (2025) conducted a qualitative meta-synthesis of women's experiences of living with chronic pain. Database searching resulted in 4,253 papers, but after removal of duplicates and those that did not meet the inclusion criteria, 70 studies were included in the review. Risk of bias was assessed using the National Institute of Care and Clinical Excellence (NICE) quality appraisal checklist for qualitative studies (NICE, 2012), with most studies judged to be of high or moderate quality. Thematic analysis of themes identified across studies showed that in addition to navigating pain, women had to balance their pain with multiple (family and work) responsibilities and experienced multiple physical, psychological and social losses. They experienced a lack of understanding from others, including healthcare professionals, in relation to the impact that chronic pain had on their lives. This led women to feel stigmatised, delegitimised and disempowered. On the positive side, women tried to empower themselves through self-management of pain and took solace in joining support groups. The authors concluded there was a need to validate women's pain experiences, raise healthcare professional understanding of the psychosocial impact of chronic pain for women and offer tailored family and community psychological support.

Interviews

Probably, the most commonly used method to collect qualitative data is the interview, which can be structured, semi-structured or unstructured. An interview is like a one-to-one conversation between the researcher and a participant, which can be conducted in person, by telephone or use an internet video platform. In semi-structured interviews, the interviewer will have a series of questions that are used to start the interview and keep the discussion flowing. Prompts may be used to explore areas in more depth and to ensure that all areas relating to the research question are discussed. Unstructured interviews can start with just one question, with the answer helping to shape the discussion, but this technique is rarely used in health psychology, as it is very easy to drift off topic. In addition, not having a series of questions can mean that participants may not discuss points that are pertinent to the research question. Interviews permit the discussion of sensitive topics and provide rich insights into participants' experiences, beliefs and points of view that would not be possible to explore using questionnaires. The downside of using interviews is that they can be time consuming to organise and conduct, with data from each interview requiring verbatim transcription (written account made of the audio-recorded discussion). Interviews are open to bias, which can be on the part of the researcher in the way they phrase questions, tone of voice used or body language, which can intentionally or unintentionally influence participants' responses. Participants can be open to social desirability bias, where answers provided are based on views that are socially acceptable, rather than being totally honest.

Focus groups

A focus group is a small group discussion that is focused on a particular area or topic and involves participants having discussions with each other. The researcher running the focus group is called a moderator and their role is to start the discussion, keep the discussion flowing and if participants stray off the topic, the moderator can bring them back on course, using predetermined questions. The moderator will also have a series of probes that can be used, to explore opinions, beliefs and/or experiences further. The benefits of focus groups are the collective aspect of the discussion, which permits multiple perspectives from participants that may align or differ. Focus groups usually have between 6 and 12 participants in an informal face-to-face setting, while smaller groups are advocated if the focus group is conducted online. At the start of a focus group, the moderator usually sets the 'ground rules' for the discussion and invites everyone to introduce themselves. Ground rules are important so that everyone has a chance to air their views and take turns in talking without others talking over them or dominating the discussion. The moderator can also encourage quieter members of the group to contribute. Once a focus group starts, the moderator's involvement may become minimal, just interjected with prompts as and when required. Focus groups permit a lot of data to be collected in a short time; discussions between participants can result in rich data that include exchanges of information and ideas from multiple perspectives. However, due to the potential for people to have differing ideas and strong opinions, focus group moderators need to be experienced in handling and managing conflicts that may arise when participants disagree. Transcription of focus group audio recordings is time-consuming and the person undertaking transcription will need to be able to match each part of the discussion to each participant. Depending on the nature of the topic being discussed within a focus group, it may be necessary to ask participants to sign a confidentiality agreement in which they agree not to disclose information shared within the group with anyone else.

Thematic analysis

The aim of this type of analysis is used to identify patterns in qualitative data from interviews, focus groups and documents. There are different types of thematic analysis and one of the most commonly used is that proposed by Braun and Clarke (2022) who have provided a good practice guide that includes explorations of common data analytical problems. Thematic analysis is concerned with meaning contained within the data and this requires familiarity with all data by reading through transcripts, identifying and coding important segments of interest (this will be determined by the research question) within transcripts. Codes that have something in common are grouped together to form broad themes and these are reviewed to make sure that they are clear and not overlapping with other themes. The themes are then named and when writing up the findings, participant quotations from transcripts are used to validate themes.

Photo-elicitation

Photo-elicitation may be useful when researching chronic diseases. In this technique, people are asked to keep records of their illness journey, including their diagnosis, treatment and recovery, which may include photographs and patient diaries. These records can be collected from more than one person to explore and analyse patterns that may inform further data collection. Kuo et al. (2022) used photographs and a focus group to understand and determine the health needs of older adults who were living with at least two of the following conditions, high blood pressure, high cholesterol or diabetes. Training was provided for participants on how to take photographs using a computer tablet and participants were asked take photographs of daily life relating to disease management for three months. Researchers analysed these photographs using content analysis (see below) to develop questions for the focus group, which was concerned with physical activity, healthy diet, regular routine, social connections and smart management of healthy behaviours. Participants reported that using photo diaries helped them think about what they did on a day-to-day basis, while the researchers concluded that such reflections could be used to prompt positive health behaviours for other older adults. Most study participants were women, the study was based in Taiwan and only explored three health conditions, hence results may not be generalisable to other populations.

Content analysis

This type of analysis involves the transformation of qualitative data (words or themes) into quantitative (numerical) data by looking at how often specific words, phrases or patterns within transcripts or health information appear. It may also explore concepts and patterns in photographs, but it is more commonly used in documentary analysis (Elo & Kyngäs, 2008). The use of content analysis as a means of exploring transcripts and dairies has been criticised by purist qualitative researchers as removing the richness of data by reducing meaning and experiences to numbers (Mays & Pope, 2000).

Trustworthiness in qualitative data

By now you will have noticed that qualitative data involves subjectivity; this is a strength as a disease can affect an individual's identity, emotions and meanings of disease, which can impact on quality of life. Qualitative research data are about people's subjective experiences and the researcher's analysis involves subjective interpretation, which is guided by their epistemology, own experiences and analytical techniques. This has resulted in qualitative research being regarded by some as less rigorous than quantitative research. To manage subjectivity, researchers explore the validity of their research in relation to four aspects of **trustworthiness**, credibility, dependability, transferability and confirmability (Lincoln & Guba, 1985). Credibility of results refers to whether the researcher's interpretation of the data is a true reflection of participants' accounts. This can be explored by inviting participants to comment on whether the researcher's findings concur with and are representative of their views. Findings can be corroborated by triangulation with other sources of data, for example, patient records, diaries and information collected from family members or friends. The use of more than one researcher to code and analyse data can add credibility to findings, any discrepancies can be explored by other members of the research team and then discussed to arrive at a meaningful and representative interpretation of data. Dependability is concerned with consistency of the research process by ensuring that there is a documented account of how data were collected, analysed and decisions made; this is commonly referred to as the 'audit' trail. This includes information about how themes were derived from the analysis and the use of selected quotations from participants to validate themes. The audit trail permits others to understand the processes involved and how findings were reached. Transferability is concerned with how well the findings may apply to other contexts and other populations. A 'thick' description of participants is required, which includes the country and area in which the study was conducted, recruitment, inclusion/exclusion criteria, ages, gender, details about the disease and symptoms, socioeconomic status, educational level, etc. The final aspect is confirmability, which requires the previous three aspects to be evident within a study along with reflexivity. The latter is concerned with what the researcher brings to the research study in terms of their own knowledge, ways of working and experiences, as these can impact on how data are interpreted and reported. Reflexivity should be involved at every stage of the research process, from initial conception of the research question, data collection processes, interpretation of results and write-up of the study. Reflexivity is about assessing own preconceptions, assumptions and beliefs that may bring bias into research.

BOX 3.2
CRITICAL THINKING

Qualitative research explores experiences, meanings and helps us understand why and how things happen in healthcare and health behaviours.

How might a researcher's own views and background influence what they study, the questions they ask and their findings?

Can qualitative research be as valid as quantitative research?

Mixed methods

Researchers may favour one methodology over another, with quantitative research being viewed as being 'more scientific' and rigorous than qualitative; however, the two can not only coexist, but they can also be combined. RCTs are the 'gold standard' in being able to control for sources of bias; nevertheless, there is a need to consider the 'patient's/participant's voice'. An RCT would not be able to provide rich insights into how an individual copes with the side effects of treatments, medications and chronic conditions. Quantitative and qualitative methodologies can be combined into what is known as **mixed methods**. The ontology of mixed methods includes the relative and realist perspectives, the epistemology is one of pragmatism, combining objective and subjective ways of gaining data. This involves both methodologies to explore measurement and meaning of a disease that can include biomedical tests, surveys and interviews or focus groups. Data are analysed using quantitative and qualitative methods and integrated in a way that has been predetermined in the planning stages of the research study.

Using mixed methods permits researchers and health professionals to maximise the strengths and minimise the weaknesses of each methodology and there are a range of mixed methods designs. Precedence can be given to one methodology over another or they can both have equal status. Rather than reporting quantitative and qualitative data as totally separate studies, integration of results is required. We will look at the four basic designs, which differ in relation to which methodology takes precedence and/or where the mixing of data takes place.

Convergent parallel design

Quantitative and qualitative data are gathered and analysed separately to each other in the convergent parallel design, then results are interpreted and discussed together. Buckley et al. (2021) explored how the cancellation of sporting events due to COVID-19 lockdowns impacted body image, relationships with food and eating disorders in former and current athletes. They used a convergent parallel design, collecting data simultaneously using open- and closed survey questions. Standardised questionnaires were used to measure eating attitudes and disordered eating, self-perceived changes in body image and relationships with food. Qualitative data collection consisted of a series of open-ended questions that asked how body image and food had changed during lockdowns. The researchers found that just over 21% of participants showed symptoms of disordered eating and it was more common in former athletes. The disruption to training due to lockdowns led to perceived loss of control and heightened body preoccupation. Reductions in energy expenditure due to changes in training triggered binge eating, guilt, shame and anxiety overweight gain or muscle loss and triggered negative body image feelings, even without there being any physical bodily changes. The use of quantitative data helped to explain the prevalence of disordered eating and body image due to the lockdowns and qualitative data explained why and how these issues were happening.

Explanatory sequential design

When one methodology takes precedence over another, the design is referred to as being sequential. An explanatory sequential design means that quantitative data are collected first, the results are analysed and the outcome is used to inform the second part of the study, which is qualitative in nature. Mixing of methods takes place prior to the qualitative part of the study and in the discussion of findings. Fischer et al. (2019) examined sexual function, quality of life (QoL) and experiences of women with ovarian cancer. Standardised questionnaires were used to measure cancer-related QoL, sexual functioning, relationship quality, sexual distress, depression and health status. Analysis of questionnaire data showed that women experienced poorer QoL, higher rates of sexual dysfunction, greater sexual distress, lower relationship satisfaction and increased levels of depression compared to population norms for people without cancer. These results were used to inform focus group questions used in the qualitative part of the study. Thematic analysis of focus groups resulted in six major themes, which included the impact of cancer in changing satisfaction with relationships; sexual problems; issues with body image; communication difficulties with healthcare professionals; emotional responses; and the types of coping strategies used to manage the challenges of ovarian cancer. The use of an explanatory sequential design meant that researchers were able to use questionnaires to gain a broad measure of the impact that ovarian cancer had on sexual functioning. These results helped researchers to probe more deeply into women's feeling and experiences, which could not be fully explored and understood by questionnaire data alone.

Exploratory sequential design

An exploratory sequential design is similar to the previous one, in that data are collected sequentially, the main difference being that qualitative data are collected first, analysed and then used to inform the quantitative part of the study. This type of design is often used when researchers wish to design a new questionnaire. Yazdi-Feyzabadi et al. (2021) wanted to develop a questionnaire to assess perceived reasons for patient nonadherence to doctor's instructions at medical outpatient clinics. Initially, researchers explored previous literature and identified 30 items from established questionnaires to include in their new measure. The qualitative phase of the study involved semi-structured interviews with patients, doctors and outpatient managers to gain insights into perceived reasons for nonadherence and data were subjected to content analysis, resulting in 48 items. These items and the ones from previous questionnaires were compared, duplicated items removed and the remaining 57 items were integrated to inform the development of a new questionnaire. The new questionnaire was tested with participants in a quantitative survey, subjected to psychometric analysis and wording refined through participant feedback. The newly developed questionnaire consisted of 18 items that covered interpersonal psychological factors, interpersonal cognitive factors, provider factors and socioeconomic factors that could impact nonadherence to medical instructions. This type of mixed methods design helped to ensure that questionnaire items were grounded in participant experiences, culture and context, reflecting real-world patient and provider experiences.

Embedded mixed methods design

In the embedded mixed methods design, one methodology takes precedence and the other is embedded, that is, it supports the dominant method that is used in the main part of the study. The supporting aspect of the study can occur before, during or after the main study. Roslan et al. (2021) explored the prevalence of burnout during the COVID-19 pandemic in Malaysian healthcare workers. Quantitative methods took precedence, with data collected using a survey that consisted of a standardised burnout scale that measured personal, work-related and patient-related burnout. To capture participants' experiences, open-ended questions were embedded within the survey to permit participants to elaborate on what caused burnout, symptoms experienced, coping strategies and how burnout affected work or life. The results were combined in the discussion, which showed that more than 50% of healthcare staff who completed the survey had experienced burnout, this was related to screening and treating patients for COVID-19, staff medical conditions and not having adequate psychological support at work. Qualitative themes confirmed that workload, strained relationships at work, concerns about infecting family members and uncertainty about the pandemic influenced experiences of burnout. Symptoms of burnout included physical, emotional exhaustion and cynicism, which resulted in physical health symptoms (headache, sleep problems, muscle pains and heart palpitations), occupational impacts (lower focus, productive and enthusiasm for work), psychological irritability anxiety and anger and social symptoms (strained family relationships and reduced QoL). The quantitative survey questions provided information about the prevalence of burnout, while embedded open questions permitted researchers to triangulate data and gain rich insights into the personal experiences of burnout that would not have been possible by just using one method.

Decolonisation of research

There seems to be an implicit assumption that Western research approaches and methods are the only correct way to investigate health problems. These determine what is construed as valid research, who can conduct that research, what topics ought to be investigated and the questions that need to be asked. This often dismisses Indigenous ways of knowing, perpetuating the legacy of colonisation. Decolonisation of research means making space for Indigenous and marginalised world views and ways of making sense of data. The inclusion of Indigenous perspectives is essential in order that research be centred on Indigenous knowledge and world views, which reflect and serve the needs of Indigenous communities and use Indigenous research methodologies. Thambinathan and Kinsella (2021, p. 1) pointed out that most of the research on Indigenous Peoples is based on "pre-existing colonial, Eurocentric paradigms created by Western scholars". In decolonising research, it is important to realise that it is not just the specific method of data collection or the type of data that is of importance, a more fundamental issue concerns the perspective from which a research study is conceived, along with the implications of such research. Historically, research has been 'done to' rather than 'for' those from marginalised groups; they have, in the past, been the 'subjects' of research, with researchers often working from a position of power, applying colonialised knowledge. Writing from the perspective of the 'colonised', Smith, an Indigenous Māori professor (2012, p. 1), stated that: "the term 'research' is inextricably linked to European imperialism and colonialism. The word itself 'research', is probably one of the dirtiest words in the indigenous world's vocabulary".

There are examples of healthcare professional and researcher involvement in unethical and harmful health practices in the name of research (see the section on Ethics later in this chapter), including the infamous Tuskegee Syphilis and Willowbrook Farm studies. Western-based research has also viewed Indigenous Peoples and their cultures through a negative lens (Bishop, 1997; Sue & Sue, 2022), which has resulted in stigmatising attitudes and discrimination from the non-Indigenous population.

This means that Western researchers need to acknowledge that other ways of knowing exist. There is no single best way or model to decolonise research, but as the starting point, researchers need to critically reflect on their own assumptions in relation to epistemology and the underlying power dynamics within the research process. Researchers bring their own biases and ways of thinking to the research process, which can directly impact the types of questions asked and ultimately the findings of their research. There is a need to go beyond mere acknowledgement of culture differences and similarities and to recognise that research is a partnership, which is inclusive and Indigenous Peoples have the right to self-determination. This is not a new idea brought about by decolonisation, the importance of this was highlighted over 50 years ago by Tapp et al. (1974) who provided guidelines for engaging in cross-cultural research, which stated that researchers must work in a culturally informed way and through partnership working that is collaborative.

Creating research partnerships with Indigenous researchers, Elders, Knowledge Keepers, traditional healers and community members, helps to gain an 'insider's perspective' (Trimble & Fisher, 2005), values Indigenous ways of knowing and listens to their research needs and priorities. Ethical guidelines and sensitivities will need to be acknowledged and discussed to protect individual, collective and traditional knowledge, ensuring that national Indigenous frameworks are followed and that the land and the spirit world are acknowledged. Many of these ethical considerations will not be evidenced within Western thinking (Thambinathan & Kinsella, 2021), hence researchers will require training in these areas.

Designing a culturally grounded intervention must start from the bottom-up that involves using specific cultural values and intergenerational knowledge systems of the community. Therefore, interventions must utilise culture-specific ways of knowing (Lee et al., 2013; Okamoto et al., 2014). There may be a need to engage in training and knowledge gathering to understand the norms, lived experiences due to historical subjugation, discrimination and stigma associated with colonialisation. Types of data gathered may include historical and traditional knowledge that is reflected in storytelling, lived experiences, ceremonies, dance, healing practices, photography and art. Erb and Stelkia (2023) report that yarning (story telling) by Elders and Knowledge Keepers is a common way of sharing information, intergenerational learning and it is a commonly used Indigenous research method (Iseke, 2013).

Yarning can be used as a method on its own or can be combined with other methods (see Chapter 6 in relation to health literacy). It has been suggested that yarning is akin to collecting interview data, but the former does not always involve the usual questioning and answering, with interruptions to seek clarification. This is especially the case when yarning with an Indigenous Elder, as it is disrespectful to interrupt them (Bessarab & Ng'andu, 2010). Due to the problems involved in keeping to the topic under discussion and needing to probe areas of interest, Western academics have challenged the idea that yarning is a valid way of collecting research data. Questions have also been posed as to how to differentiate yarning associated with just having a conversation (social yarning) from research yarning. Bessarab and Ng'andu (2010) explain that just as in

Western conversations, yarning can have different purposes, it can be social and informal, cover a range of general points such as the weather, news, advice, etc., and is often used by researchers as a way of building trust before formal collection of data. The move from social to research yarning is usually indicated by the researcher introducing the research topic and there is also a formal ending where the participant is thanked for their time.

During research yarning, collaborative ideas may be shared and thoughts about research described. In telling 'their story', the participant may talk about emotional or traumatic events that are deeply personal. In this situation, the researcher pauses the research focus of the yarn and just listens, this can help the participant to feel understood and listening can validate their experiences, but this is not the same as counselling. Yarning may, on the surface, look the same as the Western conception of interviewing, but the former is more relaxed and conversational. Yarning has a focus on building trust, which is guided by cultural respect and the participant usually takes the lead. Interviewing is much more structured with pre-planned questions and the researcher takes the lead, interviewing often strive for standardisation and may feel quite formal and one sided to participants. Kennedy et al. (2022) conducted a narrative review of yarning methods that had been used across 46 research studies with Aboriginal and Torres Strait Islanders. They concluded that yarning was a culturally safe method of data collection but cautioned that some studies did not clearly explain how yarning was used or if researchers had training in Indigenous and or qualitative methods. Furthermore, Kennedy et al. suggested that to combat colonisation of research, Aboriginal and Torres Strait Islanders' voices need to be heard in leading the research agenda and research processes, as only then can research with these Peoples be considered as collaborative (Kennedy et al., 2022)

There is a need to acknowledge that Western and Indigenous perspectives on research can coexist, be valued and respected. This has been acknowledged in the Two-Eyed Seeing (TES) model described by the Indigenous Elder Albert Marshall (Bartlett et al., 2012). TES recognises that research and health intervention development can be informed by one eye seeing Western knowledge, the other seeing Indigenous knowledge and that there are benefits from using this multi-science approach (see Chapter 7). The Medicine Wheel (described in Chapter 2) can be used by researchers to incorporate Indigenous knowledge and facilitate translation of the research or intervention processes within Indigenous conceptualisations. For example, in the Anishinaabe tradition, the Medicine Wheel starts in the East and moves clockwise to the South, West and North. The East can be used to focus on the historical context of a research study or intervention and to question current knowledge, like a conceptual framework. The South can be used to understand different perspectives and transform knowledge, in a similar way to **theory building**. The West can be used to create standards based on Indigenous knowledge, such as building an **evaluation framework**. The North can be used to emphasise reflection, wisdom and advocacy, which is comparable to analysis and reflexivity in academic research (Mashford-Pringle & Shawanda, 2023). Situating research processes within the Medicine Wheel can help researchers contextualise and explain research studies to support Indigenous ways of knowing.

Participatory research methods are used to co-create knowledge, resources and interventions. This involves the setting of mutual priorities and endpoint outcomes, emphasising mutual respect (David-Chavez et al., 2020). In conducting research with the Māori in New Zealand, Oetzel et al. (2017) outlined an enhancing wellbeing model (He Pikinga Waiora) that ensured Indigenous values were incorporated into the development of health interventions. The He Pikinga

Waiora is based on four principles that include **cultural centredness**, **community engagement**, **systems thinking** and **integrated knowledge translation**. Harding and Oetzel (2019) found that the first two aspects of this model helped enhance Māori health outcomes for chronic disease interventions. However, changing healthcare systems thinking to value Indigenous world views and the integration of Western and Indigenous knowledge, without full consideration of the **social determinants of health**, can have implications for the sustainability of interventions (see Chapter 7). Research with Indigenous and marginalised groups needs to be constructivist in nature, which must involve a thorough interaction between the researcher and the individual or groups but power dynamics and colonial influences must be addressed. It is essential that researchers and healthcare professionals understand how colonial experiences and intergenerational trauma continue to impact Indigenous Peoples around the globe (Smith, 2021).

BOX 3.3
CRITICAL THINKING

Some forms of bias are easier to identify than others, for example, the bias inherent within different research designs.

Think about who decides which research questions are worth studying and whose voices may be missing or ignored.

How might culture affect what is considered as 'valid' evidence in research?

Ethical aspects of research

Within the US, research participation by African American people is much lower than their White counterparts (Scharff et al., 2010). There are many reasons for this, with mistrust of researchers and healthcare systems being major barriers (Corbie-Smith et al., 2004; Freimuth et al., 2001). Two examples will be used to show how African Americans and a minoritised vulnerable group were experimented on and exploited in the name of 'medical science'.

The Tuskegee Syphilis Study involved poor American farm labourers who were misled and experimented on by the medical establishment. Researchers were interested in studying the disease course of syphilis; in 1932, around 600 men were unknowingly recruited into a medical experiment, without their consent or knowledge and were deceived by the offer of free medical treatment. When the men entered the study, there was no cure for syphilis, 399 men had the disease, rather than informing them of their diagnosis, they were just told they had 'bad blood'. The men's health was monitored during the study, they were prescribed aspirin and supplements, but in the 1940s syphilis became treatable by antibiotics. The men were never treated and the study continued until 1972, by which time many of them had died of the disease, had gone blind and developed other health problems directly related to syphilis. In addition, the disease had been passed on to many of their wives and children. This study was only stopped when a venereal disease investigator in the US Public Health Service discovered what had been happening and reported it to managers, even then no attempt was made to stop the experiment, it was ended only when the investigator leaked details to the press (Crash Course, 2021).

In another shocking series of medical experiments, children with learning disabilities were deliberately infected with hepatitis A. This infectious disease of the liver causes jaundice, stomach pain, fatigue, weight loss and diarrhoea; it is usually spread through ingestion of faeces from an infected person. The children were living in Willowbrook State School in New York, which was designed to accommodate 4,000 children, but during the experiments, in the 1960s and 1970s, 6,000 children resided in unsanitary conditions with inadequate staffing and care, adding to the inevitability that they would be infected with hepatitis. In one of the most deplorable studies designed to observe the course of the hepatitis A, Dr Krugman infected healthy children by mixing infected faeces with their food, which was justified by saying that the children would have become infected any way! A series of other hepatitis-based experiments also took place at Willowbrook, without informing parents or obtaining their consent and no ethical approval was sought for these shocking unethical studies (Willowbrook State School, 2022).

Code of research ethics

These are just two examples of medically unethical studies, which serve to illustrate the importance of considering the ethical implications in research. Most professional bodies have a code of research ethics that must be adhered to when working with human research participants. Within the UK, the British Psychological Society (BPS), which is the professional body for psychologists, has their own Code of Human Research Ethics (2021) that applies to all students who are undertaking BPS-accredited courses and everyone who is a member of the said Society. This Code sets out four ethical principles that must be adhered to when conducting psychological research. These are respect for the autonomy, privacy and dignity of persons; scientific value, social responsibility; maximising benefit and minimising harm.

Respect for privacy and dignity encompasses informed consent, the right to withdraw from research, the debriefing of participants after the study has finished, the right to privacy and confidentiality. Deception in research should be avoided, unless it is absolutely necessary and if used, the need must be justified. Participants must be protected from harm and if participants request advice, researchers must not give advice that they are not trained to give. Scientific value involves conducting research in a manner that is methodologically sound and rigorous; this also includes research that is being conducted as part of student training. Social responsibility relates to ensuring that any psychological knowledge generated from research is used for beneficial purposes. Research conducted by students may not add to the scientific knowledgebase, but it should be beneficial to students in providing training in research skills. Maximising benefit and minimising harm are top priorities, as research participants should not be put at greater risk of harm than they would encounter in everyday life. This means that research studies need to be risk assessed and risks weighed against any beneficial impacts a study may have.

There are various frameworks and ethical requirements for undertaking research with Indigenous Peoples in Australia, Canada, New Zealand and the

US, while there are specific country-based differences, they all have some similarities. These countries have core ethical principles about Indigenous self-determination, cultural protocols, reciprocity and community involvement when conducting research with Indigenous Peoples. Self-determination is about Indigenous People leading and being co-leaders in research that is going to affect them. This involves the use of cultural protocols that respect local customs, knowledge systems and languages. There must be reciprocity, in that the research being conducted has some benefit to those who are involved in it, research should not just be for the benefit of researchers. The specific Indigenous community must be engaged in research planning and processes, from inception to dissemination, including having rights over how data are used and shared. Finally, an ethical review must include institutional and ethical reviews from the Indigenous community where the research will be conducted.

The replication crisis and open science

Psychology is a science, as such when conducting research, we need to ensure that we follow the scientific method in gathering data, analysis and reporting in a systematic and methodical way. When a researcher sets out to conduct a research study, they engage in a series of steps that must be sufficiently documented to ensure that the study can be replicated by someone else. This means that scientific theories and research are open to retesting, scrutiny and may require updating in light of emerging evidence.

The replication crisis

The **replication crisis** refers to the inability of researchers to reproduce results similar to those obtained in previously conducted studies, calling into question the credibility and accuracy of previous research. It may be possible that previous research was not documented sufficiently to enable exact replication. There may have been unaccounted for bias within studies, which could indicate that the methodological quality of a study was not as good as it ought to have been, or in the worst-case scenario, the data had been falsified. Being unable to replicate results may also be due to something called **p-hacking**. Instead of specifying and statistically testing a hypothesis, researchers may have undertaken multiple analyses in the hope of finding something that was statistically significant. Another issue that can contribute to the replication crisis is **HARKing**, which refers to forming a hypothesis after the results are known, rather than testing the pre-specified hypothesis.

Open science

One solution to prevent p-hacking and HARKing is to **pre-register studies** prior to data collection. Researchers submit the protocol (detailed description) of the study that includes details about the research design, number of participants, who can and cannot take part in the study (inclusion and exclusion criteria), where people will be recruited from and what outcome measures will be used, details of any treatment or intervention, the hypothesis (hypotheses – plural) and exact information about data analysis. This means that the research must be conducted in accordance with the pre-registered report, which is in the public domain. Pre-registration of the study methods and data analysis plans are part of **open science**, which is about transparency in research. It includes making research and its outputs, such as publications, details of methodologies and data, open to sharing. One such platform for this is the Open Science Framework (n.d.), which is a free resource that can be used to find out about ongoing research, it also contains a data deposit area providing access to anonymised datasets and a place to share research papers.

Chapter summary

Define and explain key concepts and purposes of epidemiological data?

Epidemiological data can help to identify causes of disease. Incidence data indicate the number of new cases and prevalence statistics assist in tracking disease trends at specific time points. These data are important in assessing how disease prevention measures are working and planning current and future healthcare needs.

How do ontology and epistemology influence how we collect data and what data we collect?

Ontology is about what we believe exists and can be studied, whereas epistemology is concerned with how we gain knowledge. These two principles affect the types of data we collect and how we collect them. Using a realist ontology the best way to collect data is through objective measures the use of the scientific method and quantitative data. This contrasts with a relativist approach that acknowledges the existence of multiple realities, which can be influenced by subjectivity, culture and experience. Explored through qualitative data collection methods.

Explain what is meant by the hierarchy of research designs and how does this help our critical understanding of study bias?

This ranks studies based on the strength of evidence, which is influenced by the bias inherent within studies and the generalisability of results. Case studies sit at the bottom of the hierarchy with systematic reviews and randomised controlled trials being viewed as having the lowest levels of bias. Knowledge about the types of bias inherent within-study designs helps us judge how reliable study findings are.

Discuss the importance of standardisation, validity and reliability when selecting questionnaires

Standardisation ensures that all participants receive the same questionnaires, in the same way with the same instructions. Validity means the questionnaire measures what it was designed to measure, that it covers all aspects of the construct being measured. Reliability of questionnaires means results are reliable over time and the items within questionnaire are measuring the same construct. These three factors are used to ensure that the data collected via questionnaires are as accurate as possible.

Outline methods of qualitative data collection and assess the importance of trustworthiness in qualitative data

Common qualitative methods include interviews, focus groups, photo-elicitation and documentary analysis. When analysing qualitative data, researchers must assess the trustworthiness of the study by ensuring the findings are credible, dependable, transferable and confirmable, and the researcher must acknowledge the bias they bring to a study by engaging in reflexivity.

Discuss the value of using mixed methods

Mixed methods combine quantitative and qualitative data in the one study. The method that takes precedence and where the mixing occurs is dependent on the specific mixed methods design. Mixed methods provide a more complete analysis of healthcare issues as it can gather data that show statistical outcomes and experiences, thus it is possible to understand not just what happens but why.

Explain why decolonisation of research is important

This permits recognition of power imbalances in the production of knowledge. It recognises Indigenous values and non-Western perspectives, through respectful collaboration with Indigenous people as partners and leaders in research. This promotes inclusivity and facilitates research that is culturally relevant to the needs of the groups that are included in research studies.

Why do we need research ethics?

Past unethical studies have resulted in harm to participants; research ethics are a fundamental aspect of any study to protect participants' rights, safety, wellbeing and prevent exploitation or misuse of data. Ethical principles ensure that researchers respect participant's autonomy, privacy and dignity. Research studies need to have scientific value to be conducted in a socially responsible way and maximise benefit, while minimising harm.

Explain why the replication crisis has implications for open science

The replication crisis showed that it was impossible to repeat studies and get the same or similar results, which called into question the credibility and accuracy of previous research. It is unclear whether this was due to poor reporting of study procedures, data analysis or falsification of results. Open science is a way of ensuring transparency in research by sharing of data, methods and results, which can help others verify results. Pre-registration of studies can help to avoid p-hacking and HARKing.

Keywords

Epidemiology: The study of how diseases occur, spread, affect people and are controlled.
Prevalence: The number of people with a disease at a given time.
Incidence: The number of new cases of a disease at a given time.
Ontology: What exists, what we believe is real can be studied.
Epistemology: How we gain knowledge about things
Objective measurements: Data that are collected in a way that is unbiased, not affected by thoughts, emotions or opinions.
Subjectivity: Results that are influenced by personal thoughts, emotions or opinions.
Quantitative methods: Ways to collect numerical data that are analysed using statistical methods.
Hypothesis: A statement or prediction that is testable using statistical methods.
Qualitative methods: Ways to collect words, pictures and documents to understand meaning and experiences.
Research question: An exploratory statement that a qualitative study will address.
Central tendency: A summary statistic, usually the mean, mode or median.
Standard deviation: A statistic that shows how scores or values are spread out from the mean.
Validity: The extent to which a questionnaire measures what it is supposed to measure.
Reliability: How consistent the score of a questionnaire is over time and how well items in a questionnaire are related.
Longitudinal study: A study conducted over a period of time with the same people providing data at different time points, used to see if outcomes change over time.
Placebo: An inert substance, such as a tablet that contains no active ingredient.
Inclusion criteria: The specific characteristics that a person must meet to take part in a study. The specific characteristics that studies must meet to be included in a systematic review.
Exclusion criteria: The specific characteristics that prevent a person from taking part in a study. The specific characteristics that prevent studies from being included in a systematic review.
Narrative synthesis: A nonstatistical way of summarising the findings of a systematic review.

Meta-analysis: A method that combines the statistical results of studies that have been included within a systematic review.
Primary outcome measure: The measure that the researcher considers to be the most important of several outcomes in a study.
Meta-synthesis A method that combines and synthesises the findings from individual qualitative studies that have been included with a systematic review.
Purposeful sampling: Selecting participants on the basis that they have specific knowledge or experience of the topic or area that they study is addressing.
Trustworthiness: Four aspects of trustworthiness, credibility, dependability, transferability and confirmability are used to assess the validity of qualitative studies, with the addition of reflexivity,
Mixed methods: The use of quantitative and qualitative methods in the same study.
Yarning: An Indigenous method of qualitative data collection that uses a respectful conversational technique.
Theory building: A process in which ideas and explanations are synthesised to understand behaviour.
Evaluation framework: A structured plan used to check whether a research project or intervention achieved the intended goals.
Participatory research methods: Research that is conducted in collaboration with participants, who may help with the planning, study design, data collection, analysis and or dissemination.
Cultural centredness: Research that places people's values, culture and knowledge at the heart of research.
Community engagement: Working with communities in a culturally respectful way which can include research and/or intervention development.
Systems thinking: Looking at how various aspects of systems within a group or society are interconnected.
Integrated knowledge transition: Working in partnership with communities or organisations to ensure that knowledge gained through research is shared throughout the research process and not just at the end of a study.
Social determinants of health: Non-medical factors that can have impacts on health, for example, poverty, educational level housing and access to healthcare.
Replication crisis: The inability of researchers to repeat a study and get the same or similar results.
p-hacking: Conducting multiple statistical analyses to find a result that is significant, rather than testing the originally specified hypothesis.
HARKing: When researchers change the hypothesis of a study after seeing the results.
Pre-registration: Placing the study methods and data analysis plans or the protocol for a systematic review in an open research forum.
Open science: Making science more transparent and accessible by sharing data, methods, and results openly.

Key Readings

Greenhalgh T. (1997). How to read a paper. Getting your bearings (deciding what the paper is about). *British Medical Journal, 315*(7102), 243–246. https://doi.org/10.1136/bmj.315.7102.243

Renjith, V., Yesodharan, R., Noronha, J. A., Ladd, E., & George, A. (2021). Qualitative methods in health care research. *International Journal of Preventive Medicine, 12*, 20. https://doi.org/10.4103/ijpvm.IJPVM_321_19

Segerstrom, S. C., Diefenbach, M. A., Hamilton, K., O'Connor, D. B., Tomiyama, A. J., & Behavioral Medicine Research Council (2023). Open science in health psychology and behavioral medicine: A statement from the Behavioral Medicine Research Council. *Annals of Behavioral Medicine, 57*(5), 357–367. https://doi.org/10.1093/abm/kaac044

Thambinathan, V., & Kinsella, E. A. (2021). Decolonizing methodologies in qualitative research: Creating spaces for transformative praxis. *International Journal of Qualitative Methods, 20*, 1–9. https://doi.org/10.1177/16094069211014766

Reflective Questions

1. Why are some quantitative research methods viewed as superior to others?
2. How useful is epidemiological evidence in health psychology?
3. What factors would you consider when choosing a questionnaire?
4. Of what benefit are systematic reviews in health psychology?
5. What evidence would you look for within a paper to determine if the findings from a qualitative study were trustworthy?
6. What makes yarning different from a regular interview?

Video resources

If you are interested in learning more about critical appraisal tools, this is a useful website – Critical Appraisal Skills Programme UK. (2024). *CASP qualitative studies checklist*. https://casp-uk.net/casp-tools-checklists/qualitative-studies-checklist/

This video provides information about the Tuskegee experiment:

Crash Course. (2021, December 24). *The Tuskegee experiment: Crash course in Black American history #29* [video]. https://www.youtube.com/watch?v=56gqCXlUCoE

References

Al Maqbali, M., Gracey, J., Dunwoody, L., Rankin, J., Hacker, E., & Hughes, C. (2020). Healthcare professionals' knowledge on cancer-related fatigue: A cross-sectional survey in Oman. *Nursing & Health Sciences, 22*(3), 732–740.

Bao, Y., Bertoia, M. L., Lenart, E. B., Stampfer, M. J., Willett, W. C., Speizer, F. E., & Chavarro, J. E. (2016). Origin, methods, and evolution of the three nurses health studies. *American Journal of Public Health, 106*(9), 1573–1581. https://doi.org/10.2105/AJPH.2016.303338

Bartlett, C., Marshall, M., & Marshall, A. (2012). Two-eyed seeing and other lessons learned within a co-learning journey of bringing together indigenous and mainstream knowledges and ways of knowing. *Journal of Environmental Studies and Sciences, 2*, 331–340. https://doi.org/10.1007/s13412-012-0086-8

Barrett, D., & Noble, H. (2019). What are cohort studies? *Evidence-Based Nursing, 22*(4), 95–96. https://doi.org/10.1136/ebnurs-2019-103183

Bessarab, D., & Ng'andu, B. (2010). Yarning about yarning as a legitimate method in indigenous research. *International Journal of Critical Indigenous Studies, 3*(1), 37–50. http://doi.org/10.5204/ijcis.v3i1.57

Biring, S., Burton, A. E., Dunwoody, L., & Kevern, P. (2025). Women's experiences of living with chronic pain: A qualitative meta-synthesis. *British Journal of Health Psychology, 30*, e70023. https://doi.org/10.1111/bjhp.70023

Bishop, R. (1997). Māori people's concerns about research into their lives. *History of Education Review, 26*, 25–41.

Braun, V., & Clarke, V. (2022). Toward good practice in thematic analysis: Avoiding common problems and be(com)ing a *knowing* researcher. *International Journal of Transgender Health, 24*(1), 1–6. https://doi.org/10.1080/26895269.2022.2129597

British Heart Foundation (2025). *Global heart and circulatory diseases factsheet.* Retrieved September 8, 2025, from https://www.bhf.org.uk/-/media/files/for-professionals/research/heart-statistics/bhf-cvd-statistics-global-factsheet-jan26.pdf?rev=db96d3d8fa944b3ea427c2dddb1e9075&hash=54CF3CCE6AD161C1E06B136449C9B10B

British Psychological Society. (2021). *BPS code of human research ethics* (4th ed.). https://doi.org/10.53841/bpsrep.2021.inf180

Buckley, G. L., Hall, L. E., Lassemillante, A. M., & Belski, R. (2021). Disordered eating & body image of current and former athletes in a pandemic; a convergent mixed methods study - What can we learn from COVID-19 to support athletes through transitions? *Journal of Eating Disorders, 9*(1), 73. https://doi.org/10.1186/s40337-021-00427-3

Colditz, G. A., Philpott, S. E., & Hankinson, S. E. (2016). The impact of the Nurses' Health Study on population health: Prevention, translation, and control. *American Journal of Public Health, 106*(9), 1540–1545. https://doi.org/10.2105/AJPH.2016.303343

Corbie-Smith, G., Moody-Ayers, S., & Thrasher, A. D. (2004). Closing the circle between minority inclusion in research and health disparities. *Archives of Internal Medicine, 164*(13), 1362–1364. https://doi.org/10.1001/archinte.164.13.1362

Crash Course. (2021, December 24). *The Tuskegee experiment: Crash course in Black American history #29* [video]. https://www.youtube.com/watch?v=56gqCXlUCoE

David-Chavez, D. M., Valdez, S., Estevez, J. B., Meléndez Martínez, C., Garcia, A. A. Jr., Josephs, K., & Troncoso, A. (2020). Community-based (rooted) research for regeneration: Understanding benefits, barriers, and resources for Indigenous education and research. *AlterNative, 16*(3), 220–232. https://doi.org/10.1177/1177180120952896

Dawber, T. R., Meadors, G. F., & Moore, F. E. Jr (1951). Epidemiological approaches to heart disease: The Framingham Study. *American Journal of Public Health and the Nation's Health, 41*(3), 279–281. https://doi.org/10.2105/ajph.41.3.279

D'Souza, G., Kreimer, A. R., Viscidi, R., Pawlita, M., Fakhry, C., Koch, W. M., Westra, W. H., & Gillison, M. L. (2007). Case-control study of human papillomavirus and oropharyngeal cancer. *The New England Journal of Medicine, 356*(19), 1944–1956. https://doi.org/10.1056/NEJMoa065497

Dyrstad, S. M., Hansen, B. H., Holme, I. M., & Anderssen, S. A. (2014). Comparison of self-reported versus accelerometer-measured physical activity. *Medicine & Science in Sports & Exercise, 46*(1), 99–106. http://doi.org/10.1249/MSS.0b013e3182a0595f

Elo, S., & Kyngäs, H. (2008). The qualitative content analysis process. *Journal of Advanced Nursing, 62*(1), 107–115. https://doi.org/10.1111/j.1365-2648.2007.04569.x

Erb, T., & Stelkia, K. (2023). Best practices to support the self-determination of Indigenous communities, collectives, and organizations in health research through a provincial health research network environment in British Columbia, Canada. *International Journal of Environmental Research and Public Health, 20*(15), 6523. https://doi.org/10.3390/ijerph20156523

Fischer, O. J., Marguerie, M., & Brotto, L. A. (2019). Sexual function, quality of life, and experiences of women with ovarian cancer: A mixed-methods study. *Sexual Medicine, 7*(4), 530–539. https://doi.org/10.1016/j.esxm.2019.07.005

Freimuth, V. S., Quinn, S. C., Thomas, S. B., Cole, G., Zook, E., & Duncan, T. (2001). African Americans' views on research and the Tuskegee Syphilis Study. *Social Science & Medicine, 52*(5), 797–808. https://doi.org/10.1016/s0277-9536(00)00178-7

GRADE Working Group. (2004). Grading quality of evidence and strength of recommendations. *British Medical Journal, 328*(7454), 1490. https://doi.org/10.1136/bmj.328.7454.1490

Greenhalgh, T. (1997). How to read a paper. Getting your bearings (deciding what the paper is about). *British Medical Journal, 315*(7102), 243–246. https://doi.org/10.1136/bmj.315.7102.243

Harding, T., & Oetzel, J. (2019). Implementation effectiveness of health interventions for indigenous communities: A systematic review. *Implementation Science, 14*(1), 76. https://doi.org/10.1186/s13012-019-0920-4

Higgins, J. P. T., Savović, J., Page, M. J., Elbers, R. G., & Sterne, J. A. C. (2019). Chapter 8: Assessing risk of bias in a randomized trial. In J. P. T. Higgins, J. Thomas, J. Chandler, M. Cumpston, T. Li, M. J. Page, & V. A. Welch (Eds.), *Cochrane handbook for systematic reviews of interventions* (version 6.5, 2024). Cochrane. https://www.cochrane.org/handbook

Hollands, L., Calitri, R., Haslam, C., Lamont, R. A., Mounce, L., & Tarrant, M. (2024). A UK national cross-sectional survey of stroke support groups: Exploring the role of social identification and group processes in reducing loneliness. *BMC Public Health, 24*(1), 2992. https://doi.org/10.1186/s12889-024-20432-w

Hopkinson, L. D., Jafari, S., Frempong, E., & Zarghom, S. (2025). Onset of chronic pain triggered by a lifestyle-change-based weight loss and exercise regimen. *British Medical Journal Case Reports, 18*(4), e263172. https://doi.org/10.1136/bcr-2024-263172

Iseke, J. (2013). Indigenous Storytelling as Research. *International Review of Qualitative Research, 6*(4), 559–577. https://doi.org/10.1525/irqr.2013.6.4.559

Kennedy, M., Maddox, R., Booth, K., Maidment, S., Chamberlain, C., & Bessarab, D. (2022). Decolonising qualitative research with respectful, reciprocal, and responsible research practice: A narrative review of the application of Yarning method in qualitative Aboriginal and Torres Strait Islander health research. *International Journal for Equity in Health, 21*(1), 134. https://doi.org/10.1186/s12939-022-01738-w

Kuo, M. C., Chen, C. M., Wu, F. G., Chen, C. H., Yin, Z. X., & Wang, C. Y. (2022). Use of photo diary and focus group to explore needs for digital disease management program among community older adults with chronic disease. *Health & Social Care in the Community, 30*(3), 926–936. https://doi.org/10.1111/hsc.13241

Lee, R. M., Vu, A. M., & Lau, A. (2013). Culture and evidence-based prevention programs. In F. T. L. Leong & Yamada, A-M. (Eds.), *Handbook of multicultural mental health: Assessment and treatment of diverse populations* (2nd ed., pp. 527–546). Elsevier.

Lincoln, Y. S., & Guba, E. G. (1985). Chapter 11: Establishing trustworthiness. In: *Naturalistic inquiry* (pp. 289–331). Sage.

Mashford-Pringle, A., & Shawanda, A. (2023). Using the Medicine Wheel as theory, conceptual framework, analysis, and evaluation tool in health research. *SSM - Qualitative Research in Health, 3*, 100251. https://doi.org/10.1016/j.ssmqr.2023.100251

Mays, N., & Pope, C. (2000). Qualitative research in health care. Assessing quality in qualitative research. *British Medical Journal, 320*(7226), 50–52. https://doi.org/10.1136/bmj.320.7226.50

McCloy, K., Hughes, C., Dunwoody, L., Marley, J., & Gracey, J. (2022). Effects of mindfulness-based interventions on fatigue and psychological wellbeing in women with cancer: A systematic review and meta-analysis of randomised control trials. *Psycho-Oncology, 31*(11), 1821–1834. https://doi.org/10.1002/pon.6046

McCloy, K., Hughes, C., Dunwoody, L., Marley, J., Cleland, I., Cruciani, F., & Gracey, J. (2025). Management of fatigue in gynaecological cancer: A feasibility study of an app-based exercise and mindfulness intervention. *Gynecologic Oncology Reports, 60*, 101807. https://doi.org/10.1016/j.gore.2025.101807

Miller, T. M., Abdel-Maksoud, M. F., Crane, L. A., Marcus, A. C., & Byers, T. E. (2008). Effects of social approval bias on self-reported fruit and vegetable consumption: A randomized controlled trial. *Nutrition Journal, 7*, 18. https://doi.org/10.1186/1475-2891-7-18

Mullan, J., Semple, C., Blackburn, N., & Lorimer, J. (2022). *Evaluating the effects of lymphoedema management strategies on functional status and health-related quality of life following treatment for head and neck cancer patients*. PROSPERO. https://www.crd.york.ac.uk/PROSPERO/view/CRD42022378417

Mullan, L. J., Blackburn, N. E., Gracey, J., Dunwoody, L., Lorimer, J., & Semple, C. J. (2025). Evaluating the effects of lymphoedema management strategies on functional status and health-related quality of life following treatment for head and neck cancer: A systematic review. *Journal of Cancer Survivorship, 19*(1), 121–139. https://doi.org/10.1007/s11764-023-01453-7

National Institute for Health and Care Excellence (NICE). (2012). *Appendix H: Quality appraisal checklist - Qualitative studies*. In *Process and methods guide* (PMG4). https://www.nice.org.uk/process/pmg4/chapter/appendix-h-quality-appraisal-checklist-qualitative-studies

Oetzel, J., Scott, N., Hudson, M., Masters-Awatere, B., Rarere, M., Foote, J., Beaton, A., & Ehau, T. (2017). Implementation framework for chronic disease intervention effectiveness in Māori and other indigenous communities. *Globalization and Health, 13*(1), 69. https://doi.org/10.1186/s12992-017-0295-8

Okamoto, S. K., Kulis, S., Marsiglia, F. F., Holleran Steiker, L. K., Dustman, P., Steiker, L. K. H., & Dustman, P. (2014). A continuum of approaches toward developing culturally focused prevention interventions, from adaptation to grounding. *The Journal of Primary Prevention, 35*(2), 103–112. https://doi.org/10.1007/s10935-013-0334-z

Open Science Framework (n.d.). *The Open Science Framework*. Retrieved September 13, 2025, from https://osf.io/

Roslan, N. S., Yusoff, M. S. B., Razak, A. A., & Morgan, K. (2021). Burnout prevalence and its associated factors among Malaysian healthcare workers during COVID-19 pandemic: An embedded mixed-method study. *Healthcare, 9*(1), 90. https://doi.org/10.3390/healthcare9010090

Scharff, D. P., Mathews, K. J., Jackson, P., Hoffsuemmer, J., Martin, E., & Edwards, D. (2010). *More than Tuskegee: Understanding mistrust about research participation. Journal of Health Care for the Poor and Underserved, 21*(3), 879–897. https://doi.org/10.1353/hpu.0.0323

Smith, L. T. (2021). *Decolonizing methodologies: Research and Indigenous Peoples*. Zed Books.

Sue, D. W., Sue, D., Neville, H. A. & Smith, L. (2022). *Counseling the culturally diverse: Theory and practice* (9th ed.). Wiley.

Tapp, J. L., Kelman, H. C., Triandis, H. C., Wrightsman, L. S., & Coelho, G. V. (1974). *Continuing concerns in cross-cultural ethics: A report. International Journal of Psychology, 9*(3), 231–249. https://doi.org/10.1080/00207597408247108

Thambinathan, V., & Kinsella, E. A. (2021). Decolonizing methodologies in qualitative research: Creating spaces for transformative praxis. *International Journal of Qualitative Methods, 20*, 1–9. https://doi.org/10.1177/16094069211014766

Trimble, J. E., & Fisher, C. B. (Eds.). (2005). *The handbook of ethical research with ethnocultural populations and communities*. Sage Publications.

Tsao, C. W., & Vasan, R. S. (2015). Cohort profile: The Framingham Heart Study (FHS): Overview of milestones in cardiovascular epidemiology. *International Journal of Epidemiology, 44*(6), 1800–1813. https://doi.org/10.1093/ije/dyv337

Willowbrook State School. (2022, March 15). *The path forward: Remembering Willowbrook – Full documentary* [Video]. YouTube. https://www.youtube.com/watch?v=ev80qEtp2u4

Yazdi-Feyzabadi, V., Nakhaee, N., Mehrolhassani, M. H., Naghavi, S., & Homaie Rad, E. (2021). Development and validation of a questionnaire to determine medical orders non-adherence: A sequential exploratory mixed-method study. *BMC Health Services Research, 21*(1), 136. https://doi.org/10.1186/s12913-021-06147-3

4 Physiological knowledge for health psychology

Chapter contents

- The human brain and nervous system.
- Physiological stress pathways.
- The cardiovascular system.
- The respiratory system.
- The immune system.
- Cancer.
- Diabetes mellitus.
- Obesity and eating.

Chapter objectives

After reading this chapter, you should be able to answer the following questions

- Describe the structure and function of the central and peripheral nervous systems.
- Outline the main functions associated with each of the four lobes of the brain.
- Explain the two stress pathways.
- Summarise the functions of the cardiovascular system and associated diseases.
- Describe the respiratory system and the main factors associated with chronic obstructive pulmonary disease.
- Summarise the main categories and causes of common cancers.
- Distinguish between type 1 and type 2 diabetes.
- Discuss the potential causes of obesity.

You may be wondering why it is necessary to have knowledge of physiological processes when you are studying health psychology. In Chapter 2, you were introduced to the biopsychosocial, ecological and Indigenous models of health, which outlined links between psychological, social, cultural factors, health and disease. To fully understand the impact of these factors and how they may impact health and disease, you need to learn about the components of the nervous system and how they interact with the endocrine and immune systems, the structure and function of the cardiovascular and respiratory systems and physiological aspects of diabetes and obesity.

DOI: 10.4324/9781003423157-4

The human brain and nervous system

The human nervous system is made up of the **central nervous system** (CNS) and the peripheral nervous system (PNS). The CNS consists of the brain and spinal cord, which act as the body's command centre by processing and interpreting information. The brain is responsible for thinking, emotions, memory, coordination of bodily functions and receives messages from all around the body via the spinal cord, which consists of a dense network of nerve fibres along the spinal column. The PNS consists of nerves that are attached to the spinal cord and brain. The PNS has two parts, the **autonomic nervous system** (ANS) and the somatic nervous system (SNS) and both interact with the CNS. The SNS receives information from all around the body and sends messages from the brain to control skeletal muscles. The ANS is self-regulating, in that it is not under conscious control; it regulates the internal organs and glands. It has two separate aspects, the sympathetic and the parasympathetic divisions, and they tend to have opposite effects on internal organs (see Figure 4.1).

The brain

The brain contains billions of nerve cells, processes information from the senses, controls movement and regulates involuntary functions, for example, heart rate, blood pressure and breathing. It has specialised areas that take part in emotion regulation, decision-making, thoughts, memories, processing of language, movement, etc. Communication between the brain and rest of the body takes place via

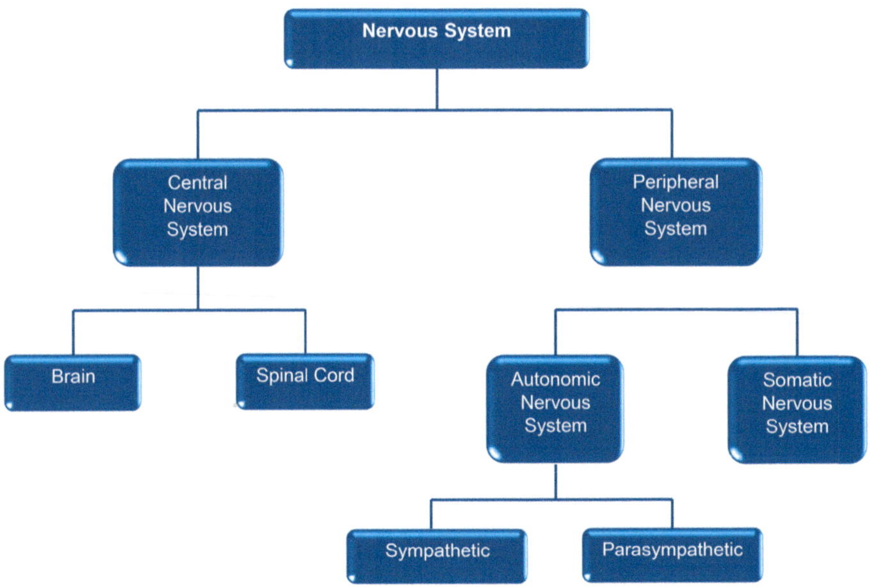

Figure 4.1
The nervous system

Source: Author

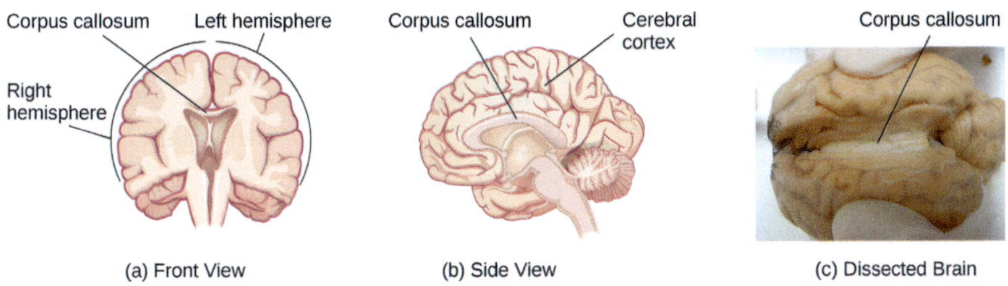

Figure 4.2
The cerebral cortex and corpus callosum

Source: Spielman et al. (2020)[1] OpenStax (CC BY 4.0)

the nervous system, through a complex network of cells, called neurons. These neurons transport information via chemical signals and electrical impulses. Sensory information (sight, hearing, taste, smell and touch) comes to the brain from the eyes, ears, tongue, nose and skin, where information is interpreted by the brain.

The brain is formed of many structures that have specialised functions. The cerebrum is the largest part of the brain; it has an outer layer called the **cerebral cortex** (the grey matter) which contains billions of brain cells. It has an undulating surface, which is covered in folds and wrinkles (called gyri), which look a bit like crumpled up paper. The longitudinal fissure divides the cerebrum into two halves, the right and left hemispheres, which are connected by the **corpus callosum**, permitting chemical and electrical communication between the two hemispheres (see Figure 4.2). While the left and right hemispheres may look the same, they control different processes. For most people, the right side of the body is controlled by the left hemisphere of the brain and the left side by the right hemisphere. For example, the right motor cortex area on the right hemisphere controls function and sensation on the left side of the body. This helps to explain why someone who acquires an injury to the right side of the brain will have functional deficits on the left side of their body.

Lobes of the brain

The frontal lobe

Each cerebral hemisphere contains four lobes (see Figure 4.3), which are the frontal, parietal, temporal and occipital. The **frontal lobe** is responsible for a wide range of functions. It is the 'executive centre' of the brain, as it plays a role in thinking, reasoning, learning, problem-solving, judgement, multitasking, along with forming and storing memories. It also contains the motor cortex, which controls voluntary movement of skeletal muscles (e.g. those involved in walking and using hands) and has a role to play in personality, emotion and social behaviour. Next to the motor cortex is Broca's area. This is usually located on the left side of the frontal lobe, which is the dominant hemisphere for most people. Damage to this area results in difficulties with language production (expressive aphasia), which is characterised by difficulty in putting words together in a sentence. Even though an individual may be able to understand spoken, written language and know what they want to say, when they try to verbalise a sentence,

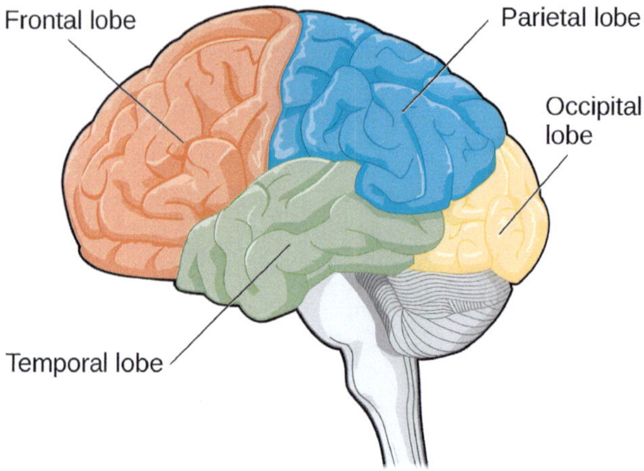

Figure 4.3
Lobes of the brain

Source: Speilman et al. (2020) OpenStax (CC BY 4.0)

words are missed out and their speech may be slow. There can be long pauses between words, as they search for the right word and speech lacks intonation. This results in difficulty in expressing thoughts and engaging in conversation, which can lead to frustration.

The parietal lobe

The somatosensory cortex on the **parietal lobe** of the brain processes sensory information, such as pain, pressure, cold, heat and touch, from various parts of the body. Movement and orientation are processed by the parietal lobe, which helps people recognise the position and movement of their arms and legs (proprioception). Other functions include the ability to follow maps, spatial orientation, spatial memory and spatial reasoning (see Box 4.1).

BOX 4.1 SPATIAL ORIENTATION

Spatial orientation involves the ability to understand where people are positioned in relation to other objects. For example, knowing if there is a car on the right or left, being able to estimate how close or far away a car is orientated and knowing that if a person moves towards the car, they will get closer to it. Spatial memory involves remembering how to get from one place to another. For example, being able to navigate from home to university, knowing how to get from the bathroom to the bedroom or remembering which kitchen cupboard contains food. Spatial reasoning is a skill that is used to visualise and manipulate objects and shapes. For example, being able to mentally rotate shapes to know what they would look like from a different angle or visualising how furniture might look like if rearranged in a room.

The temporal lobe

The **temporal lobe** is involved in hearing, memory, speech, language, visual and emotional language processes. Wernicke's area is critical for understanding language and producing speech. Damage results in difficulty in understanding the meaning of speech (receptive aphasia). While a person's speech may sound normal in terms of pace and intonation, their sentences and phrases will consist of a garble or words with no meaning. Deep within the temporal lobe is the hippocampus, which helps in the formation and retrieval of new memories. The temporal lobe also processes certain visual information, such as faces and locations. Recognising and responding to emotional cues and processing emotional experiences are other functions associated with the temporal lobe. Damage to this lobe can lead to memory impairments, difficulty in recognising other people's emotional responses and/or expressing emotions and problems with processing and interpreting sounds.

The occipital lobe

The **occipital lobe** deals with vision. This includes visual perceptions and visual memory to permit the recognition of past objects, environments and faces. It is the area where information from both eyes is integrated to enable depth perception, the ability to perceive differences between colours and shades of colour. The occipital lobe is also involved in the processes of reading and writing and provides feedback that aids in hand-eye coordination. Damage to this lobe can result in difficulty in recognising objects, loss of part of the visual field, complete loss of vision, problems with colour vision, detecting movement of objects or visual hallucinations (seeing things that are not there).

Cerebellum

There are a range of structures underneath the cerebrum (see Figure 4.4), one of which is the **cerebellum**, located at the back of the brain, just under

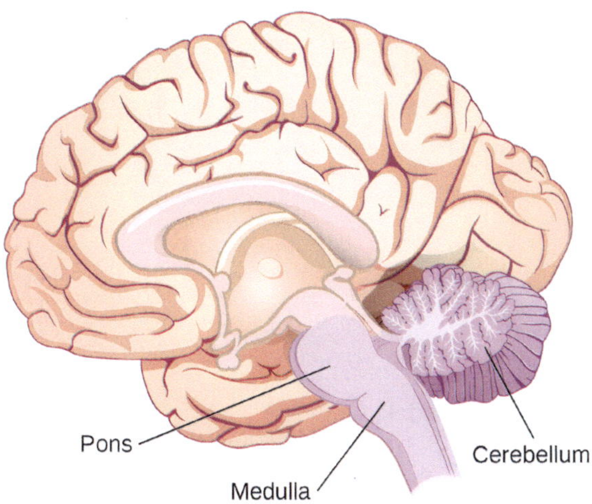

Figure 4.4
The pons, medulla and cerebellum

Source: Speilman et al. (2020) OpenStax (CC BY 4.0)

the occipital lobe. It is involved in balance, posture and ensures that voluntary muscle movement and fine motor skills are smooth and coordinated. If this area becomes damaged, an individual may exhibit tremors (shaking), clumsy movements (ataxia), inability to walk in a straight line and due to balance problems, they may walk with a wide-based gait (having a wider distance than normal between the feet when walking). It is also thought to be involved in procedural (implicit) memory, that is, the memory of how to perform actions and skills (e.g. riding a bike). The cerebellum also receives input from the visual and auditory senses to help balance and posture.

The brainstem, pons and medulla

The brainstem is located just forward of the cerebellum at the base of the brain, where it connects to the spinal cord. The pons and medulla are part of the brainstem, the pons links the hindbrain (the back of the brain) to the rest of the brain; while the medulla regulates vital functions, such as breathing, heart rate, blood pressure, as well as the cough and swallow reflexes.

Limbic system

Another series of structures located underneath the cerebrum are collectively known as the **limbic system** (see Figure 4.5) and these structures include

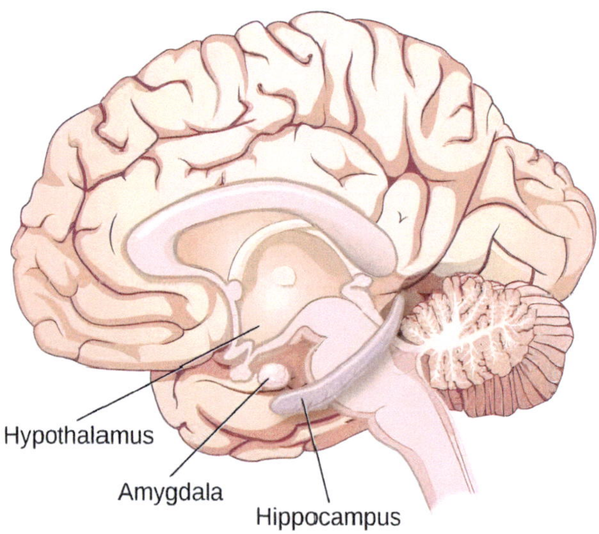

Figure 4.5
The limbic system

Source: Speilman et al. (2020) OpenStax (CC BY 4.0)

the hippocampus, amygdala and hypothalamus. The hippocampus is important in the formation and retrieval of memories, learning and spatial navigation. Close by is the **amygdala**, which helps to process emotion-related information from the senses, especially fear and anger and sends signals to the hypothalamus. The hypothalamus maintains a steady internal state (homeostasis) in controlling body temperature, regulating hunger and thirst, controlling the sleep-wake cycle, sexual behaviour and is associated with emotional responses. This structure plays a leading role in mediating the stress (fight or flight) response through stimulation of the sympathetic aspect of the autonomic nervous system (ANS) and the endocrine system via the pituitary gland.

Physiological stress pathways

We have all experienced the physiological effects of stress but may not have been aware of the underlying physiological processes that caused these effects. Have you ever wondered why your heart seems to race, you had a dry mouth or felt a bit sick after a shock or a stressful event (stressor)? This is the automatic 'fight or flight' response triggered by a stressor, it gets you ready to confront (fight) or run away (flight) from the stressor. When you are stressed, a whole chain reaction starts with the processing of emotions by the limbic system, which in turn triggers hypothalamus, the ANS and the endocrine system.

The sympathetic-adrenal-medullary response

When anxiety and fear are recognised, the amygdala sends a signal to the posterior part of the hypothalamus. The **hypothalamus** is like a 'command centre' for initiating the stress response. It activates the **sympathetic** part of the ANS, which in turn triggers the central part (medulla) of the adrenal glands, which sit on top of the kidneys. This results in the secretion of adrenaline and noradrenaline (also known as epinephrine and norepinephrine) into the bloodstream. This mobilises the body for fight or flight and is typified by increased muscle tone, heart rate, blood pressure and respiration, blood glucose becomes raised to provide energy for the muscles, pupils of the eyes dilate to permit more light into the eyes and the brain becomes more alert in order to process sensory information from the eyes, ears and nose. This is known as the sympathetic-adrenal-medullary response (SAM; see Figure 4.6), once the stressful event is over the parasympathetic part of the ANS will try to calm everything down (see Table 4.1).

The endocrine system

In addition to activating the sympathetic nervous system, the hypothalamus activates the pituitary gland, which is often referred to as the master gland, as it exerts control over the other glands that make up the endocrine

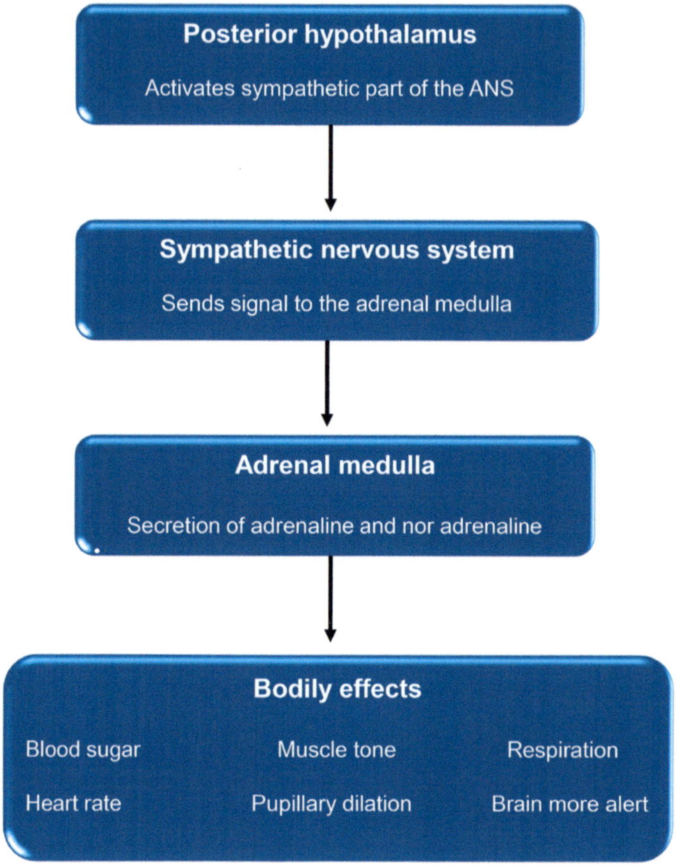

Figure 4.6 The sympathetic-adrenal-medullary response (SAM)

Source: Author

Table 4.1 Parasympathetic and sympathetic nervous system effects

Organ	Parasympathetic activity	Sympathetic activity
Heart	Slow resting	Speeds up heart rate
Breathing	Normal resting rate	Speeds up breathing
Blood vessels	Contract	Dilate
Pupils	Contract	Dilate
Salivary glands	Normal production	Decreases production
Stomach	Normal contractions	Slows down contractions
Hair follicles	Relaxed	Pilomotor response
GSR*	Normal	Increased
Adrenal glands	Normal resting state	Stimulated

*Galvanic skin response.

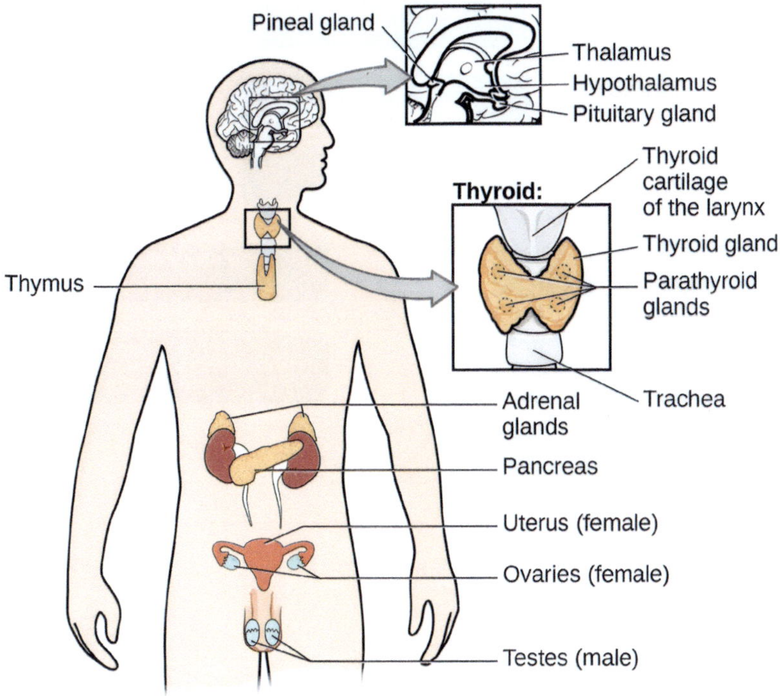

Figure 4.7
The glands of the endocrine system

Source: Speilman et al. (2020) OpenStax (CC BY 4.0)

system (see Figure 4.7). These glands secrete a variety of hormones (chemical messengers) into the bloodstream. The ones involved in the stress response are the pituitary and adrenal glands.

Hypothalamic-pituitary-adrenal-pathway

The second response to stress involves the **hypothalamic-pituitary-adrenal-pathway** (HPA; see Figure 4.8). Its effects are more prolonged than the SAM response. HPA activation happens in the background, we are unaware of it happening, as the effects are more subtle than the dramatic effects experienced during SAM activation. In tandem with SAM initiation, the anterior part of the hypothalamus sends corticotrophin-releasing factor (CRF) via the bloodstream to the anterior pituitary gland, which results in the release of adrenocorticotropic hormone (ACTH). This hormone triggers the outer section (cortex) of the adrenal glands and they in turn secrete two corticosteroids, cortisol and aldosterone. **Cortisol** results in the release of glucose (sugar) from the liver. In the short term, cortisol is beneficial, as it provides energy for the skeletal muscles, brain and reduces inflammation. Aldosterone helps to maintain blood pressure to ensure that the cardiovascular system and muscles have an adequate blood supply to respond to the stressor. Once the stressor or threat has been dealt with or it goes

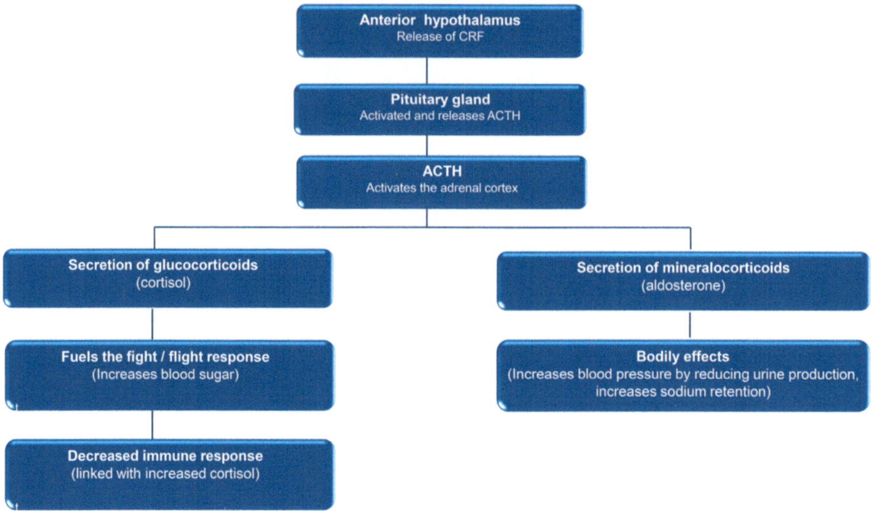

Figure 4.8
The hypothalamic-pituitary-adrenal-pathway (HPA)

Source: Author

away, the **parasympathetic nervous system** and hypothalamus help the body to return to its normal resting state (homeostasis). However, if stress is prolonged, levels of corticosteroids can remain higher than normal, but over time this is detrimental to the body and may have negative impacts on the cardiovascular and immune systems (see Chapter 8).

BOX 4.1 CRITICAL THINKING

We all experience stress, which triggers a physiological response. Think about how you feel when you are stressed.

How does your body react? E.g. faster heart rate, increased breathing rate, what physiological processes cause them?
When the stressful event is over, do you immediately feel calm? If not, what is the physiological reason for that?

The cardiovascular system

The cardiovascular system is composed of the heart, arteries and veins, where the veins carry blood to the heart and the arteries away from the heart. The heart pumps blood to and from the lungs through the pulmonary circuit and around systemic circuit to the rest of the body. The heart is a muscle with four chambers (see Figure 4.9), the top two chambers are called atria (atrium is singular) and the bottom two are the ventricles. Blood flows through the heart in one direction, which is facilitated by the heart valves. In the pulmonary circuit, deoxygenated blood from the upper body goes via the superior vena cava and via the inferior vena cava from the lower part of the body. Contraction of the right atrium moves the deoxygenated blood through the tricuspid valve at the bottom of the atrium into the right ventricle and the tricuspid valve closes. From here, blood is pumped through the pulmonary semilunar valve into the left and right pulmonary arteries into each lung to become oxygenated and to remove carbon dioxide. After being oxygenated in the lungs, blood flows through the left and right pulmonary veins into the left atrium. When the atrium contracts, it pushes oxygen-rich blood through the mitral valve (also known as the bicuspid valve) into the left ventricle. From here, the blood is pumped through the aortic semilunar valve into the aorta (the body's largest artery), then it enters the systemic circuit and is distributed through other arteries to various organs and tissues. The blood then returns to the pulmonary circuit on the right side of the heart (Figure 4.10). The heart valves ensure that blood only flows in one direction, the sounds of heart valves opening and closing constitute what we know as heartbeats or the pulse. The normal resting heart beats at around 55–85 times per minute but will beat much faster when we engage in physical activity, are excited, frightened or under stress.

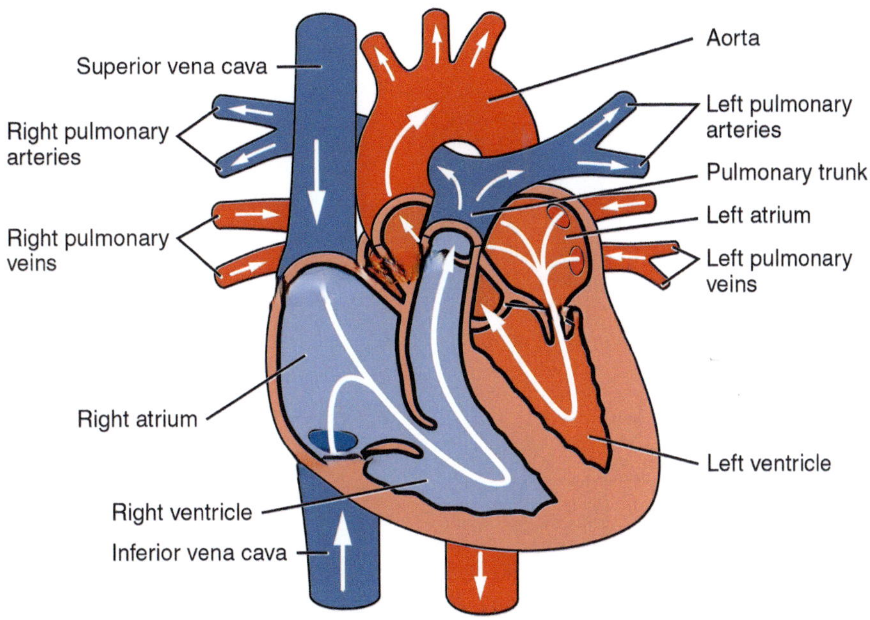

Figure 4.9
Blood flow through the heart

Source: Betts et al. (2022)[2] OpenStax (CC BY 4.0)

Blood pressure and hypertension

When the heart pumps blood to the lungs and around the body, it exerts pressure on the walls of the arteries, which is referred to as **blood pressure** (BP). When blood is pumped out of the heart, it is under high pressure, this is the systolic BP; when the heart is relaxed, blood flows into the heart and the BP is lower, this is the diastolic pressure. BP is measured in millimetres of mercury (mmHg) and recorded using two values, the systolic pressure over the diastolic pressure, for example 120/80. A normal BP ranges between 90/60 mmHg and 120/80 mmHg. A person with values between 120/80 mmHg and 140/90 mmHg is at risk of developing high BP (National Health Service, 2023a). A sustained BP of 160/100 mmHg or more is referred to as hypertension (clinically high BP). Blood pressure will normally rise when people experience stress or during exercise when muscles have a greater demand for oxygen. During these times, the heart beats faster and stronger to pump oxygenated blood and nutrients around the body. When the exercise has been completed and the demand for oxygen reduces or a stressful event or situation ends, in healthy individuals who do not have hypertension, BP returns to the normal range, but BP can remain higher than normal when exposed to chronic (long-term) stress. Other factors that can contribute to hypertension include being overweight, smoking, eating a poor diet, having a high salt intake and indulging in excess consumption of alcohol. High cholesterol, diabetes and/or kidney disease are also associated with hypertension, which can contribute to heart attacks and strokes (see Chapter 9, chronic illness).

The heart

The heart pumps oxygen and nutrient-rich blood throughout the body, but it is also a muscle, as such, it also needs its own blood supply and this is provided via the coronary arteries (see Figure 4.10).

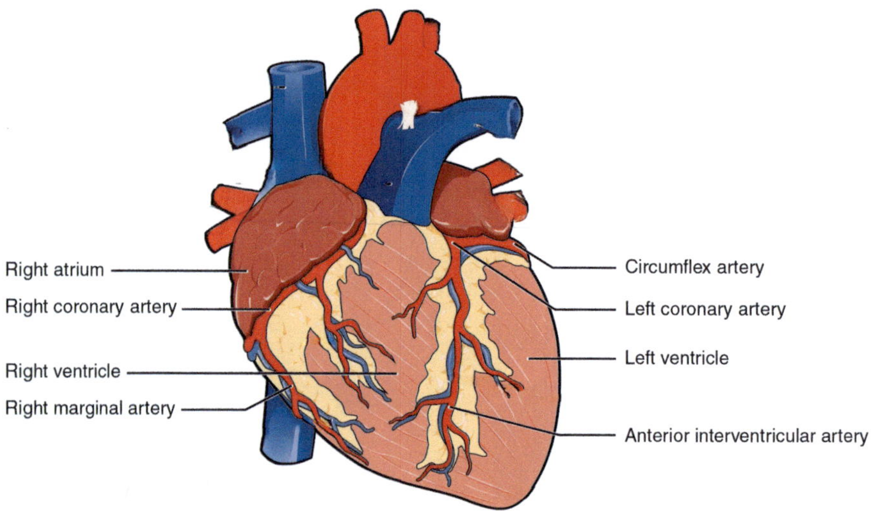

Figure 4.10
The coronary arteries

Source: Betts et al. (2022) OpenStax (CC BY 4.0)

Many years of unhealthy eating, smoking and excess alcohol consumption lead to fatty deposits in the form of cholesterol and hardened deposits called plaques to build up on the walls of the coronary arteries. These deposits cause the inner diameter of arteries to become narrowed, reducing blood flow (see Figure 4.11), which can lead to coronary heart disease (CHD). The process of plaque build-up within arteries is called **atherosclerosis**, in addition to narrowing, arteries can lose their elasticity, which is known as **arteriosclerosis**. When this happens, it becomes more difficult for arteries to expand and contract in relation to variations in BP. While the combination of atherosclerosis and arteriosclerosis results in a reduced blood flow within the coronary arteries, it can also have detrimental consequences for other arteries within the body and may lead to peripheral artery disease. People are usually unaware that they have atherosclerosis, it is a progressive disease, and along with hypertension, can go unnoticed. It may only be discovered during a health check or if an individual has chest pain, severe headaches, feels short of breath, has nosebleeds, a heart attack, stroke or vision problems. In someone who has pre-existing atherosclerosis, the physiological response to stress may result in angina or contribute to a heart attack. Globally, high blood pressure is the main risk factor for cardiovascular deaths (World Heart Report, 2023).

Angina and heart attacks

When the coronary arteries become narrowed, the blood supply to the heart is reduced, which means it does not get enough oxygen-rich blood to function

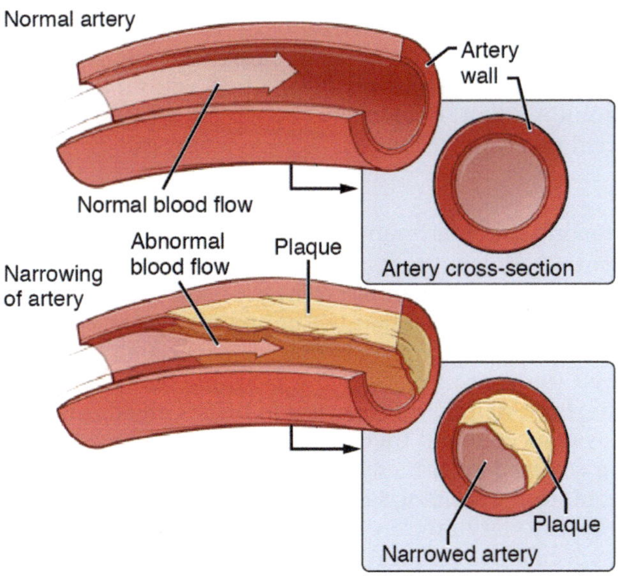

Figure 4.11
Normal artery and an artery narrowed by plaque build-up.

Source: National Heart, Lung, and Blood Institute; National Institutes of Health; U.S. Department of Health and Human Services. https://www.nhlbi.nih.gov/health/atherosclerosis

normally. This can result in symptoms of pain, feelings of pressure or squeezing located in the chest, shoulder, arm, neck jaw, back or stomach. These symptoms tend to occur during physical activity, as the heart must work harder and blood must flow more quickly to meet the increased bodily demand for oxygen. If these symptoms resolve with rest, it may be an indication of angina and medical investigations are required. Once diagnosed with angina, the individual is usually given a glyceryl trinitrate (GTN) spray, which dilates (opens) the blood vessels and increases blood flow to the heart. Angina is a warning that there is substantive narrowing in the coronary arteries that is interfering with the blood supply to the heart muscle. People with angina are at elevated risk of having a heart attack.

A myocardial infarction is the medical term for a **heart attack**; it can happen without warning and not everyone would have previously experienced angina. When atherosclerotic plaques start to form in the coronary arteries, they continue to grow, but due to the effects of hypertension on the arterial wall, a plaque may rupture or break off. When a plaque breaks off, the body's natural response is to repair the damage through blood clot formation, but the clot can break off and cause a blockage or travel to a narrowed area of artery elsewhere within the heart and block it. Both result in a lack of blood flow within the coronary arteries, causing a heart attack, which may cause irreversible damage to the heart muscle. Like angina, a heart attack produces symptoms of chest, shoulder, jaw, stomach and/or arm pain, the individual may be cold, clammy, pale and feel nauseated. Unlike angina, the pain is persistent and immediate medical intervention is required. If a heart attack is suspected, diagnosis and treatment within six hours of the onset of symptoms can have positive outcomes for the patient, minimising damage to the heart muscle (Mechanic et al., 2023). Not everyone who is having a heart attack exhibits the classic symptoms of chest, arm and jaw pain, women may have stomach or neck pain (see Chapter 9), and some people can have a 'silent' heart attack with no or very minimal symptoms. Most people who have a heart attack will survive, but recovery can range from a full resumption of normal activities to severe disability, the latter is often referred to as disease burden.

Diagnostic testing and treatment for a heart attack

Early intervention after a heart attack usually commences with prehospital emergency assessment using an electrocardiogram (ECG). During this procedure, electrodes are placed at specific points on the chest and limbs; these electrodes pick up electrical impulses that move through the heart muscle and show how well the various parts of the heart are working. This information provides basic, but essential information to help with an initial diagnosis. If a heart attack is suspected and there are no concerns about the patient having any disease associated with increased chances of bleeding, chewable aspirin is administered, to reduce blood clotting and permit blood to flow more easily around the coronary arteries. In hospital, blood tests will be conducted to assess for specific biochemical markers that indicate damage to the heart muscle.

If a patient experiences chest pain, but has not had a heart attack, they may be invited to undergo a 'treadmill test', this examines the heart's response to being physically stressed (by an increased bodily need for oxygen). There is a standard protocol to follow when conducting a treadmill test, the patient and the electrical activity of their heart are closely monitored while their heart is incrementally stressed during walking. The heart may also be examined using an ultrasound scan, which shows blood flow through the heart, how well the heart valves are working, and it is possible to image the coronary arteries to explore for bulging or ballooning of the arterial wall (called an aneurysm). A more invasive test called a coronary angiogram is often used to visualise any blockages within the coronary arteries. It involves a very thin tube (catheter) inserted into a wrist or groin artery, a special dye is introduced into the catheter, which permits visualisation of the arteries along with any narrowing or blockage using a type of X-ray. It is possible to treat blockages or narrowing during this procedure by using a balloon-type device that is inflated and used to compress the fatty material/clot against the artery wall. A short length of mesh called a stent may be inserted to hold the artery open and improve blood flow (the medical terminology for this is percutaneous coronary intervention (PCI), coronary stenting or coronary angioplasty). Sometimes it is not possible to compress the fatty material/clot or insert a stent, and the patient may be deemed suitable for coronary artery bypass surgery (CABG). During this procedure, the blocked arteries are bypassed using veins and arteries that are harvested from the patient's leg and/or chest. It is quite common for patients to have a double, triple or quadruple bypass, but this depends on how many arteries are blocked. A CABG is a very invasive type of surgery that involves the chest being opened, the heart exposed and stopped; a 'heart bypass machine' is used to oxygenate the blood and pump it around the body during surgery.

Strokes

Another type of cardiovascular disease (CVD) is a **stroke**, the medical term for this is a cerebral vascular accident (CVA). Across the world, the third highest cause of disability and the second highest cause of death is stroke (Johnson et al., 2016). A stroke involves a sudden disruption of oxygen supply to brain cells, the brain cells cannot survive without oxygen and will start to die very quickly. A stroke can be ischaemic or haemorrhagic, in the former, a blood clot (thrombosis) blocks a blood vessel within brain, whereas in a haemorrhagic stroke, a blood vessel in the brain bursts, blood is very toxic to brain cells, and they quickly die. The main cause of a haemorrhagic stroke is hypertension, which causes stress on arterial walls, which may cause swelling or ballooning of the wall, which may become thinner, making it more likely to burst.

The exact nature of disability caused by a stroke depends on where the damage occurs within the brain. Strokes can cause loss of speech, vision, paralysis, and/or confusion and the person may be at risk of developing depression and dementia. Strokes are more likely to occur in people over 40 years old; they are associated with risk factors, such as smoking, hypertension, sedentary behaviour, abdominal fat and unhealthy diets, all of these are modifiable lifestyle factors. Heart attacks and atrial fibrillation (see Box 4.2) are also risk factors for having a stroke. The acronym FAST (Face, Arms, Speech, Time) has been used to remind people of the signs of a stroke: Facial droop or an inability to smile on one side of the face, Arm weakness on one side, Speech problems and Time to call an ambulance.

BOX 4.2
ATRIAL FIBRILLATION (AF)

The heart pumps blood to the lungs and body, this pumping action is controlled by electrical activity within the heart. Sometimes this electrical activity can become irregular, too fast, or too slow, affecting how well blood is pumped around and out of the heart. Atrial fibrillation (AF) occurs when the electrical activity in atria does not work properly, they quiver or twitch, so instead of blood being pumped around the heart, it gathers in the atria. When this happens, blood clots can form, they can travel to the brain, causing a stroke or a transient ischaemic attack.

Transient ischaemic attacks

Another type of CVD is a **transient ischaemic attack** (TIA) also known as a 'mini stroke'. TIAs tend to have similar symptoms to a stroke, but the blockage in the blood supply within the brain is temporary in nature, symptoms can last for a few hours, with most symptoms resolving within 24 hours. When symptoms occur, it is impossible to know whether it is a stroke or a TIA, necessitating immediate medical care. The symptoms of a TIA are caused by a blood clot partially blocking an artery, but this is transitory in nature. People who have had a TIA are at immediate risk of having a major stroke.

Diagnosis and treatment of a stroke or TIA

When a stroke or TIA is suspected, a patient will undergo a series of tests that include measurement of blood pressure, blood tests and a brain scan, the latter is used to check for damage to the brain. An ECG will also be performed to check if there are any abnormalities in the rhythm of the heart. Medical management of acute stroke due to a blood clot will usually involve intravenous administration of a 'clot busting' drug to help disperse the clot, but this must occur within 4.5 hours of the symptoms starting. If there is a large clot, endovascular thrombectomy may be used to 'mechanically' remove the clot from inside the blood vessel; it is a more invasive procedure that can be used up to 24 hours from onset of symptoms. Irrespective of the initial treatment, during the acute stage of having a stroke or TIA, the aim of ongoing management will be focused on trying to reduce the risk of further blood clots and permanent disability. Patients will be prescribed long-term medication to help reduce the 'stickiness' of the blood and advice will be provided on necessary lifestyle changes to diet, physical activity and stress management.

BOX 4.2
CRITICAL THINKING

Your heart is responsible for pumping blood around the body, how might your heart rate, blood pressure and blood vessel diameter change when you are under stress?

What role do atherosclerosis and arteriosclerosis have in heart disease?

The respiratory system

Respiratory structures

The upper part of the respiratory tract includes the nose, mouth, throat, larynx (voice box) and trachea (windpipe), whereas the lower part consists of the lungs, bronchi, bronchioles and alveoli (see Figure 4.12). When we breathe in, air travels in through the nose and/or mouth and enters the trachea, which divides into two branches called the bronchi (one goes to each lung), within the lungs the airways divide like branches on a tree becoming smaller and smaller, leading to the bronchioles,

Alveolar ducts are found at the end of the bronchioles and lead into groups of alveoli, which look like bunches of grapes and they are stretchy to accommodate the breathing in and out. This is where the inhaled air is taken up by red blood cells contained within small blood vessels called capillaries (Figure 4.13). If a foreign body, food or fluids are accidentally inhaled, they will be trapped by mucus membranes and this results in the reflexive action of coughing. Respiratory centres in the brain constantly assess levels of oxygen and carbon dioxide in the blood and automatically adjust the rate and depth of breathing, as required. Carbon dioxide is a waste product of breathing,

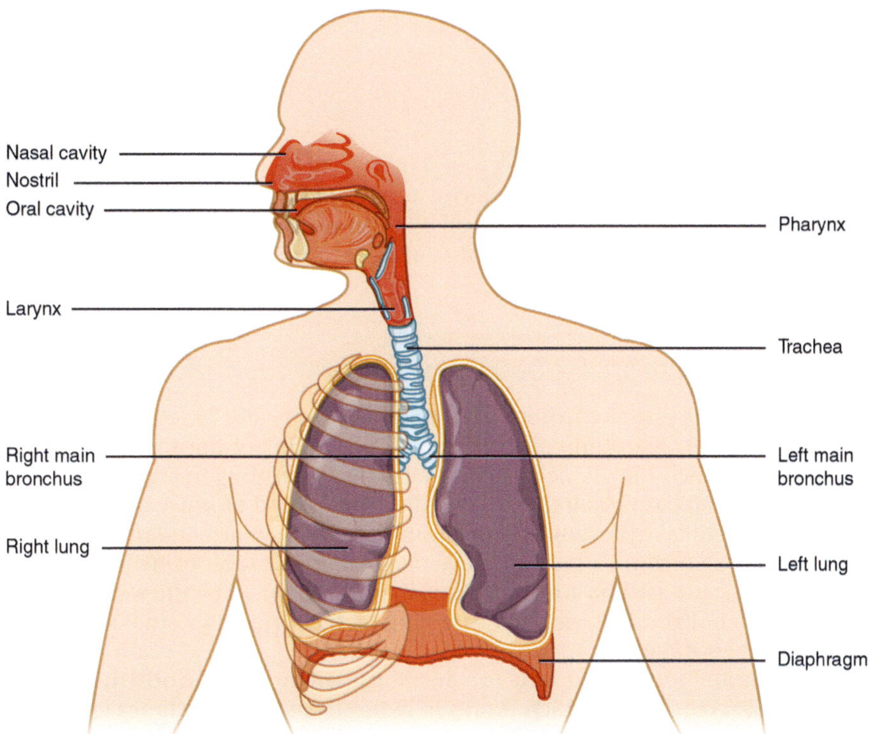

Figure 4.12 Major respiratory structures

Source: Betts et al. (2022) OpenStax (CC BY 4.0)

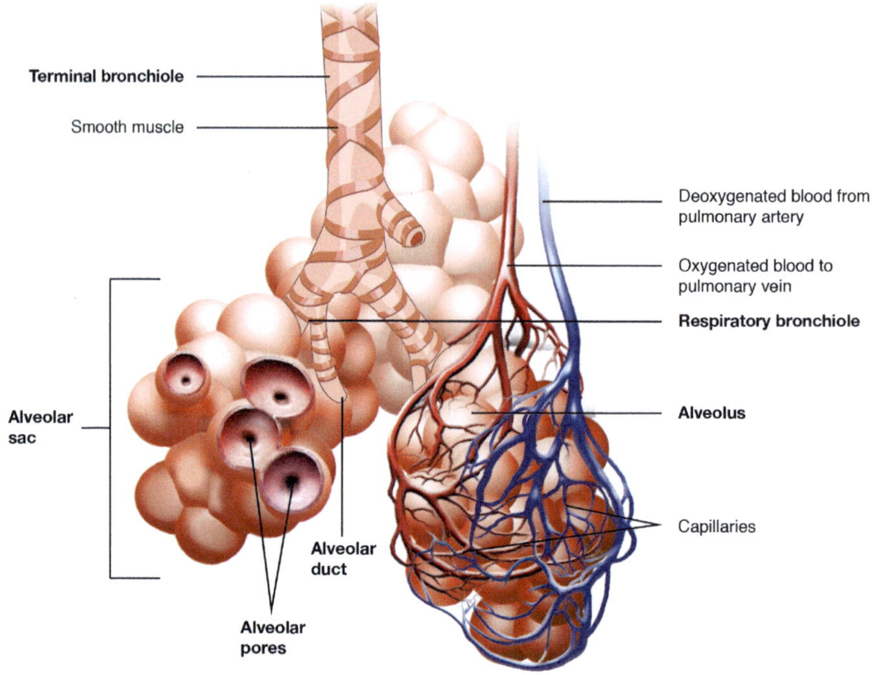

Figure 4.13 Lower respiratory tract

Source: Betts et al. (2022) OpenStax (CC BY 4.0)

which we breathe out. The respiratory system is lined with tiny hairs called cilia, which are a defence mechanism to keep out foreign materials that can interfere with breathing. The normal adult breathing rate is about 12–20 times per minute.

Asthma and chronic obstructive pulmonary disease

A common long-term (chronic) condition that impacts breathing ability is asthma. The main symptoms are inflammation, swelling of the airways and spasming of the bronchioles, which cause difficulty in breathing. In addition, inflammation in the airways results in an excessive production of mucus. Most people with asthma will take preventative medication to try to reduce inflammation and thus prevent an asthma attack and take 'reliever' medication to help reduce the impact of an acute asthma attack. Asthma may be worsened by the weather, allergens such as pollen, dust, pet hair, smoking (actual or passive smoking), stress, exercise and air pollution.

A chronic and progressive lung problem is caused by **chronic obstructive pulmonary disease** (COPD), which results in reduced ability of the lungs to oxygenate the blood. While asthma and COPD may have some similar symptoms, such as feeling short of breath and coughing, in COPD the airways, alveoli and small blood vessels within the lungs are inflamed, which is usually due to cigarette smoking. This results in narrowing of the airways and increased mucus production. The walls of the alveoli may become scarred, which can result in further narrowing and a loss of elasticity, making it difficult for people to breathe out. Some people who have never smoked can develop COPD, which can be due to air pollution and occupational causes. The impacts of COPD on breathing may result in severe disability, hospitalisations and early mortality.

Diagnosis and treatment of COPD

Diagnosis of COPD usually involves the testing of lung function through a spirometry (a special device to test how much air an individual breathes in and out and how fast air can be blown out of the lungs), imaging of the lungs by X-rays and auscultation (listening) to the individual's breathing through a stethoscope for sounds such as wheezing and crackling sounds from mucus in the lungs. Assessment of COPD may also include measurement of blood oxygen levels, examination of sputum volume and testing of sputum for infection. Shortness of breath is a common finding in COPD; it is progressive and affects the individual's ability to undertake physical activity. In severe cases, someone with COPD may be unable to undertake the normal activities of daily living, such as housework, they may need help with washing and dressing and may eventually require oxygen, even when at rest. In COPD, merely breathing takes effort and a lot of energy is used to force air out of the lungs; this can result in generalised muscle wasting, weakness and weight loss.

Treatment of COPD is palliative in nature, as the disease cannot be cured. Symptom control is the mainstay of treatment in trying to prevent exacerbations due to respiratory infections. Paramount aspects of treatment include smoking cessation, encouraging vaccine uptake of seasonal influenza (flu), COVID-19 and the respiratory syncytial virus (RSV). Like asthma, inhaled medications may be used to dilate the airways, along with corticosteroid medication to reduce airway inflammation and other medications may be prescribed to help reduce mucus production. Some people with COPD may be able to engage in pulmonary maintenance classes, which can help to keep them physically active and improve quality of life (American Lung Association, 2024).

The immune system

The role of the immune system is to defend the body against anything that can cause disease. It is a complex network of cells, tissues and organs that remain on constant alert to protect the body against pathogens, such as bacteria, viruses, parasites, fungi and/or foreign bodies. There are three primary types of blood cells, each with distinctive functions. Erythrocytes (red blood cells) carry oxygen from the lungs to all parts of the body. Thrombocytes (platelet cells) are essential for blood clotting and wound repair and **leukocytes** (white blood cells) play a key role in the immune system. Leukocytes act like an army of soldiers defending the body against threats from pathogens and foreign bodies. The key components of the immune system include the spleen, thymus, bone marrow, lymphatic system and lymphatic tissue. Pathogens can enter the body in several ways, for example, through a cut in the skin, via the mucus membranes in the nose and airways or into the digestive tract through what we eat and drink. The immune system will recognise the protein (antigen) that covers a pathogen as being 'alien', which triggers an immune response.

Innate and adaptive immune systems

We have 'innate' and 'adaptive' immune systems that work in tandem, protecting the body from pathogens. The **'innate' immune system** provides an immediate defensive response to any pathogen and a secondary line of defence is provided by the **'adaptive' immune system**, the latter is a slower response. The innate immune system includes the protective barrier of skin, the lymphatic system, mucosal tissues in the mouth, nose, airways, gastrointestinal and reproductive tracts. Specific leukocytes, namely neutrophils, monocytes, macrophages, dendritic cells and lymphocytes (B-cells, T-cells and natural killer cells), also have specific protective roles.

Leukocytes

Leukocytes have specialised functions and around 50–70% of them are neutrophils. These neutrophils can be thought of as the 'first responders'; they surround and ingest pathogens in a process known as phagocytosis, but neutrophils have a limited lifespan, they only last a few days. Macrophages are longer lasting, while they also use phagocytosis to engulf pathogens, they send chemical signals called **cytokines** to mobilise other immune cells. This results in inflammation, pain, swelling and redness of the skin, you may have experienced this with cuts and grazes. The innate immune system does not have any memory, which means that it does not recognise a pathogen from a previous encounter and will respond in the same way with repeated exposures. To help the body cope with pathogens, it sends signals via dendritic cells to alert the adaptive immune system that the body is under attack. During the period when the adaptive immune response is being activated and a more targeted response is being prepared, **natural killer cells** (NK cells) will start attacking viral pathogens. NK cells do not use phagocytes, they recognise the unusual markers on the surface of viral infected or cancerous cells and release chemicals to try and kill the cell and they can also release cytokines. If the adaptive immune system has had any previous exposure to an actual pathogen or an exposure via vaccination, it will recognise the pathogen and respond accordingly to stop it from overwhelming the body.

The main leukocytes involved in the adaptive immune response are known collectively as lymphocytes, they make up around 20–40% of leukocytes and they initially form in the bone marrow (central part of bones). B-cells continue to mature within the bone marrow, while others migrate to the thymus and become T-cells. One type of B-cell, called **antibodies**, can 'mark' pathogens for destruction. The other type of B-cell (memory B-cells (MBCs)) has a memory that recognises previously encountered antigens (see Box 4.3), which allows a rapid immune response. T-helper cells (also referred to as CD4+ cells) circulate through the blood on the lookout for pathogens and send out a chemical message to other immune cells providing the location of the pathogen, so that it can be destroyed. T cytotoxic cells kill infected viral cells and once the pathogen has been eliminated, T suppressor cells, as the name suggests, suppress the activity of other T-cells, so that the immune system returns to its normal homeostatic state.

BOX 4.3
THE DIFFERENCE BETWEEN PATHOGENS AND ANTIGENS

Pathogens cause disease by invading the body, multiplying and spreading, including viruses, bacteria, parasites and fungi. Pathogens are covered in antigens, which are proteins, and these are like a label that the immune system uses to distinguish between its own cells that are of no threat and foreign invaders that are a threat. Once the immune system detects foreign antigens, it mounts a defence by sending in white blood cells or creating antibodies to attack the antigen.

Vaccine response

Vaccines are attenuated forms of diseases that are introduced into the body to imitate an infection, which enables the adaptive immune system to respond and defend itself. Vaccines consist of antigens; the adaptive immune system identifies the antigen and responds as if it is a real disease. T-helper cells locate the antigen before activating other immune cells. B-cells make antibodies (proteins) that specifically target, bind to and neutralise the antigen. Cytotoxic T-cells attack and destroy any bodily cells that are infected with the antigen. The adaptive immune system creates a memory of the vaccine-specific antigen in the MBCs and T-cells. If the antigen is encountered again, the immune system can recognise it, respond and neutralise it quickly, which can either prevent or reduce the severity of the disease. Not everyone who receives a vaccine will respond in the same way, as age, genetics and chronic diseases may impact the ability of the immune system to mount a defence, moreover vaccine efficacy can also wane over time. People who have weakened immune systems due to disease or medical treatments, such as chemotherapy, may show a reduced response to vaccination.

The lymphatic system

The lymphatic system is a central aspect of the immune system; it contains lymphatic fluid that circulates around the body in vessels in a similar way to blood circulates in the arteries and veins. Lymphatic fluid carries lymphocytes and other white blood cells that help combat infection. Lymphatic fluid drains into oval-shaped structures called lymph nodes, which filter the fluid, trapping pathogens, dead cells and cancer cells. The 'cleaned' fluid circulates through the lymphatic system into the bloodstream. Lymph nodes can also act as a reservoir for cancer cells, and they help the spread of cancer by transporting cells via the lymphatic fluid and blood to other parts of the body.

BOX 4.3
CRITICAL THINKING

What is the difference between the innate and adaptive immune systems?

Cancer

Types of cancer

People tend to think that cancer is one disease, but there are over 200 types of cancer (Cancer Research UK, n.d.). The type of cancer that a person is diagnosed with depends on the place and type of cells the cancer had started in. Body cells are quite specialised and associated with specific structures and body parts, for example, muscle, nerves, blood, skin, etc. Body cells generate and die at specific rates, which are dependent on the type of cell, nutrients received and the balance between immature and mature cells. Normal cells do not migrate to other locations within the body, for example, a cell that has developed normally within breast tissue will not move into the bones. However, cancer cells do not obey the 'rules' to stop growing or to stay in one place. Once cancer cells grow, they can form into a mass called a tumour (see Box 4.4), which will require its own blood supply, it does this by sending out messengers to blood vessels in the area to get **capillaries** to provide oxygen and nutrients for growth. This blood supply also acts as a conduit for cancer cells to spread (metastasise). There are five main types of cancers (Table 4.2), among which carcinoma is the most common type.

BOX 4.4 WHAT IS A TUMOUR?

A tumour is an overgrowth of cells, which can be innocuous or malignant. Tumours that grow slowly are usually benign, they do not migrate to areas in the body and are rarely life threatening. Malignant tumours are cancerous; they can grow quite rapidly, spread to other bodily areas (metastasise) and can be life-threatening.

Table 4.2 Main categories of cancer

Main categories of cancer	Where it starts	Examples
Carcinoma	Skin or lining of internal organs	Bladder, breast, colon, liver, lung, prostate, skin.
Sarcoma	Bone, cartilage, fat, muscle or blood vessels	Osteosarcoma (bone) Liposarcoma (fat tissue)
Leukaemia	White blood cells, bone marrow	Acute lymphoblastic Chronic myeloid
Lymphoma and myeloma	Lymph nodes or lymphatic tissue of the immune system	Hodgkin lymphoma Non-Hodgkin lymphoma
Brain and spinal cord	Central nervous system	Glioblastoma Astrocytoma

What causes cancer?

There is no single cause for cancer, but we do know that cancer is associated with ageing and most cases are diagnosed in people who are over 65 years old. Around 5% of cancers are due to genetics, these cancers tend to develop earlier in life. Certain genes, such as *BRCA1* (*BReast CAncer Gene 1*) and *BRCA2* (*BReast CAncer Gene 2*), predispose individuals to develop a range of cancers, including breast and/ or ovarian cancers. Carcinogens, such as chemicals, viruses and radiation, can cause cancer by interfering with cell DNA, leading to uncontrolled cell growth. Tobacco smoke is a carcinogen, as it contains many chemicals that are harmful to the lungs, throat and mouth. Asbestos, when inhaled, can cause lung cancer. High doses of radiation over a short period can cause cancer, but the doses of radiation used during diagnostic X-rays and medical scans have little impact on the development of cancer. Some viruses can also cause cancer, for example, the human papillomavirus (HPV) is implicated in the development of cervical cancer and some head and neck cancers, whereas hepatitis B and C may predispose people to developing liver cancer. Too much exposure to the sun or sunbeds is linked to the development of skin cancer, especially with repeated sunburns in childhood and in those who have pale skin that burns easily or does not tan. Other factors, such as being overweight and sedentary, can predispose people to breast, colon and uterine cancers (Parkin et al., 2011). Eating a diet high in red and processed meats, such as ham, sausages and smoked meats, has been associated with a higher risk of colon cancer. Frequent alcohol intake is linked with the development of cancers of the mouth, throat, oesophagus, stomach and liver. The risks of these types of cancer increase when combined with smoking (World Health Organization [WHO], 2025a, 2025b).

Cancer diagnosis

Primary prevention of cancer involves the avoidance of behavioural risk factors that increase the likelihood of developing the disease and public health messaging is used to educate people about risk factors for cancer. Many countries around the world have population-based cancer screening programmes to detect cancers at an asymptomatic stage and they are targeted at anyone who meets the screening criteria (see Chapter 9). Within the United Kingdom (UK), everyone who has a cervix, aged 25–64 years, is invited for screening to detect cervical cancer and this occurs every three years until the age of 49, after this, screening is conducted every five years. Breast screening invitations occur every three years for women aged between 50 and 71 years. For bowel cancer screening, self-sampling kits are posted out to those aged between 50 and 74 years (60–74 years in Northern Ireland), every two years, this checks for very small amounts of blood in faeces, which can be an early sign of bowel cancer. Not everyone who has been invited to take part in asymptomatic screening avail of this offer; there are many reasons for this, which include the disease that is being screened for, the type of test, perceived discomfort of the screening test and fear of finding that something is wrong. Barriers to screening can include ethnicity, gender and sexual orientation, socioeconomic status, educational level and geographical location. We will explore some of these factors further in Chapter 7 in relation to health behaviours and beliefs in relation to behaviour change and in Chapter 9 in relation to chronic diseases.

Cancer may be diagnosed when a person goes to their healthcare practitioner with specific symptoms, such as finding a lump, a change in the appearance, itchiness or bleeding of a mole on the skin, bleeding when going to the toilet or while vomiting, changes to bowel habits, unexplained weight loss, feeling very tired, itchy and yellow skin, a prolonged cough, night sweats, indigestion or heartburn. This is not an exhaustive list of cancer-related symptoms and it must be remembered that most of these symptoms may be caused by factors other than cancer. For example, a person who has an infected cut on their hand may find a swollen lump underneath their arm, which may just be a swollen lymph node caused by an infection and the associated immune response. Discussion of the variety of tests used to diagnose cancer is beyond the scope of this book, but blood, other bodily fluids, tissue samples, x-rays and various types of scans may be used to determine the type and the stage of cancer.

When cancer is diagnosed, it will be described in relation to its stage and grade. This provides information on the size of the cancer, if it has spread into other bodily tissues and the chances of cure. Knowledge about staging and spread helps doctors to determine the types and number of required treatments. The three most common treatments for cancer involve surgery, radiotherapy and/or chemotherapy. When caught at an early stage and if confined to one area, the **primary site**, it may be possible to use surgery to remove the cancer or a series of radiotherapy treatments can be used to kill cancer cells. If cancer has spread to a nearby lymph node there may be a need to combine surgery with radiotherapy, but if there is wider spread (metastasis) through the lymphatic system to other lymph nodes and other parts of the body, known as a **secondary site**, chemotherapy may be required to target cancer cells throughout the body.

Cancer treatments

Surgery involves removal of the lump (tumour) and some surrounding tissue. In chemotherapy, drugs can be delivered through a vein or taken by mouth and sometimes more than one type of chemotherapy is required. While these drugs kill cancer cells, they also have negative impacts on normal cells. Chemotherapy may have unpleasant side effects, the most common being nausea, hair loss, sores in the mouth, reduced immune functioning, damage to peripheral nerves and the heart. The extent and duration of side effects depend on the drugs used, dosage and duration of treatment. Radiotherapy involves specific doses of radiation to kill cancer cells and reduce the size of tumours; it can be delivered externally where the x-ray beam is delivered through the skin to a very specific site. Internal radiation may involve drinking a radioactive liquid or having radioactive seeds placed inside the body. Radiotherapy can cause redness and soreness of the skin, fatigue, nausea, unintentional damage to bodily structures and organs near to the area being treated. For some cancers, treatment can be curative, meaning that it is completely gone, but this is dependent on the type and the stage of cancer, with no guarantees that it will never come back. Even if a cancer cannot be cured, treatments may be used to help symptom management and improve quality of life.

BOX 4.4
CRITICAL THINKING

We know that some cancers can be detected at an asymptomatic stage through cancer screening programmes.

Consider factors that may help facilitate someone to take up the offer of screening and what the barriers to screening might be.

Do you think the type of cancer being screened for is an important determinant of whether someone will attend screening?

Diabetes mellitus

The main source of energy used by the body is glucose, which comes mainly from carbohydrates in food. Food is digested and broken down into a form that the body can use and is absorbed into the bloodstream. When we eat, the pancreas (Figure 4.7) detects a rise in glucose (sugar) within the blood and releases insulin, this hormone assists the body in using glucose to produce energy for cell use. We are unaware of this automatic process but may become aware of it when blood glucose becomes too high. This is known as diabetes mellitus, which is a chronic disease.

Types of diabetes

The two main types of diabetes mellitus are known as type 1 (T1DM) and type 2 (T2DM). In T1DM, the pancreas stops producing insulin, blood glucose is uncontrolled and becomes too high (hyperglycaemia). The exact cause of T1DM is not fully understood but it is believed to involve the immune system attacking the insulin-producing cells of the pancreas. Individuals are at greater risk of developing T1DM if they have another family member who has diabetes. This type of diabetes is more likely to be diagnosed in children and young adults. T1DM is also referred to as insulin-dependent diabetes, as treatment involves taking insulin, which is injected or administered by a pump. T1DM also requires regular blood glucose monitoring.

T2DM is more common after the age of 40. Being obese and having a family history of diabetes are other common risk factors, and it is more prevalent in Indigenous Peoples and some ethnic groups. In T2DM, the pancreas may still produce insulin, but the body's cells may not fully respond to insulin, which is called insulin resistance. To compensate, the pancreas tries to produce even more insulin but it is eventually unable to keep up with demand and blood glucose rises. Onset of T2DM tends to be gradual, symptoms are not as marked as in T1DM and it can go unnoticed. It is estimated that between 25% and 33% of people who have T2DM go undiagnosed, potentially resulting in irreversible complications that include the development of CVD, kidney damage, visual impairments, lower limb amputation and nerve damage (International Diabetes Federation [IDF], 2021).

Diagnosis and treatment

T1DM is usually diagnosed as a result of symptoms, such as excessive thirst, frequent urination (sometimes bedwetting in children), feelings of extreme fatigue, falling asleep, lack of energy, constantly feeling hungry and weight loss. Such symptoms can be missed, thus diabetes may only be diagnosed when a person becomes acutely unwell and develops diabetic ketoacidosis, which is a medical emergency. Symptoms of T2DM can be more subtle than those of T1DM and may be diagnosed by 'accident' when a patient attends their healthcare professional for a routine health check or when they have blood tests after having had a heart attack, stroke, visual or urinary problems. It is also possible for people who are undiagnosed with T2DM to have symptoms similar to those of T1DM, which can include thirst, frequent urination, feeling tired and skin problems. T2DM is the most common type of the disease, accounting for 90% cases across the globe (IDF, 2021).

Attempts have been made across the world to standardise the way in which blood glucose is measured, but there are differences in the way it is expressed. Immediate (on-the-spot) measures of blood glucose are expressed in millimoles per litre (mmol/L) or milligrams per decilitre (mg/dL). Being aware of these different measures is important when evaluating interventions that try to reduce or control blood glucose (see Chapter 9). If diabetes is suspected, an 'on-the-spot' finger prick test may be used to evaluate current blood glucose, with levels ≥ 11.1 mmol/L or 200 mg/dL being an indication of diabetes. This will be followed up by a fasting (not eating or drinking any calories for at least 8 hours) blood sample. The normal fasting blood glucose for people without diabetes ranges between 3.9 mmol/L (126 mg/dL) and 5.6 mmol/L (100 mg/dL), a person with diabetes will have fasting blood glucose levels ≥ 7.0 mmol/L (≥126 mg/dL) and this requires confirmation on two separate occasions. While the 'on-the-spot' finger prick test shows current blood glucose levels, the preferred measure is HbA1c (glycated haemoglobin), which reflects blood glucose control over the past two to three months. HbA1c is a substance the body makes when it cannot use sugar properly, it sticks to red blood cells and it is expressed as millimoles per mole (mmol/mol) or as a percentage, with an HbA1c level of ≥48 mmol/mol (6.5%) indicative of diabetes.

Regardless of the type of diabetes, treatment focuses on self-management, including eating a healthy diet, engaging in regular physical activity, maintaining a healthy weight and having blood glucose checked at regular intervals. People diagnosed with T2DM are provided with education about the disease and how they can make lifestyle changes in relation to diet, physical activity, avoidance of smoking and the need to lose weight (Aschner, 2017). For some people, these lifestyle changes help to bring blood glucose down to acceptable levels, but some patients may require oral medication or insulin injections to keep blood glucose within a safe range. Due to the link between diabetes and other chronic conditions, it will also be necessary to keep a check on blood pressure, cholesterol and other medications. If blood glucose is poorly controlled, it can have a range of detrimental impacts on health, with reductions in life expectancy of around 20 years for those diagnosed with T1DM and 10 years for T2DM. The long-term consequences of high glucose can cause a range of health issues that include CVD, compromised kidney function, negative impacts on visual health, increased likelihood of lower limb amputation due to circulatory problems, nerve damage, fungal and bacterial infections, poor wound healing and joint problems.

Obesity and eating

What is obesity?

To function, the body requires a supply of energy, for most people, this is obtained through the food they eat (some people are unable to eat or digest food and receive nutrition through medical interventions). Between 1990 and 2022, the number of adults over 18 years old and categorised as obese has almost doubled (WHO, 2025b). **Obesity** is characterised by excess adipose tissue (fat) and commonly assessed by body mass index (BMI). Weight in kilograms is divided by height in metres squared (see Box 4.5), the resulting number is used to categorise an individual as being underweight, a healthy weight, overweight

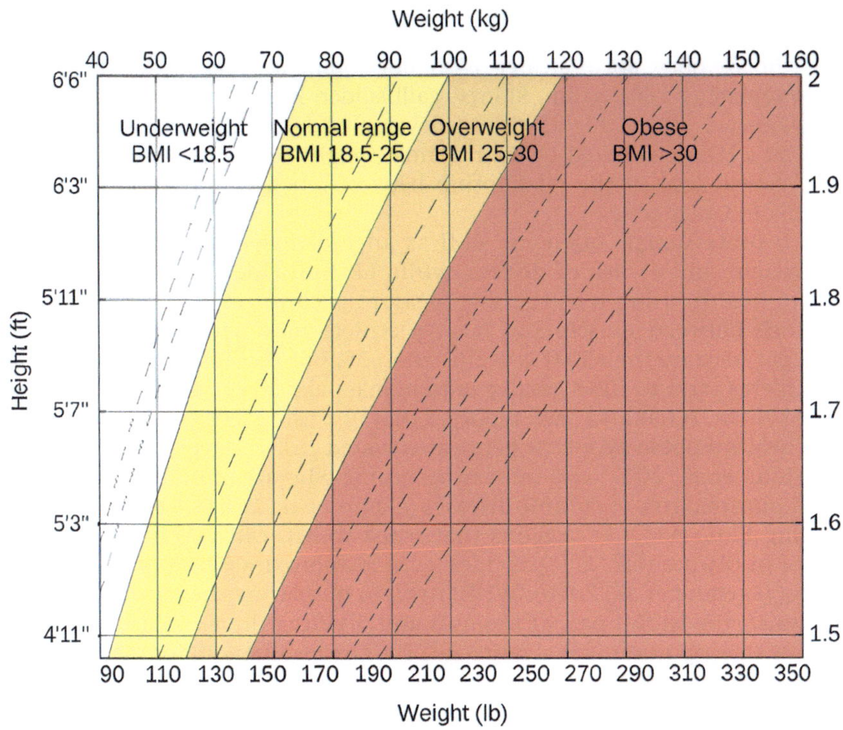

Figure 4.14 Body mass index chart

Source: Speilman et al. (2020) OpenStax (CC BY 4.0)

or obese (see Figure 4.14). People who are underweight (BMI less than 18.5) may be at risk of nutritional deficiencies. A BMI of 25–29.99 is overweight; 30–34.99 is class I obesity; 35–35.99 is class II obesity; and 40+ is class III obesity (WHO, 2000). However, as we will see in Chapter 9, these cutoff points are based on Western Eurocentric populations and lower classifications are suggested for people from other ethnic groups.

BOX 4.5
EXAMPLE OF HOW TO WORK OUT BMI

Weight = 58 kilograms and height = 1.53 metres: 1.53 m × 1.53 m = 2.34 m^2 (height in metres squared). Divide the weight by height in metres squared (e.g. 58 kilograms divided by 2.34 = 24.8). The value of 24.8 falls just within the normal weight range (BMI 18.5–24.9). Based on the National Health Service (NHS) (2023b) BMI calculator, this is considered within the healthy weight category for a female of White ethnic origin.

Why is obesity important?

People who are obese are at greater risk of developing cancers of the breast, pancreas, oesophagus, colorectum, kidney, gallbladder, liver and uterus (Pati et al., 2023). They are also at higher risk of developing hypertension, heart disease, stroke and T2DM compared to their normal weight counterparts (Owen et al., 2015). We will look at the relationship between obesity and chronic diseases more fully in Chapter 9.

Health professionals often use BMI as an indicator of whether a person is overweight and at risk of disease, while BMI provides a crude indication of risk to health, using it as the sole measure is controversial, as it does not distinguish between muscle and fat. An athlete may be classified as being overweight because their BMI is higher than 25, but this ignores the fact that most athletes tend to have greater muscle mass and lower body fat than the average person. It has also been reported that just using BMI may wrongly categorise healthy obese people at being at elevated risk of developing CVD and T2DM (Jung et al., 2017) and unhealthy people who are of normal weight, as being of minimal risk of chronic diseases (Conus et al., 2004). Rather than just measuring BMI, evidence suggests that **waist-to-hip ratio** (WHR) is a better indicator of disease risk, as it provides a crude approximation of body fat distribution (Egeland et al., 2016). WHR involves measuring the narrowest point of the waist, the widest part of the hips and dividing the waist measurement by that of the hip to provide a ratio. A WHR greater than .90 for men and .85 for women is linked with a higher risk of developing CVD and T2DM (WHO, 2011). It is also possible for someone to be within the normal range for BMI and have a WHR higher than 1, due to fat storage around the abdomen and internal organs (referred to as visceral fat). This places the person at higher risk of heart disease than people who are obese, but have a lower WHR (Lee et al., 2018).

Obesity, the search for a cause

'You are what you eat', how many times have you heard of this phrase? Also consider the common assumption that people become obese because the number of calories (energy from food) they ingest exceeds the energy they use up in everyday activities. This suggests that obesity is simply caused by overeating and if people showed more restraint in their eating habits, they would lose weight. While this sounds logical, research does not support this idea, as it cannot explain why some people regularly overeat and still do not put on weight.

Genetic and physiological theories of obesity

Someone whose parent is obese has a 40% chance of also becoming obese, this rises to 70% if both parents are obese. This suggests that genetics have a large role to play in becoming obese, but lifestyle factors of parents are shared with children, hence it can be difficult to determine whether genetics or the environment in which an individual is raised is the main contributor to obesity. One way of trying to differentiate between the various roles of nature (genetics) and nurture (environment) is to study identical twins who have been adopted into different families. Since identical twins share the same genetics, the only factor that differs should be their environment. Stunkard et al. (1990) measured the BMIs of identical twins who had lived together or were reared apart. Despite being raised in different environments, identical twins were of similar body weight, suggesting that genetic factors could be important determinants of whether a person will become obese. It has also been suggested that genetic mutations along with how genes are turned on or off can exert an influence on BMI, body fat, bodily fat distribution, eating and hormones that are associated with the risk of developing obesity (Masood & Moorthy, 2023).

The role of the hypothalamus

Earlier in this chapter, you were introduced to a structure in the brain called the hypothalamus, which has a role to play in the control of feeding behaviour. Early research with rats showed that damage to the **ventromedial hypothalamus** (VMH) resulted in overeating and obesity, hence the VMH became designated as the satiety centre (associated with feeling full). However, excessive eating and weight gain after damage to the VMH were not permanent, after several weeks, although rats weighed more than before VMH damage, eating and weight gain levelled off, suggesting satiety may be more complicated than initially thought (Hetherington & Ranson, 1940). Subsequent research showed that VMH lesions triggered an increase in insulin levels, which led to greater fat storage, highlighting interactions between the hypothalamus and hormonal activity in obesity (Bray et al., 1981). Findings that lesions to the lateral (outside) part of the hypothalamus (LH) caused cessation of eating and drinking in rats led to this being referred to as the hunger centre (Anand & Brobeck, 1951). However, later research showed that damage to the LH also caused insensitivity to sensory information about food taste and smell, which affected eating behaviour (Cho et al., 2002). Thus, the role of the hypothalamus in obesity is much more complicated than what earlier research had suggested, as hormones, habit and availability of food can all exert influences on eating.

Glucostatic theory

In 1953, Mayer proposed the glucostatic theory and suggested that the hypothalamus had a role to play in monitoring blood glucose levels. When blood glucose dropped below a specific level, the hypothalamus sent out hunger signals to encourage eating and when blood glucose increased, it signalled satiation to stop eating. In people without diabetes, blood glucose fluctuates within a normative range, dropping when food has not been consumed for a while and increasing after eating. However, the belief that feelings of hunger were based on low levels of blood glucose was unable to explain why someone with untreated diabetes who had high blood glucose still felt hungry. This created a problem for Mayer's initial theory, but the explanation was clarified to mean that the hypothalamus monitored the amount of glucose used by the body, rather than the amount in the blood and it was the usage of glucose that triggered feelings of hunger. Confirmation of glucose usage idea came from studies with rats and mice which had just eaten but had been injected with a substance that blocked the ability of cells to use blood glucose, the result was overeating (Smith & Epstein, 1969). We now know that eating, hunger and body weight are much more complicated than initially thought, especially as subsequent animal studies found contrasting results, with insulin injections resulting in increased food intake and obesity. Furthermore, there was no clear link between bodily use of glucose and reductions in eating in human studies (Levitsky et al., 2022).

The role of ghrelin in eating

When the stomach is empty, ghrelin (the hunger hormone) is released, which tells the hypothalamus to stimulate appetite. Ghrelin levels usually show a temporary decrease after eating, it works on a short-term basis, fluctuating between one meal or snack and the next. Despite the finding that people who are obese exhibit lower fasting levels of ghrelin than their lean counterparts (Cummings et al., 2001), the signal to turn off ghrelin seems to be blunted in people who are obese (English et al., 2002), meaning that satiety does not register in the brain and they tend to overeat. However, other theories have been suggested to explain overeating and obesity.

Set point theory

People tend to think that when they feel hungry, it is an indication that their body is low on energy and they need to eat, which may suggest that the body has a set point at which energy is required. The set point theory of weight works in a similar way to that of a heating thermostat. If the room temperature falls below a specific point on a thermostat, the heating goes on, when the temperature reaches the required level, the heating goes off, but if the temperature drops below the set point, the heating will go back on again. It has been proposed that weight is controlled by a type of internal thermostat that tries to maintain a person's weight at a genetically predetermined set point. This may help explain why many people who are overweight or obese try diets, lose weight, only to regain it when they stop dieting. Instead of the hypothalamus directly controlling eating, Kennedy (1953) suggested that it functions as a lipostat, monitoring the body's fat levels that have a genetically predetermined set point. If fat levels fall below the set point, the lipostat promoted eating and if higher than the set point, eating was suppressed.

The role of fat cells and leptin

The average person has a certain number and size of fat cells that are used to store calories (Hirsch et al., 1989). This store acts as an 'energy reserve' that can be used by the body when calorie intake is lower than the energy being expended. Fat cells develop during childhood and puberty, before slowing down in adulthood when the number of cells remains constant. This has implications for overeating and weight gain in childhood and adolescence, as increases in the number of fat cells may predispose the individual to become overweight or obese in adulthood. Furthermore, women who develop diabetes during pregnancy (known as gestational diabetes) tend to give birth to higher weight babies and these babies are more likely to be overweight during childhood (Leng et al., 2015). Ingesting more calories than required may increase fat cell volume, leading to consequential weight gain, but dieting to reduce weight does not impact the number of fat cells (Spalding et al., 2008). For many years, the exact nature of communication between fat stores and the brain has remained a bit of a mystery, which changed with the discovery that that mice with a genetic mutation, which prevented them from making leptin, tended to overeat and become obese (Zhang et al., 1994).

Leptin is the fullness hormone, when the body's fat stores are full, fat cells release leptin into the blood, which signals to the hypothalamus that there is a need to reduce eating. In the Zhang et al. (1994) study, the hypothalamus registered the lack of leptin as a sign that the body was lacking in fat, triggering overeating and lowering of the basal metabolic rate (BMR) (the number of calories required to maintain essential bodily functions, see Box 4.6). These findings were confirmed by giving leptin-deficient mice injections of leptin, resulting in reduced eating, increased basal metabolic rate (BMR) and a return to normal body weight. This suggested that injections of leptin could be a possible pharmacological treatment for obesity. However, human studies found that leptin injections made no difference to BMI (Lejeune et al., 2003) and that individuals who were obese had more leptin than their lean counterparts. It seems that in obesity, the hypothalamus becomes resistant to leptin, which results in a lack of satiety. In addition, leptin resistance is associated with the body trying to conserve energy by lowering the BMR, which results in fewer calories being used at rest (Obradovic et al., 2021).

BOX 4.6
BASAL METABOLIC RATE

Engaging in physical activity burns up calories, but even when we are resting, calories are required to maintain breathing, heart rate, temperature, blood circulation, digestion, immune activity, etc. The number of calories required to maintain these essential bodily functions is called the basal metabolic rate (BMR). People who have a low BMR burn fewer calories to maintain these bodily functions compared to people with a higher BMR. It was thought that people who were obese had lower BMRs, leading to storage of unused calories, helping to explain weight gain. An average person requires around 1,500 to 2,000 calories per day, but this requirement can vary according to age, current weight, biological sex, occupation, disease and physical activity. People who are obese must expend more energy to do the same activities and some have higher metabolic rates compared to their lean counterparts (Prentice et al., 1989).

Global growth in obesity

Genetic and physiological theories can help explain how people may be predisposed to developing obesity, but they cannot account for the global growth in obesity. Food preferences also impact eating behaviour. For example, even though we may not manage to finish the main course due to satiation, many of us do find room for a dessert! This suggests that while hunger and satiety do have a physiological basis, the development and maintenance of obesity seem to involve other factors, such as habit, emotional eating and stress (see Chapter 8) and/or enjoyment of food. Brain imaging studies have shown that sensory information relating to just seeing, smelling and tasting food can increase appetite, even in people who have already eaten (Sorokowska et al., 2017). This is known as **hedonic hunger**, which involves eating for pleasure, due to certain foods tasting good, rather than because of physiological hunger. The combination of fat and sugar-based foods seems to be especially appealing (Drewnowski & Greenwood, 1983), they may trigger neural responses that involve the release of dopamine, which is associated with reward and pleasure. Dopamine is a neurotransmitter that helps brain cells communicate with one another. When we get a 'hit' of dopamine, it causes a feel-good factor, our brains remember this and we may feel motivated to eat the same foods. Hence, eating can become a habit due to cravings for the dopamine hit and we may become addicted to certain foods. The hypothalamus, endocrine system and the gastrointestinal tract work in tandem with **olfactory** and taste senses to affect appetite, eating and food preferences (Holt et al., 2025). Thus, it seems that the global growth in obesity may not just be physiological, it is also fuelled by what Hill and Peters (1998) referred to as an **obesogenic environment**, which will be explored in Chapter 9.

BOX 4.5 CRITICAL THINKING

Eating is about much more than food and energy expenditure.

What influences your eating choices?
Does stress or tiredness influence what you eat?

Treatments to help people who are obese to lose weight

Obesity is a complex condition involving interactions between genetically related predispositions, psychological, social and environmental influences. After trying many dietary and exercise regimes with limited or no success, people who are obese may have a passive acceptance that there is nothing they can do to lose weight and this can be compounded by negative experiences when seeking help from GPs (general practitioners). Due to inadequate education on nutrition, obesity and dietary matters within medical training, along with limited knowledge about evidence-based clinical guidelines (Oshman et al., 2023; Schwenke et al., 2020; Wass & Finer, 2013), many GPs feel ill-equipped to provide advice and effective treatments for obesity. This coupled with an inability to devote time to patient assessment and lack of access to multidisciplinary team services to manage obesity in primary care may contribute to suboptimal care for this patient population (Oshman et al., 2023).

Several medical causes of obesity have been identified, which include endocrine diseases, for example, hypothyroidism, polycystic ovarian disease and Cushing's disease, which require medication as the mainstay of treatment. There general agreement that obesity is being fuelled by increasing sedentary lifestyles, with environmental and dietary factors interacting with genetic susceptibility, leading to weight gain (Butland et al., 2007), which means treatments for obesity must be multifaceted in nature. This includes individual lifestyle assessment, collaboratively agreed goals and patient expectations that need to be revised in the short- and longer term to sustain weight loss and prevent further weight gain. A combination of treatments may be including dietary, pharmacological, surgical and physical activity management, along with lifestyle behavioural interventions. The types of lifestyle behavioural interventions offered will depend on the individual's weight and any other diseases they have. Initial assessment is paramount, as lifestyle factors like current dietary patterns, physical activity and stress can have negative consequences for obesity. It must be remembered that obesity management is a long-term process, not a quick fix, it involves permanent changes to diet and physical activity (Butland et al., 2007).

Dietary management of obesity

Dietary management of obesity includes taking a history of previous attempts at weight loss and assessment of current dietary habits by means of a food intake record. This can be used to explore missed meals, times of eating, snacking and sources of meals, including takeaway meals, portion sizes and consumption of hidden sugars (Greenwood & Stanford, 2008). This will provide a baseline from which to provide education and help an individual make changes to their diet. Weight management goals must be collaboratively agreed with the patient and achievable. Ingesting fewer calories than are expended is a starting point, which can involve a range of dietary approaches, such as lowering fats and/or carbohydrates, while increasing fresh fruits and vegetables and using a smaller plate to cut down on portion sizes. Substituting food for low-calorie meal replacement drinks, reducing calories through calorie counting of food or changing to a Mediterranean-style diet that increases fruits, vegetables and grains can be combined with methods, including fasting or calorie restriction on some days of the week.

Physical activity

Current levels of physical activity can be measured in a variety of ways that include simple reporting of current activity in minutes of walking or distance and how difficult it felt. Physical activity can also include daily activities, such as working around the house and garden, walking to work, leisure time activities and having a physically active job. People often overestimate their physical activity, pedometers, mobile phone apps and smart watches can be used to provide an indication of the number of steps taken, minutes of physical activity and intensity based on heart rate. Such 'baseline measures' can then be used to set collaborative, tangible and progressive physical activity goals. The current advice for normal-weight adults is 30 minutes of moderate-level physical activity (at this level, the person will be slightly breathless, but still able to have a conversation) on at least five days of the week. To prevent obesity, 45–60 minutes per day are required, but people who are obese need to increase this duration to between 60 and 90 minutes (NICE, 2025). Even in patients who have not managed to lose any weight, physical activity should be encouraged, because it can have other benefits to health.

Pharmacological management of obesity

For people who have a BMI of 30 or 35+, who have made dietary and physical activity changes and are still struggling to lose weight, or who have other diseases, such are CVD or T2DM, pharmacological agents may be used as an additional treatment. Within the UK, the National Institute for Health and Care Excellence (NICE) have produced guidance for overweight and obesity management (NICE, 2025), which details that when prescribing medication to help with weight management, it is essential to support the patient with behavioural strategies to reduce calorie intake and increase physical activity. Four medications, Tirzepatide, Semaglutide, Liraglutide and Orlistat, have been licensed for use in the UK, each having specific prescribing criteria that include BMI values in the morbidly obese range and the presence of comorbidities, for example, CVD, high BP and T2DM. Some of these drugs are only available from specialist services and none can be used in pregnancy (NICE, 2025). These drugs work in one of two ways, they can suppress appetite or reduce the ability of the bowel (part of the digestive system) to absorb fat, but the drugs can have unpleasant side effects, which can lead to them being discontinued. Their use is evaluated after 12–16 weeks, a 5% reduction in weight is required for evidence of effectiveness and they will need to be prescribed on a long-term basis. If used as a sole intervention, once stopped, many people will experience weight gain. Access to these drugs can be hampered by costs to health services and in some countries, they may not be covered by medical insurance as a treatment for obesity (Henderson et al., 2024).

Surgical management of obesity

Surgery for obesity, also referred to as bariatric surgery, works by decreasing the size of the stomach, limiting the amount of food it can hold. Surgery may be considered for individuals who have had limited weight loss success with diet, exercise and obesity drugs. Within the UK, surgery may be offered to patients who have a BMI greater than 40 and to patients who have BMIs between 35 and 39.9 who also have CVD, T2DM or hypertension. There are various types of surgeries, but all of them have the goal of reducing the amount of food that can be ingested and consequent calorie intake. Patients must undergo dietary and physical activity assessments and are provided with support to adhere to lifestyle advice post-surgery and longer term (NICE, 2025). Due to reductions in food intake, bariatric surgery carries the risk of long-term vitamin and mineral deficiencies, which may necessitate long-term supplementation (Holmberg & Lagergren, 2022). Most individuals who undergo bariatric surgery do experience substantial weight loss, reduced risks of CVD and in some cases, remission of T2DM (O'Brien et al., 2019), but for some, initial weight loss may not be maintained (Velapati et al., 2018). This highlights the need for ongoing post-surgical lifestyle interventions that focus on habitual eating and dietary preferences (Kalarchian et al., 2012).

It is essential that a patient-centred approach is taken when helping people manage obesity, so that they are advised of treatment options and involved in decision-making in how to manage their weight. Obesity is a disease rather than a lifestyle choice, it has negative consequences for morbidity, quality of life and mortality, but with appropriate treatment and support, obesity, like many chronic diseases, it can be prevented and even reversed (Kopelman & Finer, 2001).

Chapter summary

Describe the structure and function of the central and peripheral nervous systems

The central nervous system consists of the brain and spinal cord, which process information and bodily responses. The peripheral nervous system is connected to the spinal cord and consists of the sensory and autonomic nervous systems. The autonomic nervous system is self-regulating and has an important role to play in the management of stress responses.

Outline the main functions associated with each of the four lobes of the brain

The frontal lobe is the executive centre of the brain as it undertakes a wide range of functions; it also contains the motor cortex, essential for voluntary movement of skeletal muscles and is involved in language production. The parietal lobe processes information from the senses, bodily movement and orientation, along with spatial information. The temporal lobe is involved in hearing, memory, speech, language and comprehension. The occipital lobe deals with visual perceptions and visual memory and integrates information from both eyes.

Explain the two stress pathways

When we experience stress, the amygdala signals to the posterior hypothalamus, which in turn activates the sympathetic nervous system. This triggers the adrenal medulla to secrete adrenaline and noradrenaline to get the body ready for fight or flight. At the same time, the anterior hypothalamus releases corticotrophin-releasing factor (CRF); this activates the pituitary gland, which releases adrenocorticotropic hormone that stimulates the adrenal cortex to release cortisol and aldosterone, which readies the body for action.

Summarise the functions of the cardiovascular system and cardiovascular diseases

The heart pumps oxygenated blood from the lungs around the body and deoxygenated blood back into the lungs to be oxygenated. Blood vessels usually dilate and contract, but arteriosclerosis makes them less flexible. Atherosclerosis leads to narrowing of the arteries, which can cause hypertension and angina. If a piece of plaque breaks off the artery wall, a clot will form, which can block the artery or a piece of clot can break off, leading to a heart attack, stroke or transient ischaemic attack.

Describe the respiratory system and the main factors associated with chronic obstructive pulmonary disease

When we breathe in, air travels through the upper respiratory system (nose and mouth, trachea) and into the lower respiratory system (lungs, bronchi, bronchioles and alveoli). The latter are stretchy to accommodate breathing in and out. This is where oxygen is absorbed into red blood cells and transported around the body. Chronic obstructive pulmonary disease is mainly caused by smoking, it creates inflammation in the alveoli and small blood vessels, resulting in narrowing of the airways and increased mucus production. This disease cannot be cured, but symptoms can be managed.

Summarise the main categories and causes of common cancers

There are five main categories of cancer: brain and spinal cord, carcinoma, sarcoma, leukaemia, and lymphoma and myeloma. There is no single cause for cancer, but lifestyle behaviours, such as smoking, obesity, diet, alcohol, ultraviolet radiation and exposure to environmental pollutants, have a role to play. Genetic factors, along with exposure to viruses such as HPV and hepatitis, can also predispose people to developing cancer.

Distinguish between type 1 and type 2 diabetes

Type I diabetes is more commonly diagnosed in young people and thought to be due to the immune system attacking insulin-producing cells in the pancreas. Type 2 diabetes is the most common form of the disease worldwide and is linked to lifestyle factors, such as obesity, overeating and having a sedentary lifestyle. In type 2 diabetes, the body may still produce insulin, but bodily cells may not respond properly, known as insulin resistance.

Discuss the potential causes of obesity

Various causes have been offered for obesity, which have included early physiological studies implicating the hypothalamus, glucostatic theory, set point theory, the role of fat cells and leptin and the basal metabolic rate. However, the global growth in obesity suggests that other factors, such as lifestyle and living in an obesogenic environment are important.

Keywords

Central nervous system: The brain and spinal cord.

Autonomic nervous system: A self-regulating system that regulates internal organs and glands and is involved in the stress response.

Cerebrum: Largest part of the brain, which has an outer layer called the cerebral cortex, which is responsible for most of the higher brain functions. It has two hemispheres, each having four lobes.

Corpus callosum: Connects the two hemispheres of the brain.

Cerebellum: Part of the brain associated with balance, coordination and fine motor movements.

Limbic system: Contains the hippocampus, amygdala and hypothalamus that are involved in emotion, motivation, learning and memory.

Amygdala: Found within the limbic system, it processes information related to fear, stress and emotion.

Hypothalamus: It maintains homeostasis, regulates hunger, thirst, controls the sleep-wake cycle sexual behaviour and plays a major role in the stress response.

Sympathetic-adrenal-medullary response: The body's immediate reaction to stress, controlled by the sympathetic nervous system, and involves the adrenal medulla to secrete adrenaline and noradrenaline during the fight or flight response.

Endocrine system: A network of glands that produce hormones. The pituitary and adrenal glands are involved in the stress response and the pancreas in diabetes.

Hypothalamic-pituitary-adrenal-pathway: The slower stress pathway that involves the hypothalamus, the pituitary gland and the adrenal cortex that secretes cortisol to help manage longer-term stress.

Cardiovascular system: The heart, arteries and veins that transport oxygen and nutrients around the body.

Blood pressure: The pressure of blood on the walls of arteries.

Atherosclerosis: The build-up of fatty deposits (plaques) on the walls of arteries that reduces the internal diameter of the artery, restricting blood flow and contributing to cardiovascular disease.

Arteriosclerosis: An ageing process whereby the arteries become less flexible.

Heart attack: Occurs when the blood supply to a part of the heart muscle has been blocked.

Angina: Chest pain caused by reduced blood supply to the heart muscle.

Stroke: The blood supply within the brain is compromised by a blockage due to a clot or less commonly a haemorrhage. Both result in the death of brain cells and cause some type of loss of function depending on where within the brain that the stroke occurs.

Transient ischaemic attack: A temporary blockage to the blood supply in the brain.

Upper respiratory system: The nose, mouth, throat, throat and larynx.

Lower respiratory system: The trachea, bronchi, bronchioles, alveoli and lungs.

Chronic obstructive pulmonary disease: A progressive lung disease that causes breathing difficulty, mucus production, breathlessness and fatigue.

Erythrocytes: Red blood cells that carry oxygen.

Leukocytes: White blood cells that are part of the immune system.

Innate immune system: The body's first line of defence against pathogens includes the skin, lymphatic system, mucosal membranes in the mouth, nose, airways, gastrointestinal tract, reproductive system and specific leukocytes.

Adaptive immune system: Creates immunity after exposure to specific pathogens.

Neutrophils: Fast-acting cells that surround and ingest pathogens.

Macrophages: Engulf pathogens through phagocytosis and signal other immune responses.

Natural killer cells: Cells that destroy virus-infected cells and cancerous cells through the release of chemicals.

Antibodies: Recognise and attack specific pathogens.

T-helper cells: Help to coordinate the immune response and send messages to other immune cells by indicating the location of pathogens.

Primary cancer site: The original site where the cancer first developed.

Secondary cancer site: Cancer that has spread from the primary site to other parts of the body.

Type 1 diabetes: The pancreas does not produce insulin, thought to be due to the immune system attacking cells within the pancreas. An individual will be dependent on insulin to metabolise glucose.

Type 2 diabetes: The body becomes resistant to the effects of insulin; this type of diabetes is thought to be related to lifestyle factors such as obesity.

Obesity: Excess accumulation of fat that is a risk to health.

Body mass index: A ratio of weight to height that can be used to classify people as being underweight, normal weight, overweight and various classes of obesity.

Waist-to-hip ratio: The waist measurement is divided by the hip measurement and provides a crude approximation of fat distribution.

Ventromedial hypothalamus: The front, middle part of the hypothalamus, implicated in eating behaviours.

Lateral hypothalamus: Outside part of hypothalamus linked with satiety.

Hedonic hunger: Eating for pleasure rather than because of feelings of hunger

Obesogenic environment: An environment that encourages eating of unhealthy foods and sedentary behaviour.

Key Readings

Betts, G. J., Young, K. A., Wise, J. A., Johnson, E., Poe, B., Kruse, D. H., Korol, O., Johnson, J. E., Womble, M., DeSaix, P., Blaker, W., Bowers, J., Barlow, M., Hortsch, M., Bradshaw, E., Tallman, K., Campbell., B., Tarapore, R., Jablanovic, B., ... Elf, P. (2022). *Anatomy and physiology 2e* (p. 15.3). OpenStax. https://openstax.org/books/anatomy-and-physiology-2e/pages/1-introduction

Holt, R. R., Schmitz, Hf H., Mhawish, R., Komarnytsky, S., Nguyen, T., Caveney, P. M., & Munafo, J. P. (2025). Comfort foods in the twenty-first century: Friend or foe? *Annual Review of Food Science and Technology, 16*(1), 433–458. https://doi.org/10.1146/annurev-food-111523-122109

O'Connor, D. B., Thayer, J. F., & Vedhara, K. (2021). Stress and health: A review of psychobiological processes. *Annual Review of Psychology, 72*, 663–688. https://doi.org/10.1146/annurev-psych-062520-122331

Reflective Questions

1 Explain how the body responds physiologically to stress.
2 Do you think that pharmacological drugs can control obesity on their own?
3 Consider lifestyle factors that are associated with the development and progression of chronic diseases, such as CVD, T2DM and obesity.

Notes

1 Access for free at https://openstax.org/books/psychology-2e/pages/1-introduction
2 Access for free at https://openstax.org/books/anatomy-and-physiology-2e/pages/19-1-heart-anatomy

References

American Lung Association. (2024). *Pulmonary rehabilitation*. Retrieved March 1, 2025, from https://www.lung.org/lung-health-diseases/lung-procedures-and-tests/pulmonary-rehab

Anand, B. K., & Brobeck, J. R. (1951). Hypothalamic control of food intake in rats and cats. *The Yale Journal of Biology and Medicine, 24*(2), 123–140.

Aschner, P. (2017). New IDF clinical practice recommendations for managing type 2 diabetes in primary care. *Diabetes Research and Clinical Practice, 132*, 169–170. https://doi.org/10.1016/j.diabres.2017.09.002

Betts, G. J., Young, K. A., Wise, J. A., Johnson, E., Poe, B., Kruse, D. H., Korol, O., Johnson, J. E., Womble, M., DeSaix, P., Blaker, W., Bowers, J., Barlow, M., Hortsch, M., Bradshaw, E., Tallman, K., Campbell, B., Tarapore, R., Jablanovic, B., & ...Elf, P. (2022). *Anatomy and physiology 2e* (p. 15.3). OpenStax. https://openstax.org/books/anatomy-and-physiology-2e/pages/1-introduction

Bray, G. A., Inoue, S., & Nishizawa, Y. (1981). Hypothalamic obesity: The autonomic hypothesis and the lateral hypothalamus. *Diabetologia, 20*(1), 366–377. https://doi.org/10.1007/BF00254505

Butland, B., Jebb, S., Kopelman, P., McPherson, K., Thomas, S., Mardell, J., & Parry, V. (2007). *Foresight – Tackling obesities: Future choices* project report (2nd ed.). Government Office for Science. https://assets.publishing.service.gov.uk/media/5a759da7e5274a4368298a4f/07-1184x-tackling-obesities-future-choices-report.pdf

Cancer Research UK (n.d.). What is cancer. Retrieved March 14, 2025, from https://www.cancerresearchuk.org/about-cancer/what-is-cancer

Cho, Y. K., Li, C. S., & Smith, D. V. (2002). Taste responses of neurons of the hamster solitary nucleus are enhanced by lateral hypothalamic stimulation. *Journal of Neurophysiology, 87*(4), 1981–1992. https://doi.org/10.1152/jn.00765.2001

Conus, F., Allison, D. B., Rabasa-Lhoret, R., St-Onge, M., St-Pierre, D. H., Tremblay-Lebeau, A., & Poehlman, E. T. (2004). Metabolic and behavioral characteristics of metabolically obese but normal-weight women. *The Journal of Clinical Endocrinology & Metabolism, 89*(10), 5013–5020. https://doi.org/10.1210/jc.2004-0265

Cummings, D. E., Purnell, J. Q., Frayo, R. S., Schmidova, K., Wisse, B. E., & Weigle, D. S. (2001). A preprandial rise in plasma ghrelin levels suggests a role in meal initiation in humans. *Diabetes, 50*(8), 1714–1719. https://doi.org/10.2337/diabetes.50.8.1714

Drewnowski, A., & Greenwood, M. R. (1983). Cream and sugar: Human preferences for high-fat foods. *Physiology & Behavior, 30*(4), 629–633. https://doi.org/10.1016/0031-9384(83)90232-9

Egeland, G. M., Igland, J., Vollset, S. E., Sulo, G., Eide, G. E., & Tell, G. S. (2016). High population attributable fractions of myocardial infarction associated with waist-hip ratio. *Obesity, 24*(5), 1162–1169. https://doi.org/10.1002/oby.21452

English, P. J., Ghatei, M. A., Malik, I. A., Bloom, S. R., & Wilding, J. P. (2002). Food fails to suppress ghrelin levels in obese humans. *The Journal of Clinical Endocrinology and Metabolism, 87*(6), 2984. https://doi.org/10.1210/jcem.87.6.8738

Greenwood, J. L., & Stanford, J. B. (2008). Preventing or improving obesity by addressing specific eating patterns. *Journal of the American Board of Family Medicine, 21*(2), 135–140. https://doi.org/10.3122/jabfm.2008.02.070034

Henderson, K., Lewis, Sloan, C. E., Bessesen, D. H., & Arterburn, D. (2024). Effectiveness and safety of drugs for obesity. *British Medical Journal, 384*, e072686. https://doi.org/10.1136/bmj-2022-072686

Hetherington, A. W., & Ranson, S. W. (1940). Hypothalamic lesions and adiposity in the rat. *The Anatomical. Record, 78*, 149–172. https://doi.org/10.1002/ar.1090780203

Hill, J. O., & Peters, J. C. (1998). Environmental contributions to the obesity epidemic. *Science, 280*(5368), 1371–1374. https://doi.org/10.1126/science.280.5368.1371

Hirsch, J., Fried, S. K., Edens, N. K., & Leibel, R. L. (1989). The fat cell. *The Medical Clinics of North America, 73*(1), 83–96. https://doi.org/10.1016/s0025-7125(16)30693-9

Holmberg, D., & Lagergren, J. (2022). What do we know about long-term effects of bariatric surgery? *The British Journal of Surgery, 110*(1), 1–2. https://doi.org/10.1093/bjs/znac327

Holt, R. R., Schmitz, H. H., Mhawish, R., Komarnytsky, S., Nguyen, T., Caveney, P. M., & Munafo, J. P. (2025). Comfort foods in the twenty-first century: Friend or foe? *Annual Review of Food Science and Technology, 16*(1), 433–458. https://doi.org/10.1146/annurev-food-111523-122109

International Diabetes Federation. (2021). *IDF diabetes atlas* (10th edn). Retrieved March 7, 2025, from https://www.diabetesatlas.org

Johnson, W., Onuma, O., Owolabi, M., & Sachdev, S. (2016). Stroke: A global response is needed. *Bulletin of the World Health Organization, 94*(9), 634–634A. https://doi.org/10.2471/BLT.16.181636

Jung, C. H., Lee, W. J., & Song, K. H. (2017). Metabolically healthy obesity: A friend or foe? *The Korean Journal of Internal Medicine, 32*(4), 611–621. https://doi.org/10.3904/kjim.2016.259

Kalarchian, M. A., Marcus, M. D., Courcoulas, A. P., Cheng, Y., Levine, M. D., & Josbeno, D. (2012). Optimizing long-term weight control after bariatric surgery: A pilot study. *Surgery for Obesity and Related Diseases, 8*(6), 710–715. https://doi.org/10.1016/j.soard.2011.04.231

Kennedy, G. C. (1953). The role of depot fat in the hypothalamic control of food intake in the rat. *Proceedings of the Royal Society of London. Series B, Biological Sciences, 140*(901), 578–596. https://doi.org/10.1098/rspb.1953.0009

Kopelman, P. G., & Finer, N. (2001). Reply: Is obesity a disease? *International Journal of Obesity and Related Metabolic, 25*(10), 1405–1406. https://doi.org/10.1038/sj.ijo.0801791

Lee, J. J., Pedley, A., Hoffmann, U., Massaro, J. M., Levy, D., & Long, M. T. (2018). Visceral and intrahepatic fat are associated with cardiometabolic risk factors above other ectopic fat depots: The Framingham Heart Study. *The American Journal of Medicine, 131*(6), 684–692.e12. https://doi.org/10.1016/j.amjmed.2018.02.002

Lejeune, M. P., Hukshorn, C. J., Saris, W. H., & Westerterp-Plantenga, M. S. (2003). Effect of dietary restraint during and following pegylated recombinant leptin (PEG-OB) treatment of overweight men. *International Journal of Obesity and Related Metabolic Disorders, 27*(12), 1494–1499. https://doi.org/10.1038/sj.ijo.0802431

Leng, J., Li, W., Zhang, S., Liu, H., Wang, L., Liu, G., Li, N., Redman, L. M., Baccarelli, A. A., Hou, L., & Hu, G. (2015). GDM women's pre-pregnancy overweight/obesity and gestational weight gain on offspring overweight status. *PLoS One, 10*(6), e0129536. https://doi.org/10.1371/journal.pone.0129536

Levitsky, D. A., Barre, L., Michael, J. J., Zhong, Y., He, Y., Mizia, A., & Kaila, S. (2022). The rise and fall of physiological theories of the control of human eating behavior. *Frontiers in Nutrition, 9*, 826334. https://doi.org/10.3389/fnut.2022.826334

Masood, B., & Moorthy, M. (2023). Causes of obesity: A review. *Clinical Medicine, 23*(4), 284–291. https://doi.org/10.7861/clinmed.2023-0168

Mayer, J. (1953). Glucostatic mechanism of regulation of food intake. *The New England Journal of Medicine, 249*(1), 13–16. https://doi.org/10.1056/NEJM195307022490104

Mechanic, O. J., Gavin, M., & Grossman, S. A. (2023). Acute myocardial infarction. In *StatPearls*. StatPearls Publishing. https://www.ncbi.nlm.nih.gov/books/NBK459269/

National Health Service (2023a). *Blood pressure test*. Retrieved March 14, 2025, from https://www.nhs.uk/conditions/blood-pressure-test/

National Health Service (2023b). *Calculate your body mass index (BMI)*. Retrieved September 17, 2025, from https://www.nhs.uk/health-assessment-tools/calculate-your-body-mass-index/calculate-bmi-for-adults

National Institute for Health and Care Excellence (2025). *Overweight and obesity management* (NICE guideline NG246). Retrieved June 24, 2005, from https://www.nice.org.uk/guidance/ng246/resources/overweight-and-obesity-management-pdf-66143959958725

Obradovic, M., Sudar-Milovanovic, E., Soskic, S., Essack, M., Arya, S., Stewart, A. J., Gojobori, T., & Isenovic, E. R. (2021). Leptin and obesity: Role and clinical implication. *Frontiers in Endocrinology, 12*, 585887. https://doi.org/10.3389/fendo.2021.585887

O'Brien, P. E., Hindle, A., Brennan, L., Skinner, S., Burton, P., Smith, A., Crosthwaite, G., & Brown, W. (2019). Long-term outcomes after bariatric surgery: A systematic review and meta-analysis of weight loss at 10 or more years for all bariatric procedures and a single-centre review of 20-year outcomes after adjustable gastric banding. *Obesity Surgery, 29*(1), 3–14. https://doi.org/10.1007/s11695-018-3525-0

Oshman, L., Othman, A., Furst, W., Heisler, M., Kraftson, A., Zouani, Y., Hershey, C., Cho, T. C., Guetterman, T., Piatt, G., & Griauzde, D. H. (2023). Primary care providers' perceived barriers to obesity treatment and opportunities for improvement: A mixed methods study. *PloS One, 18*(4), e0284474. https://doi.org/10.1371/journal.pone.0284474

Owen, C. G., Kapetanakis, V. V., Rudnicka, A. R., Wathern, A. K., Lennon, L., Papacosta, O., Cook, D. G., Wannamethee, S. G., & Whincup, P. H. (2015). Body mass index in early and middle adult life: Prospective associations with myocardial infarction, stroke and diabetes over a 30-year period: The British regional heart study. *BMJ Open, 5*(9), e008105. https://doi.org/10.1136/bmjopen-2015-008105

Parkin, D. M., Boyd, L., & Walker, L. C. (2011). The fraction of cancer attributable to lifestyle and environmental factors in the UK in 2010. *British Journal of Cancer, 105*(2), S77–S81. https://doi.org/10.1038/bjc.2011.489

Pati, S., Irfan, W., Jameel, A., Ahmed, S., & Shahid, R. K. (2023). Obesity and cancer: A current overview of epidemiology, pathogenesis, outcomes, and management. *Cancers, 15*(2), 485. https://doi.org/10.3390/cancers15020485

Prentice, A. M., Black, A. E., Murgatroyd, P. R., Goldberg, G. R., & Coward, W. A. (1989). Metabolism or appetite: Questions of energy balance with particular reference to obesity. *Journal of Human Nutrition and Dietetics, 2*, 95–104. https://doi.org/10.1111/j.1365-277X.1989.tb00014.x

Schwenke, M., Luppa, M., Pabst, A., Welzel, F. D., Löbner, M., Luck-Sikorski, C., Kersting, A., Blüher, M., & Riedel-Heller, S. G. (2020). Attitudes and treatment practice of general practitioners towards patients with obesity in primary care. *BMC Family Practice, 21*(1), 169. https://doi.org/10.1186/s12875-020-01239-1

Smith, G. P., & Epstein, A. N. (1969). Increased feeding in response to decreased glucose utilization in the rat and monkey. *The American Journal of Physiology, 217*(4), 1083–1087. https://doi.org/10.1152/ajplegacy.1969.217.4.1083

Sorokowska, A., Schoen, K., Hummel, C., Han, P., Warr, J., & Hummel, T. (2017). Food-related odors activate dopaminergic brain areas. *Frontiers in Human Neuroscience, 11*, 625. https://doi.org/10.3389/fnhum.2017.00625

Spalding, K. L., Arner, E., Westermark, P. O., Bernard, S., Buchholz, B. A., Bergmann, O., Blomqvist, L., Hoffstedt, J., Näslund, E., Britton, T., Concha, H., Hassan, M., Rydén, M., Frisén, J., & Arner, P. (2008). Dynamics of fat cell turnover in humans. *Nature, 453*(7196), 783–787. https://doi.org/10.1038/nature06902

Spielman, R. M., Jenkins, W. J., Lovett, M. D., Aruguete, M., Bryant, L., Chappell, B., Dumper, K., Lacombe, A., Lazzara, J., McClain, T., Oswald, B. B., Perimutter, M., & Thomas, M. D. (2020). *Psychology* (2nd ed.). OpenStax. https://openstax.org/details/books/psychology-2e

Stunkard, A. J., Harris, J. R., Pedersen, N. L., & McClearn, G. E. (1990). The body-mass index of twins who have been reared apart. *The New England Journal of Medicine, 322*(21), 1483–1487. https://doi.org/10.1056/NEJM199005243222102

Velapati, S. R., Shah, M., Kuchkuntla, A. R., Abu-Dayyeh, B., Grothe, K., Hurt, R. T., & Mundi, M. S. (2018). Weight regain after bariatric surgery: Prevalence, etiology, and treatment. *Current Nutrition Reports, 7*(4), 329–334. https://doi.org/10.1007/s13668-018-0243-0

Wass, J., & Finer, N. (2013). Action on obesity: Comprehensive care for all. *Clinical Medicine, 13*(1), 4–5. https://doi.org/10.7861/clinmedicine.13-1-4

World Health Organization (2025a). Cancer. Retrieved March 14, 2025, from https://www.who.int/news-room/fact-sheets/detail/cancer

World Health Organization (2025b). *Obesity and overweight*. Retrieved June 6, 2025, from https://www.who.int/news-room/fact-sheets/detail/obesity-and-overweight

World Health Organization (2000). *Obesity: Preventing and managing the global epidemic: Report of a WHO consultation* (WHO Technical Report Series No. 894). Retrieved June 24, 2005, from https://iris.who.int/handle/10665/42330

World Health Organization (2011). *Waist circumference and waist–hip ratio: Report of a WHO expert consultation, Geneva, 8–11 December 2008*. World Health Organization. https://apps.who.int/iris/handle/10665/44583

World Heart Report (2023). *Confronting the world's number one killer*. World Heart Federation. Retrieved March 14, 2025, from https://world-heart-federation.org/wp-content/uploads/World-Heart-Report-2023.pdf

Zhang, Y., Proenca, R., Maffei, M., Barone, M., Leopold, L., & Friedman, J. M. (1994). Positional cloning of the mouse obese gene and its human homologue. *Nature, 372*(6505), 425–432. https://doi.org/10.1038/372425a0

5 Conceptions of health, disease and illness

What is health?

Chapter contents

- What is health.
- Disease versus illness.
- Attributions, health and illness.
- Infectious versus chronic disease.
- How social determinants of health affect different groups.
- Cultural perspectives on health and illness.
- Traditional healthcare practices and the need for cultural humility.
- Measuring health and disease.

Chapter objectives

After reading this chapter, you should be able to answer the following questions

- Explain how different groups define health and distinguish between the concepts of disease and illness.
- Describe the role of attributions in how people understand and respond to illness.
- Identify and discuss key social determinants of health.
- Explain the difference between Western and Indigenous illness representations.
- Describe how health psychologists may measure health, including population-level indicators and individual assessments.

In Chapter 2, we learned that health is more important than the absence of disease or symptoms. It includes psychosocial factors (Engel, 1977), along with multiple interpersonal, organisational, community and policy factors (McLeroy et al., 1988). How people define health is influenced by personal, family, social experiences culture and current disease status.

BOX 5.1
CRITICAL THINKING

What does health mean to you?

Spend a few minutes writing down your thoughts, ask a friend or a family member to do the same. Try this with someone who is older or younger than you. Are there any similarities or differences in what you have written?

DOI: 10.4324/9781003423157-5

What is health?

A survey of around 9,000 individuals in England, Wales and Scotland found that people struggled to define health. They referred to health as not having symptoms, pain or illness and being able to recovery quickly from any illness (Blaxter, 1990). People conceptualise heath as having enough energy to carry out daily tasks, experiencing good relationships, feeling relaxed, happy and perceiving certain lifestyle behaviours as healthy, such as vegetarianism, the avoidance of smoking and alcohol and being able to engage in regular physical activity. These findings were echoed in a study with young adults who defined health in terms of having energy, feeling happy, sleeping well, eating a good diet, living into old age and enjoying the absence of disease (Lau, 1995). From these two studies, it is apparent that from an individual point of view, health is multidimensional and often includes activities that prevent disease, permit people to do the things they want to do and is associated with having a good quality of life. An individual may still consider themselves to be quite healthy, even though they have a heart problem, diabetes or cancer. This shows that there is no straightforward dichotomy between health and disease. People who have chronic diseases may have 'good' days when they are symptom free and 'bad' days when symptoms interfere with activities. Thus, health and disease are best viewed on a continuum (Antonovsky, 1987); both are dynamic, in that they can change over time, they are subjective and can be affected by past experience, age, social and cultural experiences. Taking these factors into account, Bircher (2005, p. 335) defined health as "a dynamic state of wellbeing characterised by a physical, mental and social potential, which satisfies the demands of a life commensurate with age, culture, and personal responsibility".

Disease versus illness

You will have noticed that this chapter's title included the terms disease and illness, and maybe wondered if there is any difference between the two. While the terms disease and illness are often used interchangeably to describe some interruption in a person's normal health status (Lach, 2013), they do have different conceptions. **Disease** is biomedical in origin. It is the term used by healthcare professionals to describe a medical condition that has a name and series of objective signs (measurable indications that can be determined by someone other than the patient) that are indicative of some deviation from normal functioning. Signs include things like an elevated temperature, high blood pressure, very fast pulse rate or blood test values that are outside the normal range. Diseases have universality, in that they are characterised by specific biomedical outcomes; they may have a specific natural history (how they develop) and are associated with patient-reported symptoms (Helman, 1981).

Illness is a much broader concept than disease. It involves social construction, as it includes the patient's perception of a disease. This includes physical, emotional and psychological factors. Illness is more about the individual's experience and less about the specific medical diagnosis, that is not to say giving a name to symptoms is unimportant. When a person feels unwell and goes to the doctor, they will talk about their symptoms and convey information about the impact that symptoms are having on their daily lives. They will report how they feel, how intense a pain or symptom is, where the problem is located, along with how it has impacted their sleep, emotions and/or ability to engage in everyday activities. The patient may have some insight into what their symptoms mean; they may have researched them on the internet and/or sought advice from family and friends and have expectations of what the doctor should do. A doctor is trained to initially think about disease from a biomedical perspective by listening to the patient's symptoms, look for objective signs that could indicate specific diseases and compare these with their knowledge from training and professional experience. This culminates in a diagnosis or the need for more detailed biomedical information about the patient via tests and/or investigations. The process a doctor engages in to arrive at a diagnosis is called clinical reasoning. Hence, a doctor's perception of disease is quite different to that of a patient. Take, for example, a 60-year-old individual who has had a heart attack caused by an almost total blockage in one or more of their coronary arteries. Due to the restricted blood supply to the heart muscle, the patient is experiencing episodes of chest pain and is at risk of having a more serious heart attack. The patient requires surgery to bypass the blockage, but they are on a waiting list and their activities are severely restricted due to episodic chest pain. After surgery, when the patient has recovered, they believe that having no heart-related symptoms means their heart disease is cured. From a biomedical perspective, the doctor knows that tests have shown that the heart attack caused damage to the heart muscle, the patient still has coronary artery disease (CAD) and they are still at risk of further blockages within the coronary blood vessels and the peripheral arteries of the lower limbs. While the patient and doctor agree that surgery was a success, the patient seems unaware that the surgery was just a palliative measure to relieve symptoms and improve quality of life, it was not a cure for the underlying arterial disease (see Chapter 9). The patient thinks that their 'new' arteries will last them another 60 years and is surprised to be told that to prevent another heart attack, they need to engage in a cardiac rehabilitation programme. This will help them to gradually increase their physical activity within safe limits, adopt healthy eating habits, adhere to prescribed heart medication, stop smoking and reduce their stress levels.

There are differences in how people with the same symptoms arrive at different interpretations of illness, which is due to variations in symptom appraisal and coping. Two patients who have experienced a heart attack will have the same type of biological marker (although the exact values will differ) in their blood. They may undergo the same diagnostic scans, receive similar medication to reduce blood pressure and cholesterol, but each patient's subjective experiences of dealing with a heart attack and subsequent coping will differ. Past experience, knowledge about health, the patient's family, cultural background, occupation, ethnicity and socioeconomic status can influence health beliefs (perceptions, attitudes and values about health) and have implications for health-related behaviours. One patient may view their heart attack as a chance to revise their priorities in life. They may appreciate life more than before the heart attack, work at maintaining better relationships with family (Lee et al., 2022) and friends, set new goals, take responsibility for their health by revising their diet and increasing physical activity. Often family members have a key role in helping the patient's recovery from a heart attack through the provision of support and encouragement for them to become more physically active (Birtwistle et al., 2021). In contrast to this, another patient may appraise a heart attack as a threat to ongoing health, fear another heart attack is imminent, become depressed and think that life as they know it, is over. Overprotective family members can reinforce these behaviours by discouraging physical activity due to fears of causing the patient to suffer another heart attack; this can increase the patient's feelings of helplessness and contribute to cardiac invalidism (Furze et al., 2002; Gonzales & Henning-Smith, 2017). Beliefs about disease have implications for rehabilitation and recovery; they may also influence symptom interpretation and may encourage or dissuade help-seeking behaviours, which can have implications for diagnosis and recovery.

Attributions, health and illness

When making **attributions** (causes) about becoming sick, the starting point is often 'what have I done to cause this?' The individual may search for explanations relating to their own behaviours and habits, such as smoking, drinking too much alcohol, getting upset and stressed over trivial things that happen in everyday life. Alternatively, external factors may also be considered as the cause of illness, such as the cold weather being responsible for aching joints. An individual's job may be considered as the cause of illness, for example, being asked to do too much work in a given time or being bored at work and/or antagonistic relationships between work colleagues, all of which may contribute to stress-related physical health problems (see Chapter 8). Depending on culture and beliefs, disease may also be attributed to God, predestination, desecration of sacred lands and disturbance of the spirit world (Helman, 2014).

The actions that people engage in when they are sick or try to remain healthy are influenced by attributions of the causes of illness and health and we all hold certain biases. In the self-serving bias, we tend to take credit for our successes, for example, 'I was able to lose weight because I have great will power', but when unsuccessful, there is a tendency to attribute the cause to external factors, such as 'I was unable to lose weight because I have been really busy at work, had to take work home and had no time to prepare healthy meals'. Sometimes other people make incorrect or biased attributions; for example, a healthcare professional may make a fundamental attribution error by thinking, 'that patient is overweight because they are lazy, they eat too much and do not care about looking after their health'. This ignores situational factors such as the patient's medical condition having caused weight gain or the patient being unable to exercise because of pain or disability or that prescribed medication may have caused dramatic weight gain, or for financial or social reasons the patient may not be able to make healthy food choices. The core aspect of the fundamental attribution error in this example is that the healthcare professional has attributed being overweight to some aspect of the patient's character, ignoring the potential impact of situational factors. This can have detrimental consequences in healthcare settings, especially when health professionals make biased attributions due to culture, ethnicity, sexual or gender stereotypes.

The prevalence of lung cancer is higher for Indigenous Peoples within Australia, Canada, New Zealand and the US compared to that for the non-Indigenous populations and survival from lung cancer is lower for Indigenous patients. Many lay people believe that the only cause of lung cancer is smoking, which is a view shared by many health professionals (Cataldo et al., 2012). This can lead to a fundamental attribution bias that lung cancer is a self-inflicted disease; therefore, it is the individual's own fault they developed cancer and they are not deserving of treatment. While smoking is the main cause of lung cancer, passive smoking, air pollution, exposure to asbestos fibres, radon gas and occupational exposure to chemicals also have a role to play in causing lung cancer (NHS, 2022). Indigenous Peoples often experience additional attribution biases, such as not valuing health and healthcare services, ignoring symptoms and delay seeking medical help (Carter-Harris, 2015). This attribution bias may culminate in a late diagnosis of cancer, which may result in poor outcomes (Moore et al., 2014). Such biased views ignore situational barriers for cancer care that are commonly experienced by Indigenous populations. These barriers include reduced treatment rates, suboptimal care that does not align with cancer care guidelines, mistrust of Western healthcare, language and geographical difficulties, cultural beliefs about healing and the importance of traditional Indigenous treatments (Australian Institute of Health and Welfare & National Indigenous Australians Agency, 2024; Huot et al., 2019; Nguyen et al., 2020). It is also evident that broader structural factors can impact on health, these include systemic discrimination targeted at minority groups, resource allocation that impacts the provision of health education and healthcare, lack of adequate housing, clean drinking water and sanitation. Disparities in health and disease around the world consistently show that those living in impoverished conditions have poorer health. The types of diseases that impact an individual's quality of life and those that cause premature death vary according to whether they live in a high- or low-income country.

Infectious versus chronic disease

Statistics from the Word Health Organization ([WHO], 2024) showed that chronic diseases, such as cardiovascular disease (CVD), most cancers, chronic respiratory and kidney diseases, were the most common causes of premature deaths in high-income countries in 2021. Conversely, communicable diseases were the major causes of premature deaths in low-income countries, for example, lower respiratory infections, malaria, diarrhoeal diseases, tuberculosis and HIV/AIDS (human immunodeficiency virus/acquired immunodeficiency syndrome) (WHO, 2024). Such differences can be explained by a lack of access to clean drinking water, poor sanitation, limited access to nutritious food, poverty, lack of healthcare infrastructure and limited access to healthcare within low-income countries. In high-income countries, lifestyle behaviours, such as poor diet, being sedentary, alcohol use and smoking, are major contributors to the development of chronic disease. In addition, there is more health messaging about chronic disease prevention and management in high-income countries, with greater access to disease screening, medical facilities and treatments, hence these diseases are managed as long-term conditions. In contrast, low-income countries have double the burden, with high rates of communicable diseases and a rapid increase in chronic diseases. There is limited disease screening in low-income countries to facilitate early diagnosis and limited access to medical care, meaning that people only seek care when symptoms are severe, resulting in poorer survival rates and premature deaths. That said, even within high-income countries, some people have worse health outcomes than others, with **social determinants of health** (SDOH) making substantial contributions to health inequities (Butler-Jones & Wong, 2016).

BOX 5.2
CRITICAL THINKING

We have all experienced illness at some time in our lives and we usually engage in a range of behaviours to try to determine what our symptoms mean. Think about a recent illness you have experienced, what do you perceive to be the cause of the illness? Did you discuss your disease symptoms with family and/or friends or avoid telling anyone about these symptoms because you believed that it was something that you did that may have caused the symptoms?

How social determinants of health affect different groups

Social determinants of health (SDOH) include income, social support, neighbourhood conditions, education, employment, isolation, loneliness and belonging to marginalised groups (ethnic, sexual or gender minorities disabled and/or from Indigenous populations). It is important to note that each SDOH does not impact health outcomes in isolation. Having a low income does not necessarily mean that an individual will have worse health outcomes, but the intersection of having a low income, a low level of educational attainment and living in a **deprived neighbourhood** has been associated with having two or more chronic diseases (Valenzuela et al., 2024; WHO 2025a). Such disparities are worse for marginalised groups who face discrimination, which includes Indigenous Peoples, irrespective of where they live in the world.

Women

Women are disproportionately affected by poverty and discrimination (Springer et al., 2012). Globally, they can experience lifelong inequalities, as only 14 countries around the world have bestowed full legal equality between men and women (World Bank, 2023). Unpaid household and care work is usually undertaken by women, which can have negative impacts on health, leading to emotional exhaustion (Gérain & Zech, 2021) and social isolation (Hajek et al., 2021). Even though women usually live longer than men, they often experience poorer health for around a quarter of their lives and report multiple health issues (World Economic Forum, 2024). Women with disabilities are more likely to smoke, experience additional chronic health conditions and have overall poorer health than their non-disabled counterparts (Mitra et al., 2016). In addition, they are less likely to undergo breast and cervical cancer screening compared to those without a disability (Mitra et al., 2022).

LGBTQI+ individuals

Experience of discrimination and microaggressions from healthcare professionals has been reported by LGBTQI+ (lesbian, gay and bisexual with the addition of queer or questioning and intersex) communities, especially among transgender adults. In fact, transgender adults may face the additional burden of being treated badly by staff who lack awareness of transgender health issues (Gonzales & Henning-Smith, 2017; Rossman et al., 2017; Valdiserri et al., 2019). Within the US, people who identify as bisexual, transgender and gender nonconfirming have a higher prevalence of disabilities compared to cisgender and heterosexual populations (Varadaraj et al., 2021). The intersections of having a disability and belonging to LGBTQI+ communities results in worse health outcomes (Streed et al., 2021) and more unmet care needs compared to non-LGBTQI+ peers (Mulcahy et al., 2022). Due to the fear of discrimination, judgement, biased assumptions about heterosexuality and being misunderstood, LGBTQI+ people with disabilities often conceal their gender and/or sexual identity in healthcare settings. Mulcahy et al. (2023) found that patients with disabilities who self-identified as being from LGBTQI+ groups often experienced negative or unsupportive encounters with healthcare professionals.

In recognising the need to better care for LGBTQI+ patients, within the UK, the National Health Service (NHS) has implemented staff training to understand LGBTQI+ needs and improve care (Government Equalities Office, 2018). However, the same can no longer be said about the US, since January 20, 2025, President Trump's executive orders have considerably reduced policies that support the healthcare of LGBTQI+ people. Research projects have been halted or defunded and non-discriminatory protections based on sexual orientation and gender identity have ended. In addition, LGBTQI+ health disparity data have been removed from US government websites and overseas aid halted to LGBTQI+ populations worldwide, thus increasing the vulnerability of already at-risk groups (Cahill, 2025).

People with disabilities

Within the UK, the Equality Act (Parliament of the United Kingdom, 2010) refers to a disability as being mental and/or physical, which has negative impacts on an individual's daily activities and is long - lasting. People with disabilities face barriers in relation to accessing suitable housing, work, appropriate education and healthcare. The mortality rate for people who have disabilities in low- to middle-income countries and in the US is twice that of the general population (Smythe & Kuper, 2024) and individuals with Down syndrome die, on average, 28 years earlier than the general population. Higher mortality rates for people with disabilities in the US were not attributable to the primary disability itself, rather people with disabilities tended to have a higher prevalence of comorbidities (diabetes, obesity and cardiovascular disease) and were more likely to face financial barriers to accessing healthcare. Additionally, people with disabilities are more likely to be sedentary, which is a risk factor for several chronic diseases. Within the UK, Heslop et al. (2014) showed that people with **learning disabilities** (see Box 5.1) are at a greater risk of unavoidable death (37%) compared to the general population (13%). Contributory factors included inadequate care to meet specific needs, not permitting patients to make their own healthcare decisions, challenges in making **advanced care plans** (see Chapter 11) and caregivers feeling unheard. The most recent UK statistics for 2023 showed that on average, 39% of deaths of people who had a learning disability or diagnosis of autism were unavoidable (White et al., 2024).

BOX 5.1
LEARNING DISABILITIES

The Department of Health and Social Care (2001, p. 14) in the UK defines a learning disability as "a significantly reduced ability to understand new or complex information, to learn new skills (impaired intelligence), with a reduced ability to cope independently (impaired social function), which started before adulthood, with a lasting effect on development". It should be noted that while the term learning disability is used in the UK, within other countries, intellectual disability may be the preferred term.

Accessing healthcare can be challenging for people with physical disabilities due to mobility problems, lack of physical access to buildings due to infrastructure issues and sometimes the need for someone to accompany them to appointments. There are also increased daily living costs associated with a disability and transport costs can be a barrier to attending appointments. In addition, inappropriate or inadequate interactions and care from healthcare professionals are common (Hall et al., 2019; Lagu et al., 2022; Meade et al., 2015), which can result in reduced patient satisfaction with care. Having a disability is associated with greater discrimination compared to patients without a disability (Emerson et al., 2021), less access to disease preventative healthcare, a higher likelihood of being unemployed, having a lower income and inadequate access to transport (Krahn et al., 2015).

Sakellariou and Rotarou (2017) analysed secondary data from the European Health Interview Survey for people living with and without a disability in the UK. They found that people living with disabilities had to wait twice as long for medical appointments/treatments and were also 3.6 to 5.4 times more likely to face unmet health needs due to cost-related barriers for prescribed medication (the latter only applied to England, as this was the only region of the UK that had prescription charges) compared to those without disabilities. Transport issues were 4.3 times more likely for patients with severe disabilities and twice as likely for those with mild disabilities compared to the general patient population. The intersection of disability and gender showed that women faced structural barriers to accessing healthcare in relation to waiting times, costs of prescribed medication and transport. In general, people with physical disabilities had more unmet healthcare needs (dental, medical, medication) than those without disabilities (Mitra et al., 2022). This is not unique to the UK, across the globe, people with disabilities face a range of intersectional challenges that have negative impacts on their health, highlighting the need for inclusive healthcare services that are responsive to the needs of this population (Umucu et al., 2025).

People from ethnic minorities

An individual's trust in healthcare services can be undermined by discrimination, which can have negative implications for health outcomes. In a survey of over 41,000 adults in the US, just under 37% reported that they had experienced discrimination in healthcare settings (Wang et al., 2024). Discrimination was more likely to be experienced by women, non-Hispanic Black groups, non-native

English speakers, people who rented rather than owned their homes and people who had multiple chronic conditions and/or disabilities. Discrimination can discourage individuals from seeking healthcare advice and treatment, which results in opportunities for early intervention and healthcare screening being missed, contributing to further health disparities (Nguyen et al., 2018). In a large-scale survey (n = 92,321), Sabater Minarim et al. (2025) found that even though African American patients only made up 7% of the sample, almost half of them said that they had experienced healthcare discrimination, compared to 35% of White people. In addition, patients with lower levels of education were more likely to experience discrimination than those with higher education.

People from minority ethnic groups are not only at higher risk of developing chronic health conditions, but they also tend to develop them at a younger age than their White counterparts (Verest et al., 2019). Furthermore, ethnicity intersects with gender, disability, socioeconomic and geographical factors to increase the likelihood of adverse health outcomes (Taskforce on Multiple Conditions, 2021). The intersection of having a low income, belonging to an ethnic minority group, living in an area of high deprivation and having a disability is associated with residing in **food deserts**. Meaning that access to affordable and healthy food is limited, while unhealthy processed foods are more readily available. This is of particular concern, as processed foods can contribute to poorer health outcomes, such as increased rates of obesity, cardiovascular disease and diabetes (Andretti et al., 2023; Bridle-Fitzpatrick, 2015).

In the UK, people from ethnic minority backgrounds have poorer general health and higher rates of chronic illnesses compared to the White population. It is generally accepted that lifelong socioeconomic factors account for these health disparities, which are cumulative, meaning they become more pronounced in later life, especially for Bangladeshi, Indian and Pakistani populations (Evandrou et al., 2016). In 2018, Kingston et al. estimated that the number of people over the age of 65 with multiple chronic diseases will double by 2035 and addressing health inequities for ethnic minority groups will become even more urgent.

Indigenous Peoples

In addition to having higher rates of chronic illness and disability, life expectancy for individuals from Indigenous populations can be up to 20 years lower than non-Indigenous People (WHO, 2025b). So far in this chapter, our conceptualisation of health, disease and illness has been interpreted through a Western lens, which has considered the impacts of psychosocial factors and typical SDOH, such as education, income, access to healthcare, etc. The SDOH within Indigenous contexts go far beyond these typical factors to include historical injustices associated with colonisation that have led to discrimination, cultural disruption due to displacement from and dispossession of lands, removal of children to residential schools, the subjugation of Indigenous knowledge, language, the negation of traditional medicines and healing practices. This has culminated in distrust in Western medical care and poorer health outcomes to the extent that the WHO (2025a, p. 83) recognised that "Indigeneity is a social determinant of health".

Land has a special meaning to Indigenous People, and it is conceptualised as a living entity that offers sustenance and spiritual connections with ancestors. Government policies have resulted in Indigenous People being subjected to specific laws that affect their rights, tribal sovereignty and access to services. These factors have negative influences on self-determination, such as being able to have control over their own health services, education and governance, all of which are underfunded. Marginalisation of Indigenous populations has resulted in disparities across a range of areas including education, employment, housing and income, all of which have negative consequences for health.

There are ethnic differences in the prevalence of disability within the US, with the highest age-adjusted rates (see Box 5.2) reported for American Indian and Native Alaskans (30%), followed by Black African Americans (25%), Whites (20%) and Asian populations (10%) having the lowest rates (Centers for Disease Control, 2025). Indigenous People tend to make lower use of disability services compared to their non-Indigenous counterparts, which may be symptomatic of intersectional discrimination (Avery, 2018). Being from an Indigenous community and having a disability have resulted in heightened minority stress, with Temple et al. (2020) reporting that 42% Aboriginal and Torres Strait Islanders with disabilities experienced interpersonal racism compared to 32% without disabilities. These researchers also highlighted that those with mental health or learning disabilities faced a higher risk of racism. Lower-use of disability services may also be compounded by a lack of culturally appropriate services (Canuto et al., 2018; Jacklin et al., 2017). Many Indigenous cultures do not have a word or concept within their languages to describe disabilities. This may reflect the view that rather than disability being something that differentiates one section of a community from another, Indigenous People tend to view disability as normal diversity (Puszka et al., 2022). Disability services do not embrace Indigenous cultural values, which can lead to further marginalisation and discrimination acting as a barrier to formal support services.

BOX 5.2
ACTUAL AND AGE-ADJUSTED RATES OF DISABILITY

Actual rates of disability give a measure of the total number of people in a given population who have a disability. This is a good measure of the overall burden of disability and can be useful in estimating the need for services. However, when comparing two population groups (e.g. group A and group B), age-adjusted rates can be even more meaningful. If population A has an older age profile, we would expect to see greater disability compared to population B, because disability increases with age. Age-adjusted rates of disability permit a comparison of trends in disability at various time points and permit a comparison of health outcomes between different groups, according to specific criteria, such as gender, ethnicity and sexual orientation.

Cultural perspectives on health and illness

Western illness representations

Leventhal (1970) proposed that when faced with a threat to health, people engage in a problem-solving approach that considers five aspects of an illness (see Figure 5.1). The initial representation is identity, which is concerned with

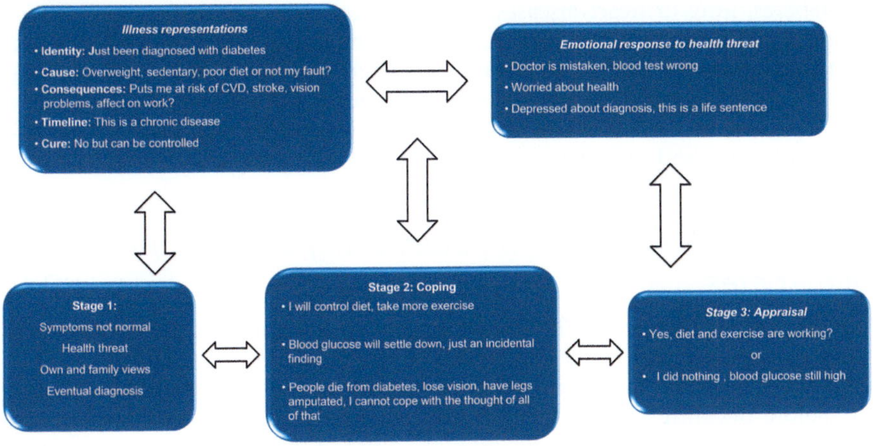

Figure 5.1
Self-Regulatory Model (SRM) of illness

Source: Based on Leventhal (1970) and Leventhal et al. (1980)

getting a name for symptoms, such as a lump could be cancer, a sore throat and runny nose could be the common cold, and chest pain could be heart disease. Only when the symptoms have a name can the cause of an illness be considered. It may be attributed to genetics, a virus, lifestyle or environmental factors. When searching for a cause, individuals may question whether it is something they have done, something they have eaten or perhaps something they have not done that has caused the illness or symptoms. Attribution of cause is important, as it may help or hinder the individual from seeking medical help. For example, the cause of a chronic cough (lasting more than three months) accompanied by feeling breathless may be attributed to personal or external factors. A smoker may view the cause as due to cigarette smoking and avoid seeking medical help because they feel that they will be blamed for their symptoms. A non-smoker may be more likely to seek medical help, as they attribute their symptoms to external factors over which they have no control, such as viruses, bacteria or disease. Having a name for symptoms enables the individual to explore potential consequences of the disease to assess the impact it will have on physical abilities, emotional well-being, social activities, and if it has financial consequences due to an inability to work and the costs of care. The consequences of any disease can affect quality of life, but more so for chronic diseases, as they tend to be associated with disability and increased need for healthcare (Watson et al., 2025). The timeline of an illness is concerned with how long it will last, for example, the common cold is considered as an acute self-limiting disease that may only require self-medication. A longer-lasting acute disease, such as pneumonia (lung inflection), will require time off work and antibiotic therapy, whereas, a chronic condition, such as cardiovascular disease, will be lifelong, requiring lifestyle changes, medication and medical checkups. Other conditions, such as allergies, can be cyclical in nature, for example, hay fever, which is caused by seasonally high pollen counts. The final aspect of illness representations is concerned with whether the illness can be cured or controlled and by whom. Most acute illnesses (e.g. common cold, flu, stomach upsets) can be cured by self-management, but chronic conditions, such as diabetes, lung or heart diseases, cannot be controlled without some lifestyle changes on the part of the patient, ongoing medical monitoring and intervention (e.g. taking prescribed medication, engaging in or refraining from certain activities) from healthcare professionals. Emotional responses to disease, such as fear, denial, anxiety, anger and depression, may develop in tandem with illness representations and may have positive or negative impacts on coping.

Self-Regulatory Model of illness using the example of diabetes

When people experience illness symptoms, they form lay (non-healthcare-trained) beliefs about what the symptoms mean. These beliefs are based on own knowledge, previous experiences and views expressed by friends and family. Before deciding to seek medical help, people usually take a commonsense problem-solving approach to try and make sense of their symptoms. In addition, symptoms may be compared to the experiences of others and explored via the internet or in books. Lay beliefs about symptoms are central to an individual's health decision-making and were conceptualised by Leventhal (1970) and Leventhal et al. (1980) in the Self-Regulatory Model (SRM) of illness (Figure 5.1). Stage 1 of the model is concerned with the recognition of symptoms not being normal for that individual. Medical help is usually sought when symptoms persist, become troublesome, interfere with everyday life or the individual and/or family become concerned about them. Leventhal et al. (1980) proposed that becoming ill was a threat to an individual and they engaged in a problem-solving approach to try and understand the nature and extent of the threat, that could guide their coping and health behaviours.

Vague feelings of fatigue, increased thirst and weight loss can be symptomatic of a range of diseases or due to everyday activities, such as not drinking enough water, working hard and not eating regular meals. However, family members may prompt an individual to go to their doctor, as they perceived these symptoms as a threat to the patient's health. Based on these symptoms and tests, an individual receives a diagnosis of type 2 diabetes (T2DM). In this condition, the body cannot process sugar (glucose) properly due to an insufficiency of insulin or the insulin may not be working effectively. Persistently high blood glucose can cause serious health problems (see Chapters 4 and 9). Having a name for symptoms helps the individual to look for a cause, such as a family history of T2DM, being overweight, being sedentary or eating foods that are high in sugar. Receiving a diagnosis of T2DM may cause anxiety about disease consequences, such as heart disease, eye problems and circulatory problems, especially in the lower limbs. In addition, the individual is concerned about the potential impact of diabetes on day-to-day life, social activities, being able to lose weight, adhere to a healthy diet and engage in more physical activity. It may not be possible to cure T2DM, but it can be controlled through lifestyle choices, medication and regular monitoring of blood glucose. This knowledge can help an individual to take control of their diabetes, but some people may struggle with lifestyle changes and feel that no matter what they do, their blood glucose will always be high.

Stage 2: Coping

Stage 2 of the SRM involves doing something about the disease through approach or avoidance coping strategies. Decisions on coping are influenced by the individual's disease representations and emotions. Approach coping in T2DM includes health-related activities, such as attending regular checkups, taking prescribed medication, engaging in physical activity, adhering to a healthy diet, monitoring blood glucose, joining a self-help group or diabetes education class and following other treatment advice. These coping strategies may help the patient reduce anxiety about managing blood glucose and help prevent longer-term side effects of T2DM. Avoidance coping may involve the denial of having diabetes, thinking that it is a minor problem that is not important or engaging in wishful thinking that test results were wrong or that it is a temporary problem that will settle down on its own. This type of coping can result in uncontrolled high blood glucose levels, nonadherence to medication and/or advice about diet and physical activity, which may in turn result in nonattendance at medical appointments, that can contribute to longer-term negative health outcomes (Adler et al., 2024).

Stage 3: Appraisal

In stage 3 of the SRM, the individual assesses whether their coping strategies have been effective in keeping blood glucose levels within prescribed limits. If coping strategies were effective, it will empower the individual to continue to take control of their health. Individuals, who engage in avoidance coping strategies, may try to ignore symptoms associated with high blood glucose, but their symptom burden may increase, which may put them at higher risk of depression and anxiety, which can lead to feelings of hopelessness. This is quite a fluid model, as symptoms can change for the better or worse, likewise for consequences, controllability, cure and timelines. Depending on the seriousness of the disease, this can have beneficial or potentially detrimental implications for recovery (Hagger et al., 2017).

Some individuals tend to ignore symptoms, they try to carry on with their everyday activities as normal and refuse to seek medical advice. Others tend to be hypervigilant about their health and exhibit health-related anxiety (see Box 5.3). The SRM is just one explanation of how people think about, interpret symptoms and how that can affect health-related behaviours. We will explore theories and models of health behaviour in a more detailed manner in Chapter 7.

BOX 5.3
HIGH HEALTH ANXIETY OR MUNCHAUSEN'S SYNDROME?

Some individuals are hypervigilant to bodily symptoms, schedule frequent appointments with their doctor and undergo many medical tests, Even when tests show up no abnormality, they still continue to seek reassurance about their health and remain concerned about having a serious disease. For example, a headache and feeling a bit nauseous may be interpreted as symptoms of a brain tumour, rather than a migraine headache; chest pain due to indigestion may be interpreted as a heart attack. Individuals who have excessive worry or fear about developing serious illness, even though there are no biomedical signs to suggest this is the case may be diagnosed with high anxiety about their health, known as illness anxiety disorder (previous called hypochondriasis). In contrast, some people tend to ignore, minimise or delay seeking help for symptoms, even when they are serious. For example, chest pain may be shrugged off as being due to indigestion or a strained muscle, along with the denial that symptoms could be indicative of a heart problem. These individuals may view being ill as a weakness and avoid medical checkups and invitations to attend screening for disease at an asymptomatic stage. This can lead to a later diagnosis of disease, which in the case of some cancers can mean treatment benefits are limited and due to disease spread, there may even be no possibility of cure.

Health anxiety is different to Munchausen's syndrome (known as factitious disorder), the latter is a psychological disorder. For example, someone with Munchausen's syndrome will go to their doctor complaining of symptoms of a urinary tract infection (UTI), including pain lower down in the abdomen, a frequent need to urinate and a burning sensation when urinating. To check if the patient has a UTI, the doctor will request a urine sample. A patient with Munchausen's syndrome will prick their finger with a sharp implement to cause bleeding and add blood to their urine sample to falsify signs of an infection. The aim of this behaviour is to get attention, sympathy and to be cared for. While people with high health anxiety will make frequent appointments with their doctor and undergo some tests, someone with Munchausen's syndrome often 'shops around' several doctors and hospitals to get attention, care a multiplicity of medical tests and even unnecessary surgery.

Indigenous illness representations

Culture influences people's beliefs about health and disease. There are fundamental differences in the beliefs about health and illness advocated by Western-trained healthcare professionals compared to Indigenous patients, extended families, communities and traditional healers. The SRM views health and disease in terms of biomedical and psychological factors; it is focused on how individuals interpret and respond to illness and the role of the environment is not considered. In addition, Western healthcare is based on an individualistic approach to health, but Indigenous healthcare practices are holistic, with health and disease being a community concern. Indigenous Peoples conceive health as promoting wellness, preventing illness and use the term wellbeing instead of health. Wellbeing is multidimensional in nature, it includes physical, emotional, mental and spiritual health that is intertwined with self-determination, respect, trust and involves the whole community. In addition, the intergenerational connections with Elders who are the 'keepers' of culture, traditional knowledge, language and history are viewed as essential in helping protect the health of future generations (Salmon et al., 2018; Smythe & Kuper, 2024). Thus, Western notions of self-care and independence have limited relevance to Indigenous Peoples (Angell, 2016). The definition of health offered by the WHO (1948), being "a state of complete physical, mental and social wellbeing and not just the absence of health" is not sufficient to capture the meaning of Indigenous health. An updated view on Indigenous health was offered by the WHO (2000), which included the four interconnected dimensions of emotional, physical, spiritual and mental health, along with connection to the land and self-determination being associated with health and disease attributed to oppression. The WHO also recognised the collective and intergenerational aspects of health as being deeply rooted in traditional knowledge that has been passed down by Elders through storytelling, ceremonies, cultural values, traditional health

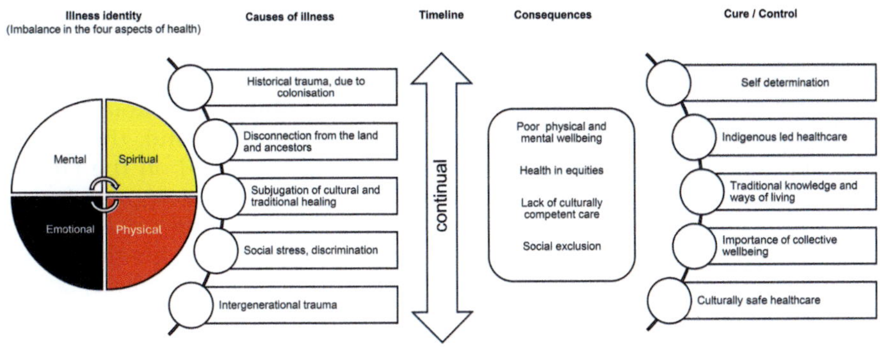

Figure 5.2
Indigenous illness representations

Source: Author

practices and ways of living. To illustrate Indigenous illness representations, they have been mapped onto the five aspects proposed by Leventhal (1970) (see Figure 5.2). It should be noted that this is the author's interpretation of illness representations, based on interrogation of the literature, as to date there are no direct framework comparisons available between Western and Indigenous illness representations. However, there are Indigenous models of health, such as the Medicine Wheel and Te Whare Tapa Whā (see Chapter 7), which are holistic and rooted in Indigenous values that have been used to inform health interventions.

Understanding and use of Indigenous models can help health professionals to enhance their cultural competence and deliver healthcare in a more holistic, culturally sensitive and responsive manner. The role of family, community and traditional healing practices are fundamental aspects of health for Indigenous People. The concepts of health and illness are often intertwined with the spirit world, an important aspect of holistic healing that can impact the wellbeing of the whole community. Spiritual factors are not confined to religious beliefs, they refer to connectedness to the natural world and with ancestors. Thus, unlike Western views, responsibility for health is not just about the individual getting better from illness, with treatment delegated to medical doctors, health involves having respect for others, animals and the land. Health also includes hunting practices that involve giving thanks to the animal and the earth for providing food, along with community connectedness (Adelson, 2005). Traditional practices are part of healthcare for many Indigenous People and involves consulting with traditional healers and community Elders. To prevent and treat illness, practices, such as spiritual rituals, prayers, massage, incantations, songs, cultural ceremonies, dietary guidelines and herbal remedies, may be used. Kinship and healing practices involve connection with ancestors who lived on the land, thus being connected to the land and caring for it is central to Aboriginal health (Morgan et al., 1997) and illness may be due to sacred customs being infringed upon, such as improper handling of human remains or disrespect for sacred places.

To some extent, there is still underrecognition of the importance of traditional Indigenous healthcare practices within mainstream healthcare provision, thus limiting culturally informed and appropriate healthcare. That said, since 2013, the First Nations Health Authority in British Colombia, Canada has worked in partnership with Indigenous representatives to reduce the burden of chronic diseases and has incorporated specific traditional Indigenous healing alongside culturally safe Western medical care. In New Zealand, the culturally based service, Whānau Ora (healthy families), is centred on the family, rather than individual health, and adopts a **strengths-based approach** (see Box 5.4) by building on what families already do well. For example, a 10-week community-based fitness programme was used to support families to become more active by training together for a triathlon. During the programme, family members learned about fitness, nutrition and goal setting, ending with a triathlon event that also celebrated culture and health. This initiative encouraged intergenerational participation, which helped strengthen family ties, increased self-esteem, community engagement and promoted healthy lifestyles. The success of this community-based intervention was sustained and it became an annual event (Reweti, 2019). Whānau Ora is a success because it promotes collaborative and holistic health and it is based on Māori cultural values that were not achievable by Western approaches that emphasised individual health behaviours.

These examples illustrate that Indigenous culture and values are being incorporated into mainstream health contexts. However, the legacy of colonisation still results in inequities that include discrimination and more recently, climate change, all of which have negative consequences on emotional, physical, spiritual and mental health (Pérez Ramos et al., 2022) of Indigenous populations around the world.

BOX 5.4

STRENGTHS- AND DEFICIENCIES-BASED APPROACHES TO HEALTH

Western medicine often takes a **deficiencies-based approach to health**, identifying and focusing on problems that need to be fixed and the negative health consequences of not taking action. A strengths-based approach focuses on what people can do to improve health, based on their current capabilities. Physical activity has been shown to help prevent disease and has beneficial effects on a range of chronic diseases (Warburton & Bredin, 2017), with a target of 150 minutes of moderate physical activity (this intensity is typically described as being out of breath, but still able to have a conversation) per week or 75 minutes of physical activity per week at vigorous intensity. A deficits-based approach proposes that to have any benefit to health, you must adhere to these recommendations. Such messaging is demoralising to people who are physically inactive, but they can be helped by taking a strengths-based approach to encourage any type, duration and intensity of any physical activity as being better than doing nothing (UK Chief Medical Officers, 2019). Strengths-based physical activity messaging may also involve building on current strengths, such as you can walk for 10 minutes, let's set a goal for 15, or asking about what the individual's goal is in terms of physical activity and trying to involve family members and/or the community (Warburton & Bredin, 2019).

BOX 5.3
CRITICAL THINKING

Western health focuses on the individual and the disease, compared to Indigenous views that emphasise the community, harmony and connection to the land. How might these different perspectives affect how people think about health and disease?

Traditional healthcare practices and the need for cultural humility

Western healthcare professionals who lack cultural awareness and sensitivity may overlook the importance of traditional and holistic health models that are so central to Indigenous People; this can lead to distress, feelings of distrust, marginalisation and underutilisation of medical care. Health services need to become more integrative by listening to the needs of Indigenous People and involving them in the design and delivery of care, with greater consideration of integrating Indigenous and Western healthcare practices. For example, when investigating the potential causes of illness, Putsch and Joyce (1990) contrasted the differing diagnostic questioning used in Western and Indigenous practices. Western healthcare professionals used extensive questioning focused on physiological symptoms and universal metrics, such as physical examinations, laboratory tests, scans, blood pressure measurement, etc. This contrasted with Indigenous healers and patients who made use of observation, visions and storytelling. Patients from Indigenous backgrounds may find the type and extent of questioning that happens during Western health consultations as confusing and uncomfortable. This is because the conceptions of health and illness are quite different. When describing symptoms, Indigenous patients may refer to feelings of disharmony with self, family, community or the land, that their spirit feels heavy and they may talk about imbalances in emotional, mental, physical and spiritual wellbeing.

Culturally sensitive care

It is essential that healthcare professionals are trained to deliver culturally sensitive care and attempt to reduce health disparities in treatment (de Freitas et al., 2023). This does not just apply to Indigenous Peoples, as Yu et al. (2023) reported the need for healthcare professionals to provide culturally safe healthcare treatments for people from LGBTQI+ communities. Without culturally sensitive care, people from minority groups may delay or avoid treatment and their symptoms may go undiagnosed or be dismissed. There is a need for training to ensure that identity is respected using correct pronouns, the acknowledgement of spiritual or cultural needs and training in intersectionality. Health professionals also need to engage in self-reflection to reduce conscious and unconscious biases.

Patients' views of health and healthcare

Healthcare interventions and services must be suited to the cultural context and to the people who use them. There is a move to try and capture the views of people who use healthcare services, as the perspectives of healthcare professionals alone are insufficient to represent patient views. In Western health-related research, obtaining patients' views on the design and delivery of healthcare has been referred to as **patient and public involvement** (PPI). To enhance patient-centred care, the inclusion of 'expert patients' or 'experts by experience' must also feature in healthcare professional training (Saif et al., 2024). Patients with lived experience of a disease provide insights that cannot be gained from textbooks, this includes the sharing of experiences of bias, the importance of empathy and the need for healthcare to be a collaborative process.

Measuring health and disease

In this chapter, you have learned that health is a multidimensional concept influenced by a range of factors that incorporate more than just the absence of disease. Health can be measured in a variety of ways, including objective physical assessments, such as blood pressure, blood tests, scans, weight, temperature, respiration rate and so on. These measures will provide indications of the presence or absence of disease signs, a name for symptoms and how serious or progressive a disease (prognosis) will be. However, these measurements do not provide insights into the impact of disease on the individual in terms of the subjective symptom burden and health-related quality of life (HRQoL).

Questionnaires

Various questionnaires have been designed to measure general and specific HRQoL and disease burden. A commonly used measure of HRQoL is the Short Form-36 (SF36) (Ware & Sherbourne, 1992). This self-administered questionnaire contains 36 items that measure various aspects of functioning (social, physical), role limitations (associated with physical and emotional problems), mental health, general perceptions about health, energy and pain. There is also a question about general health over the past year. HRQoL can also be assessed using disease-specific measures, such as the Functional Assessment of Cancer Therapy General (FACT-G; Cella et al., 1993). This 27-item scale assesses four aspects of HRQoL (physical, social and family, emotional and functioning) in people who have cancer. The 13-item Functional Assessment of Chronic Illness Therapy – fatigue scale (FACIT-F; Cella et al., 2002) can be used to assess the impact of cancer-related fatigue on daily activities. There are also a range of measures for specific types of cancer and their symptoms, different cancer treatments, palliative care and spiritual wellbeing and satisfaction with treatment; many of these measures have been translated into and validated in languages other than English. The health measures that a researcher or a health professional uses, need to be suited to the population, culture and the concept of health being assessed (general or disease specific). In addition, the health measure must be standardised, valid and reliable (see Chapter 3).

When measuring Indigenous health, it is essential that scales are **culturally grounded**, community informed and consider the four domains of health (spiritual, emotional, physical and mental). The differences between Western and Indigenous conceptions of health mean using existing HRQoL measures that have been developed and validated using Western cultural values will probably not be applicable to Indigenous populations. In a systematic review of HRQoL measures used in research with Indigenous populations, Angell et al. (2016) found that out of 41 studies, only 3 used an Indigenous specific measure. The remainder adapted the existing questionnaire by making changes to language or omitting questions that were deemed as not suitable. Gupchup et al. (2001) adapted the 20-item Asthma Quality of Life Questionnaire (AQLQ; Marks et al., 1992) by conducting a focus group with three Indigenous patients who had a diagnosis of asthma. The patients were asked to consider the relevance of questions and whether any adjustments were required to the language used in each question. Some questions required minor wording modifications and others included more information to make the questions more relevant to Indigenous patients. For example, a question concerned with 'tightness in chest' was revised to include the words 'stinging and itching'. A question asked if asthma prevented the patient from 'achieving what they wanted from life' was amended to 'doing things that are part of my life'. When asked to think about the impact on social life, Indigenous patients suggested that the word 'community' was added; 'hobbies and recreations' were substituted by 'community and cultural activities'. The question about asthma causing 'restrictions to life' was changed to 'feeling misunderstood by family or community'. This resulted in a new measure, the Asthma Quality of Life Questionnaire for Native American Adults (AQLQ-NAA), which placed greater prominence on community and social, rather than individual restrictions of asthma. The AQLQ-NAA was tested with a sample of Indigenous patients who had asthma and was found to have good internal consistency and construct validity. However, Peters and Peterson (2019) take the view that such adaptations are problematic, as they use Western 'dominant' scientific conceptions and knowledge about health. This perpetuates colonisation, leading to Indigenous health knowledge and culture being subjugated, reinforcing health inequities for Indigenous communities. Furthermore, the differential conceptions of health between Western and Indigenous cultures may not be accounted for by subtle changes to language used in questionnaire items; this can lead to test bias and misinterpretation of Indigenous health, especially when comparisons are made across populations (Sharma et al., 2024).

Functional tests

An individual's **functional ability** can be assessed in several ways, including interviews, physical tests and completion of self-report questionnaires. In chronic respiratory, cardiovascular and neuromuscular diseases, a commonly used measure of functional ability is the six-minute walk test (6MWT). This provides a measure of how far a person can walk on a hard surface within a six-minute period. It can be used to assess disease progression or as a baseline measure prior to surgery or as part of pre- and post-outcomes used within an intervention. A subjective assessment of perceived exertion, ranging from no exertion to maximal exertion, can be combined with the 6MWT (Borg Scale; Borg, 1998). In older adults, grip strength may be used as a proxy measure of overall muscular strength and as a measure of frailty and muscle loss. In a seated position, the individual is asked to squeeze a handheld device that measures the maximum force they can squeeze with. Three trials are undertaken, with the highest measures used. Low grip strength is associated with longer recovery from hip fracture surgery in the elderly (Pérez-Rodríguez et al., 2020) and a greater chance of mortality in cardiovascular, respiratory diseases and a range of cancers (Celis-Morales et al., 2018).

Population measures

Within countries, patient surveys may be used by specific health providers to gain insights into patient lifestyle behaviours, prevalence of chronic diseases and social determinants of health. Some health providers will invite patients to complete satisfaction surveys to assess what is working well and what needs to improve within an organisation. Population-based health measures (e.g. life expectancy, morbidity, mortality) may be used to assess trends in disease, monitor health disparities across different countries, analyse income levels and study health measures between minority groups. This information may be used to identify areas of health need and resource allocation, assessment of what works best and for whom. These measures tend to be used by the WHO and governments to understand health patterns.

Chapter summary

Explain how different groups define health and distinguish between the concepts of disease and illness

People often find it difficult to define health, usually describing it as not being sick and being able to do the things they want to do. The WHO (1948) defines health as a state of complete physical, mental and social wellbeing, not merely the absence of disease or infirmity. In contrast, many Indigenous Peoples include spiritual dimensions, the land and ancestors in their understanding of health. Disease refers to a medical condition that is diagnosed through objective signs and biomedical tests, whereas illness is concerned with the subjective effects of symptoms, including personal, social and cultural experiences.

Describe the role of attributions in how people understand and respond to illness

Attributions are the explanations that people arrive at for the cause of illness, but attributions can be open to bias. Individuals may attribute illness to genetics, their own actions or the actions of others. Such beliefs can influence whether someone seeks help, follows medical advice or feels personally responsible for their illness. Likewise, healthcare professionals may sometimes blame patients for being ill.

Identify and discuss key social determinants of health

Social determinants of health include non-medical factors that can influence health outcomes. They include income, educational level, employment, social support, neighbourhood conditions and access to healthcare. Belonging to marginalised groups, such as ethnic, sexual, gender, disabled or Indigenous populations, can also affect health. When multiple social determinants of health intersect, they can exert a negative influence on access to healthcare and health outcomes.

Explain the difference between Western and Indigenous illness representations

Western illness representations are individually focused and can be conceptualised using the Self-Regulatory Model, where illness symptoms are viewed as a threat. People seek to identify the name, cause, consequences, timeline and cure/controllability of an illness. Once the illness has a name, treatment usually involves medical treatment and lifestyle changes. Approach or avoidant coping may be used and then appraised. Indigenous illness representations emphasise the four aspects of health (emotional, physical, mental and spiritual), with cause being due to the enduring effects of colonisation that includes discrimination and stigma. The consequences of being ill can be exacerbated by health inequities and the lack of culturally safe care. The focus is on collective health and healing involves traditional practices.

Describe how health psychologists may measure health, including population-level indicators and individual assessments

Health can be measured in various ways, including asking directly about health, self-report questionnaires that assess general or specific health-related quality of life and how specific diseases impact daily life. Functional measures, such as the 6-Minute Walk Test (6MWT), grip strength and perceived exertion, provide an objective indication of physical ability. At a population level, health can be assessed using epidemiological information on prevalence and mortality.

Keywords

Disease: A medical condition diagnosed through objective signs and biomedical tests.

Illness: The subjective effects of symptoms.

Attributions: The explanations that people arrive at for the cause of illness.

Social determinants of health: Non-medical factors, such as income, education, employment, social support and belonging to minoritised groups that influence people's health and access to care.

Deprived neighbourhoods: Areas in which residents have poor housing, low incomes, high unemployment, lower educational levels and limited access to services.

Learning disabilities: A significantly reduced ability to understand new or complex information, to learn new skills, with a reduced ability to cope independently, which started before adulthood, with a lasting effect on development.

Advanced care planning: An individual's record of their preferences for future healthcare and treatment.

Food deserts: Areas where people have limited access to affordable, healthy and nutritious food due to a lack of supermarkets or shops that sell fresh foods.

Strengths-based approach to health: Building on the skills, resources and abilities of what people and communities already do well to empower them to achieve positive health outcomes.

Deficiencies-based approach to health: Focuses on an individual's and/or community's problems or limitations, with the aim of fixing deficits.

Patient and public involvement: Active participation of patients, carers and the public in helping to design, change and evaluate healthcare services and/or research.

Culturally grounded: Interventions or practices that are based on the values, beliefs and traditions of a specific cultural group.

Functional ability: An individual's ability to engage in physical tasks, such as walking, muscular strength and activities required for daily living.

Key Readings

Bircher J. (2005). Towards a dynamic definition of health and disease. *Medicine, Health Care, and Philosophy*, *8*(3), 335–341. https://doi.org/10.1007/s11019-005-0538-y

Evandrou, M., Falkingham, J., Feng, Z., & Vlachantoni, A. (2016). Ethnic inequalities in limiting health and self-reported health in later life revisited. *Journal of Epidemiology and Community Health*, *70*(7), 653–662. https://doi.org/10.1136/jech-2015-206074

Krahn, G. L., Walker, D. K., & Correa-De-Araujo, R. (2015). Persons with disabilities as an unrecognized health disparity population. *American Journal of Public Health*, *105*(2), S198–S206. https://doi.org/10.2105/AJPH.2014.302182

Sabater Minarim, D., Morgan, K. M., Buckley, K., Riviere, P., Ochoa, C., Deshler, L. N., Duran, E. A., Mehtsun, W. T., Rose, B. S., & Banegas, M. P. (2025). Racial and ethnic disparities in perceived healthcare discrimination and health outcomes. *Journal of General Internal Medicine*. https://doi.org/10.1007/s11606-025-09627-y. Advance online publication.

Reflective Questions

1 Why might focusing only on physical symptoms not be enough to fully understand someone's illness?
2 How do social determinants of health impact disease?
3 How do Western and Indigenous conceptions of health and disease differ?

Video resources

Medical deception: Understanding Munchausen's syndrome/factitious disorder.
Website: https://www.youtube.com/watch?v=vrF-F_ZeRy8

References

Adelson, N. (2005). The embodiment of inequity: Health disparities in aboriginal Canada. *Canadian Journal of Public Health, 96*(2), S45–S61. https://doi.org/10.1007/BF03403702

Adler, A. I., Coleman, R. L., Leal, J., Whiteley, W. N., Clarke, P., & Holman, R. R. (2024). Post-trial monitoring of a randomised controlled trial of intensive glycaemic control in type 2 diabetes extended from 10 years to 24 years (UKPDS 91). *Lancet*, *404*(10448), 145–155. https://doi.org/10.1016/S0140-6736(24)00537-3

Andretti, B., Cardoso, L. O., Honório, O. S., de Castro Junior, P. C. P., Tavares, L. F., da Costa Gaspar da Silva, I., & Mendes, L. L. (2023). Ecological study of the association between socioeconomic inequality and food deserts and swamps around schools in Rio de Janeiro, Brazil. *BMC Public Health, 23*(1), 120. https://doi.org/10.1186/s12889-023-14990-8

Angell, B., Muhunthan, J., Eades, A. M., Cunningham, J., Garvey, G., Cass, A., Howard, K., Ratcliffe, J., Eades, S., & Jan, S. (2016). The health-related quality of life of Indigenous populations: A global systematic review. *Quality of Life, 25*(9), 2161–2178. https://doi.org/10.1007/s11136-016-1311-9

Antonovsky, A. (1987). The salutogenic perspective: Toward a new view of health and illness. *Advances, 4*(1), 47–55.

Australian Institute of Health and Welfare & National Indigenous Agency (2024). *Health performance framework - Summary report August 2024*, AIHW, Australian Government. Retrieved May 21, 2025, from https://www.indigenoushpf.gov.au/report-overview/overview/summary-report

Avery, S. (2018). *Culture is inclusion: A narrative of Aboriginal and Torres Strait Islander people with disability*. First Peoples Disability Network (Australia).

Bircher, J. (2005). Towards a dynamic definition of health and disease. *Medicine, Health Care, and Philosophy, 8*(3), 335–341. https://doi.org/10.1007/s11019-005-0538-y

Birtwistle, S. B., Jones, I., Murphy, R., Gee, I., & Watson, P. M. (2021). Family support for physical activity post-myocardial infarction: A qualitative study exploring the perceptions of cardiac rehabilitation practitioners. *Nursing & Health Sciences, 23*(1), 227–236. https://doi.org/10.1111/nhs.12806

Blaxter, M. (1990). *Health and lifestyles*. Routledge.

Borg, G. (1998). *Borg's perceived exertion and pain scales*. Human Kinetics.

Bridle-Fitzpatrick, S. (2015). Food deserts or food swamps?: A mixed-methods study of local food environments in a Mexican city. *Social Science & Medicine, 142*, 202–213. https://doi.org/10.1016/j.socscimed.2015.08.010

Butler-Jones, D., & Wong, T. (2016). Infectious disease, social determinants and the need for intersectoral action. *Canada Communicable Disease Report, 42*(1), S1-18–S1-20. https://doi.org/10.14745/ccdr.v42is1a04

Cahill, S. R. (2025). A severe dismantling of LGBTQI+ health equity and equality: Impact of new U.S. policies on the global response to HIV. *Journal of the International AIDS Society, 28*(5), e26485. https://doi.org/10.1002/jia2.26485

Canuto, K., Brown, A., Wittert, G., & Harfield, S. (2018). Understanding the utilization of primary health care services by Indigenous men: A systematic review. *BMC Public Health, 18*(1), 1198. https://doi.org/10.1186/s12889-018-6093-2

Carter-Harris, L. (2015). Lung cancer stigma as a barrier to medical help-seeking behavior: Practice implications. *Journal of the American Association of Nurse Practitioners, 27*(5), 240–245. https://doi.org/10.1002/2327-6924.12227

Cataldo, J. K., Jahan, T. M., & Pongquan, V. L. (2012). Lung cancer stigma, depression, and quality of life among ever and never smokers. *European Journal of Oncology, 16*(3), 264–269. https://doi.org/10.1016/j.ejon.2011.06.008

Celis-Morales, C. A., Welsh, P., Lyall, D. M., Steell, L., Petermann, F., Anderson, J., Iliodromiti, S., Sillars, A., Graham, N., Mackay, D. F., Pell, J. P., Gill, J. M. R., Sattar, N., & Gray, S. R. (2018). Associations of grip strength with cardiovascular, respiratory, and cancer outcomes and all cause mortality: Prospective cohort study of half a million UK Biobank participants. *British Medical Journal, 361*. https://doi.org/10.1136/bmj.k1651

Cella, D., Lai, J. S., Chang, C. H., Peterman, A., & Slavin, M. (2002). Fatigue in cancer patients compared with fatigue in the general United States population. *Cancer, 94*(2), 528–538. https://doi.org/10.1002/cncr.10245

Cella, D. F., Tulsky, D. S., Gray, G., Sarafian, B., Linn, E., Bonomi, A., Silberman, M., Yellen, S. B., Winicour, P., Brannon, J., Eckberg, K., Lloyd, S., Purl, S., Blendowski, C., Goodman, M., Barnicle, M., Stewart, I., McHale, M., Bonomi, P., & Harris,

J. (1993). The functional assessment of cancer therapy scale: Development and validation of the general measure. *Journal of Clinical Oncology, 11*(3), 570–579. https://doi.org/10.1200/JCO.1993.11.3.570

Centers for Disease Control and Prevention. (2025). *Socioeconomic factors at the intersection of race and ethnicity influencing health risks for people with disabilities.* Retrieved March 3, 2026, from https://www.cdc.gov/disability-and-health/articles-documents/socioeconomic-factors-race-and-ethnicity.html

Centers for Disease Control and Prevention (2022). *Disability and health data system data.* National Center on Birth Defects and Developmental Disabilities, Division of Human Development and Disability. Retrieved August 22, 2025, from https://dhds.cdc.gov

de Freitas, M. H., Vilela, P. R., & Nwora, E. I. (2023). Religiosity and Indigenous cosmology in a Brazilian Hospital setting: The challenges faced by health professionals. *International Journal of Latin American Religions, 7,* 46–77. https://doi.org/10.1007/s41603-023-00194-w

Department of Health and Social Care (2001). Valuing people: A new strategy for learning disability for the 21st Century. Retrieved September 9, 2025, from https://assets.publishing.service.gov.uk/media/5a7b854740f0b62826a041b9/5086.pdf

Emerson, E., Milner, A., Aitken, Z., Krnjacki, L., Vaughan, C., Llewellyn, G., & Kavanagh, A. (2021). Overt acts of perceived discrimination reported by British working-age adults with and without disability. *Journal of Public Health, 43*(1), e16–e23. https://doi.org/10.1093/pubmed/fdz093

Engel, G. L. (1977). The need for a new medical model: A challenge for biomedicine. *Science, 96,* 129–136. https://doi.org/10.1126/science.847460

Evandrou, M., Falkingham, J., Feng, Z., & Vlachantoni, A. (2016). Ethnic inequalities in limiting health and self-reported health in later life revisited. *Journal of Epidemiology and Community Health, 70*(7), 653–662. https://doi.org/10.1136/jech-2015-206074

Furze, G., Roebuck, A., Bull, P., Lewin, R. J., & Thompson, D. R. (2002). A comparison of the illness beliefs of people with angina and their peers: A questionnaire study. *BMC Cardiovascular Disorders, 2,* 4. https://doi.org/10.1186/1471-2261-2-4

Gérain, P., & Zech, E. (2021). Do informal caregivers experience more burnout? A meta-analytic study. *Psychology, Health & Medicine, 26*(2), 145–161. https://doi.org/10.1080/13548506.2020.1803372

Gonzales, G., & Henning-Smith, C. (2017). Barriers to care among transgender and gender nonconforming adults. *The Milbank Quarterly, 95*(4), 726–748. https://doi.org/10.1111/1468-0009.12297

Government Equalities Office. (2018). *LGBT Action Plan 2018: Improving the lives of lesbian, gay, bisexual and transgender people.* Retrieved August 22, 2025, from https://assets.publishing.service.gov.uk/media/5b39e91ee5274a0bbef01fd5/GEO-LGBT-Action-Plan.pdf

Gupchup, G. V., Hubbard, J. H., Teel, M. A., Singhal, P. K., Tonrey, L., Riley, K., Rupp, M. T., & Coultas, D. B. (2001). Developing a community-specific health-related quality of life questionnaire for asthma: The Asthma-Specific Quality of Life Questionnaire for Native American Adults (AQLQ-NAA). *The Journal of Asthma, 38*(2), 169–178. https://doi.org/10.1081/jas-100000036

Hagger, M. S., Koch, S., Chatzisarantis, N. L. D., & Orbell, S. (2017). The common-sense model of self-regulation: Meta-analysis and test of a process model. *Psychological Bulletin, 143*(11), 1117–1154. https://doi.org/10.1037/bul0000118

Hajek, A., Kretzler, B., & König, H. H. (2021). Informal caregiving, loneliness and social isolation: A systematic review. *International Journal of Environmental Research and Public Health, 18*(22), 12101. https://doi.org/10.3390/ijerph182212101

Hall, J. P., Kurth, N. K., Gimm, G., & Smith, S. (2019). Perspectives of adults with disabilities on access to health care after the ACA: Qualitative findings. *Disability and Health Journal, 12*(3), 350–358. https://doi.org/10.1016/j.dhjo.2019.01.014

Helman, C. G. (1981). Disease versus illness in general practice. *The Journal of the Royal College of General Practitioners, 31*(230), 548–552.

Helman, C. G. (2014). *Culture, health and illness: An introduction for health professionals.* Butterworth-Heinemann.

Heslop, P., Blair, P. S., Fleming, P., Hoghton, M., Marriott, A., & Russ, L. (2014). The confidential inquiry into premature deaths of people with intellectual disabilities in the UK: A population-based study. *Lancet, 383*(9920), 889–895. https://doi.org/10.1016/S0140-6736(13)62026-7

Huot, S., Ho, H., Ko, A., Lam, S., Tactay, P., MacLachlan, J., & Raanaas, R. K. (2019). Identifying barriers to healthcare delivery and access in the Circumpolar North: Important insights for health professionals. *International Journal of Circumpolar Health, 78*(1), 1571385. https://doi.org/10.1080/22423982.2019.1571385

Jacklin, K. M., Henderson, R. I., Green, M. E., Walker, L. M., Calam, B., & Crowshoe, L. J. (2017). Health care experiences of Indigenous people living with type 2 diabetes in Canada. *Canadian Medical Association Journal, 189*(3), E106–E112. https://doi.org/10.1503/cmaj.161098

Kingston, A., Robinson, L., Booth, H., Knapp, M., & Jagger, C., & MODEM project (2018). Projections of multi-morbidity in the older population in England to 2035: Estimates from the Population Ageing and Care Simulation (PACSim) model. *Age and Ageing, 47*(3), 374–380. https://doi.org/10.1093/ageing/afx201

Krahn, G. L., Walker, D. K., & Correa-De-Araujo, R. (2015). Persons with disabilities as an unrecognized health disparity population. *American Journal of Public Health, 105*(2), S198–S206. https://doi.org/10.2105/AJPH.2014.302182

Lach, K. (2013). The difference between disease and illness. *McGill Journal of Medicine, 14*(2), 20–21. https://mjm.mcgill.ca/article/view/204/61

Lagu, T., Haywood, C., Reimold, K., DeJong, C., Walker Sterling, R., & Iezzoni, L. I. (2022). 'I am not the doctor for you': Physicians' attitudes about caring for people with disabilities. *Health Affairs, 41*(10), 1387–1395. https://doi.org/10.1377/hlthaff.2022.00475

Lau, R. (1995). Cognitive representations of health and illness. In D. Gochman (ed). *Handbook of health behavior research.* Vol 1, Plenum.

Lee, S. Y., Park, C. L., & Laflash, S. (2022). Perceived posttraumatic growth in cardiac patients: A systematic scoping review. *Journal of Traumatic Stress, 35*(3), 791–803. https://doi.org/10.1002/jts.22799

Leventhal, H. (1970). Findings and theory in the study of fear communications. In L. Berkowtiz (Ed.). *Advances in experimental social psychology* (Vol. 5, pp. 119–186). Academic Press.

Leventhal, H., Meyer, D., & Nerenz, D. (1980). The common sense representation of illness danger. In S. Rachman (Ed.), *Contributions to medical psychology* (Vol. 2, pp. 7–30). Pergamon Press.

Marks, G. B., Dunn, S. M., & Woolcock, A. J. (1992). A scale for the measurement of quality of life in adults with asthma. *Journal of Clinical Epidemiology, 45*(5), 461–472. https://doi.org/10.1016/0895-4356(92)90095-5

McLeroy, K. R., Bibeau, D., Steckler, A., & Glanz, K. (1988). An ecological perspective on health promotion programs. *Health Education Quarterly, 15*(4), 351–377. https://doi.org/10.1177/109019818801500401

Meade, M. A., Mahmoudi, E., & Lee, S. Y. (2015). The intersection of disability and healthcare disparities: A conceptual framework. *Disability and Rehabilitation, 37*(7), 632–641. https://doi.org/10.3109/09638288.2014.938176

Mitra, M., Clements, K. M., Zhang, J., & Smith, L. D. (2016). Disparities in adverse preconception risk factors between women with and without disabilities. *Maternal and Child Health Journal, 20*(3), 507–515. https://doi.org/10.1007/s10995-015-1848-1

Mitra, M., Long-Bellil, L., Moura, I., Miles, A., & Kaye, H. S. (2022). Advancing health equity and reducing health disparities for people with disabilities in the United States. *Health Affairs, 41*(10), 1379–1386. https://doi.org/10.1377/hlthaff.2022.00499

Moore, S. P., Green, A. C., Bray, F., Garvey, G., Coory, M., Martin, J., & Valery, P. C. (2014). Survival disparities in Australia: An analysis of patterns of care and comorbidities among indigenous and non-indigenous cancer patients. *BMC Cancer, 14*, 517. https://doi.org/10.1186/1471-2407-14-517

Morgan, D. L., Slade, M. D., & Morgan, C. M. (1997). Aboriginal philosophy and its impact on health care outcomes. *Australian and New Zealand Journal of Public Health, 21*(6), 597–601. https://doi.org/10.1111/j.1467-842x.1997.tb01762.x

Mulcahy, A., Batza, K., Goddard, K., McMaughan, D. J. D., Kurth, N. K., Streed, C. G., Wallisch, A. M., & Hall, J. P. (2023). Experiences of patients with disabilities and sexual or gender minority status during healthcare interactions. *Journal of Public Health, 33*, 1735–1743. https://doi.org/10.1007/s10389-023-02145-3

Mulcahy, A., Streed, C. G. Jr, Wallisch, A. M., Batza, K., Kurth, N., Hall, J. P., & McMaughan, D. J. (2022). Gender identity, disability, and unmet healthcare needs among disabled people living in the community in the United States. *International Journal of Environmental Research and Public Health, 19*(5), 2588. https://doi.org/10.3390/ijerph19052588

Nguyen, N. H., Subhan, F. B., Williams, K., & Chan, C. B. (2020). Barriers and mitigating strategies to healthcare access in Indigenous communities of Canada: A narrative review. *Healthcare, 8*(2), 112. https://doi.org/10.3390/healthcare8020112

Nguyen, T. T., Vable, A. M., Glymour, M. M., & Nuru-Jeter, A. (2018). Trends for reported discrimination in health care in a national sample of older adults with chronic conditions. *Journal of General Internal Medicine, 33*(3), 291–297. https://doi.org/10.1007/s11606-017-4209-5

NHS (2022). Causes lung cancer. Retrieved August 18, 2025, from https://www.nhs.uk/conditions/lung-cancer/causes/

Parliament of the United Kingdom. (2010). *Equality Act 2010, chapter. 15, section 6*(1). Retrieved August 21, 2025, from https://www.legislation.gov.uk/ukpga/2010/15/section/6

Pérez Ramos, J. G., Garriga-López, A., & Rodríguez-Díaz, C. E. (2022). How is colonialism a sociostructural determinant of health in Puerto Rico? *AMA Journal of Ethics, 24*(4), E305–E312. https://doi.org/10.1001/amajethics.2022.305

Pérez-Rodríguez, P., Rabes-Rodríguez, L., Sáez-Nieto, C., Alarcón, T. A., Queipo, R., Otero-Puime, Á, & Gonzalez Montalvo, J. I. (2020). Handgrip strength predicts 1-year functional recovery and mortality in hip fracture patients. *Maturitas, 141*, 20–25. https://doi.org/10.1016/j.maturitas.2020.06.013

Peters, H. J., & Peterson, T. R.; Dakota Wicohan Community (2019). Developing an Indigenous measure of overall health and well-being: The Wicozani Instrument. *American Indian and Alaska Native Mental Health Research, 26*(2), 96–122. https://doi.org/10.5820/aian.2602.2019.96

Putsch, R. W. III, & Joyce, M. (1990). Dealing with patients from other cultures. In H. K. Walker et al. (Eds.), *Clinical methods: The history, physical, and laboratory examinations* (3rd ed.). Butterworths.

Puszka, S., Walsh, C., Markham, F., Barney, J., Yap, M., & Dreise, T. (2022). Towards the decolonisation of disability: A systematic review of disability conceptualisations, practices and experiences of First Nations people of Australia. *Social Science & Medicine, 305*, 115047. https://doi.org/10.1016/j.socscimed.2022.115047

Reweti, A. (2019). Tū Kahikatea: Whanaungatanga as a catalyst for whānau wellbeing. *Te Kura Nui o Waipareira, 3,* 21–34. https://wairangahau.waipareira.com/wp-content/uploads/2019/11/Waipareira-Journal_Kotahitanga-Issue-3-2019-WEB.pdf

Rossman, K., Salamanca, P., & Macapagal, K. (2017). A qualitative study examining young adults' experiences of disclosure and nondisclosure of LGBTQ identity to health care providers. *Journal of Homosexuality, 64*(10), 1390–1410. https://doi.org/10.1080/00918369.2017.1321379

Sabater Minarim, D., Morgan, K. M., Buckley, K., Riviere, P., Ochoa, C., Deshler, L. N., Duran, E. A., Mehtsun, W. T., Rose, B. S., & Banegas, M. P. (2025). Racial and ethnic disparities in perceived healthcare discrimination and health outcomes. *Journal of General Internal Medicine.* https://doi.org/10.1007/s11606-025-09627-y. Advance online publication

Saif, J., Mellor, D., Rogers, D., & Stocker, C. (2024). Integrating expert patients' perspectives on the processes of engaging them in early medical education. *Research Involvement and Engagement, 10*(1), 124. https://doi.org/10.1186/s40900-024-00655-2

Sakellariou, D., & Rotarou, E. S. (2017). Access to healthcare for men and women with disabilities in the UK: Secondary analysis of cross-sectional data. *BMJ Open, 7*(8), e016614. https://doi.org/10.1136/bmjopen-2017-016614

Salmon, M., Doery, K., Dance, P., Chapman, J., Gilbert, R., Williams, R., & Lovett, R. (2018). *Defining the indefinable: Descriptors of Aboriginal and Torres Strait Islander peoples' cultures and their links to health and wellbeing.* National Centre for Epidemiology and Population Health, Research School of Population Health, Australian National University. https://doi.org/10.25911/5bdbcdf5c89a7

Sharma, N., Walker, J. D., Wenghofer, E., Moeke-Pickering, T., & Lindenbach, J. (2024). Indigenous approaches to health assessment: A scoping review protocol. *Systematic Reviews, 13,* 78. https://doi.org/10.1186/s13643-024-02496-2

Smythe, T., & Kuper, H. (2024). The association between disability and all-cause mortality in low-income and middle-income countries: A systematic review and meta-analysis. *The Lancet. Global Health, 12*(5), e756–e770. https://doi.org/10.1016/S2214-109X(24)00042-1

Springer, K. W., Hankivsky, O., & Bates, L. M. (2012). Gender and health: Relational, intersectional, and biosocial approaches. *Social Science & Medicine, 74*(11), 1661–1666. https://doi.org/10.1016/j.socscimed.2012.03.001

Streed, C. G. Jr., Hall, J. P., Boyd, B. A., Batza, K., & Kurth, N. K. (2021). Comparative health status and characteristics of respondents of the 2019–2020 national survey on health and disability by sexual and gender minority status. *LGBT Health, 8*(8), 563–568. https://doi.org/10.1089/lgbt.2021.0075

Taskforce on Multiple Conditions (2021). Health equity and multiple long-term conditions: Evidence review. Retrieved August 22, 2025, from http://revealingreality.co.uk/wp-content/uploads/2021/07/evidence_review_final_22.07.pdf

Temple, J. B., Wong, H., Ferdinand, A., Avery, S., Paradies, Y., & Kelaher, M. (2020). Exposure to interpersonal racism and avoidance behaviours reported by Aboriginal and Torres Strait Islander people with a disability. *Australian Journal of Social Issues, 55,* 376–395. https://doi.org/10.1002/ajs4.126

UK Chief Medical Officers. (2019). *Physical activity guidelines: UK Chief Medical Officers' report.* Department of Health and Social Care. Retrieved August 26, 2025, from https://www.gov.uk/government/publications/physical-activity-guidelines-uk-chief-medical-officers-report

Umucu, E., Vernon, A. A., Pan, D., Qin, S., Solis, G., Campa, R., & Lee, B. (2025). Health inequities among persons with disabilities: A global scoping review. *Frontiers in Public Health, 13,* 1538519. https://doi.org/10.3389/fpubh.2025.1538519

Valdiserri, R. O., Holtgrave, D. R., Poteat, T. C., & Beyrer, C. (2019). Unraveling health disparities among sexual and gender minorities: A commentary on the persistent impact of stigma. *Journal of Homosexuality, 66*(5), 571–589. https://doi.org/10.1080/00918369.2017.1422944

Valenzuela, S., Peak, K. D., Huguet, N., Marino, M., Schmidt, T. D., Voss, R., Quiñones, A. R., & Nagel, C. (2024). Social deprivation and multimorbidity among community-based health center patients in the United States. *Preventing Chronic Disease, 21*, E75. https://doi.org/10.5888/pcd21.240060

Varadaraj, V., Deal, J. A., Campanile, J., Reed, N. S., & Swenor, B. K. (2021). National prevalence of disability and disability types among adults in the US, 2019. *JAMA Network Open, 4*(10), e2130358. https://doi.org/10.1001/jamanetworkopen.2021.30358

Verest, W. J. G. M., Galenkamp, H., Spek, B., Snijder, M. B., Stronks, K., & van Valkengoed, I. G. M. (2019). Do ethnic inequalities in multimorbidity reflect ethnic differences in socioeconomic status? The HELIUS study. *European Journal of Public Health, 29*(4), 687–693. https://doi.org/10.1093/eurpub/ckz012

Wang, V. H., Cuevas, A. G., Osokpo, O. H., Chang, J. E., Zhang, D., Hu, A., Yun, J., Lee, A., Du, S., Williams, D. R., & Pagán, J. A. (2024). Discrimination in medical settings across populations: Evidence from the All of Us Research Program. *American Journal of Preventive Medicine, 67*(4), 568–580. https://doi.org/10.1016/j.amepre.2024.05.018

Warburton, D. E. R., & Bredin, S. S. D. (2017). Health benefits of physical activity: A systematic review of current systematic reviews. *Current Opinion in Cardiology, 32*(5), 541–556. https://doi.org/10.1097/HCO.0000000000000437

Warburton, D. E. R., & Bredin, S. S. D. (2019). Health benefits of physical activity: A strengths-based approach. *Journal of Clinical Medicine, 8*(12), 2044. https://doi.org/10.3390/jcm8122044

Ware, J. E. Jr, & Sherbourne, C. D. (1992). The MOS 36-item Short-Form health survey (SF-36). I. Conceptual framework and item selection. *Medical Care, 30*(6), 473–483.

Watson, K. B., Wiltz, J. L., Nhim, K., Kaufmann, R. B., Thomas, C. W., & Greenlund, K. J. (2025). Trends in multiple chronic conditions among US adults, by life stage, Behavioral Risk Factor Surveillance System, 2013–2023. *Preventing Chronic Disease, 22*, 240539. http://dx.doi.org/10.5888/pcd22.240539

White, A., Sheehan, R., Ditzel, N., Ding, J., Roberts, C., Magill, N., Yu, M. K. L., Keagan-Bull, R., Chauhan, U., Tuffrey-Wijne, I., & Strydom, A.(2024). *Learning from lives and deaths - People with a learning disability and autistic people (LeDeR) report for 2023*. LeDeR Autism and Learning Disability Partnership, King's College London. Retrieved September 3, 2025, from https://www.kcl.ac.uk/ioppn/assets/pdfs/leder/leder-annual-report-2023.pdf

World Bank Group (2023). *Women, business and the law*. Retrieved August 19, 2025, from https://openknowledge.worldbank.org/entities/publication/e0437bc9-bac8-4486-959e-5be1dd45f253

World Economic Forum (2024). *Closing the women's health gap: A $1 trillion opportunities to improve lives and economies. Insight Report.* Retrieved August 19, 2025, from https://www.weforum.org/publications/closing-the-women-s-health-gap-a-1-trillion-opportunity-to-improve-lives-and-economies/

World Health Organization (1948) *Constitution of the World Health Organization.* Retrieved October 24, 2024, from https://apps.who.int/gb/bd/PDF/bd47/EN/constitution-en.pdf?ua=1

World Health Organization (2000). *Report on the international consultation on the health of Indigenous Peoples*. Retrieved August 20, 2025, from https://iris.who.int/bitstream/handle/10665/69464/WHO_HSD_00.1_eng.pdf?sequence=1&isAllowed=y

World Health Organization (2024). *The top 10 causes of death*. Retrieved October 28, 2024, from https://www.who.int/news-room/fact-sheets/detail/the-top-10-causes-of-death

World Health Organization (2025a) *World report on social determinants of health equity*. Retrieved August 19, 2025, from https://www.who.int/teams/social-determinants-of-health/equity-and-health/world-report-on-social-determinants-of-health-equity

World Health Organization. (2025b). *Global plan of action for the health of Indigenous peoples*. World Health Organization. https://www.who.int/initiatives/global-plan-of-action-for-health-of-indigenous-peoples

Yu, G., Panagioti, M., Tang, E. Y. H., Robinson, D., Husain, N., Lasrado, R., Lovell, K., Kaner, E., & Fu, Y. (2023). Establishing evidence to inform culturally competent mental health services: A mixed methods study protocol. *PloS One, 18*(3), e0282445. https://doi.org/10.1371/journal.pone.0282445

6 Adherence

Chapter contents

- What are adherence and nonadherence?
- A socio-cultural-cognitive model of adherence.
- Assessing adherence.
- Healthcare system issues and adherence.
- How to improve adherence to medication.
- Reasons for nonattendance at medical appointments.

Chapter objectives

After reading this chapter, you should be able to answer the following questions:

- Define the concept of adherence in healthcare contexts.
- Describe the socio-cultural-cognitive model of adherence that goes beyond understanding, memory and satisfaction when considering factors that influence adherence.
- Explain the concept of health literacy and discuss how it influences patient adherence.
- Identify methods used to measure health literacy and why they may not be applicable to everyone.
- Explain how culture, ethnicity and intersectionality can shape adherence.
- Outline the key components of the World Health Organization's Multidimensional Adherence Model.
- Describe strategies to improve medication adherence, included in the Hierarchical Model for Medication Adherence.
- Explain how culture, ethnicity and intersectionality can shape nonadherence at medical appointments.

What are adherence and nonadherence?

Adherence, compliance and co-operation have been used interchangeably to describe whether a person is engaging in a health-related behaviour, following guidance, or taking medication. Adherence and co-operation are the preferred terms, as compliance implies that the person is passive, yielding to pressure and following instructions of someone in authority. Adherence and co-operation are more suggestive of a person taking an active role and personal responsibility for lifestyle choices, treatment-related decisions and behaviours. Such behaviours are important in helping individuals achieve optimal health outcomes, especially as a systematic review that showed that people with two or more chronic conditions had medication nonadherence rates ranging from 44% to 77% (Foley et al., 2021).

DOI: 10.4324/9781003423157-6

BOX 6.1
CRITICAL THINKING

Have you ever been prescribed a medication, but forgot to take it, taken an incorrect dose or taken medicine at the wrong time? Think about why this happened. Is there anything that a health professional could have done to help you take the medication as prescribed?

Nonadherence to medication may have serious risks to health. For example, adherence to medication is essential for an individual who has received an organ transplant, as they must take **immunosuppressive** drugs for life to prevent organ rejection, illness and death. Yet, after kidney transplantation approximately one-third of recipients do not adhere to medication (Gandolfini et al., 2022). However, adherence may not be just as important for an individual who has been prescribed pain medication and skips occasional doses when their pain is manageable. Individuals may make a conscious decision not to take medication or follow medical advice, which is referred to as **intentional nonadherence**. Nonadherence can also be **unintentional**, which includes forgetting about an appointment, forgetting to take medication, taking the wrong dose or taking it at the wrong time. In the case of a bacterial infection, adhering to instructions is paramount. This includes taking the correct dose of antibiotics, at the prescribed time intervals and the importance of finishing the course, even if symptoms have gone or reduced. This is not only important for patient recovery, but also for helping to prevent the emergence of drug-resistant bacteria. In long-term (chronic) conditions, adherence to medical advice, medication and other treatments can help to manage symptoms and may reduce the pace of disease progression.

A socio-cultural-cognitive model of adherence

Ley (1986) proposed that adherence was dependent on three cognitive factors, which were understanding, memory and satisfaction with treatment and/or the medical encounter (see Figure 6.1). Ley believed that understanding and memory could directly impact adherence, but may affect adherence indirectly, via satisfaction. However, this model is too simplistic and requires extending, as it ignores the influence of culture, ethnic minority status and the cumulative effects of discrimination, which exert various influences on the cognitions about adherence.

Understanding

Patients do not always understand what healthcare professionals tell or ask of them. They may give incorrect answers due to uncertainty regarding the meaning of medical terminology and healthcare professionals may credit patients with knowledge they do not have. This was exemplified by Weinman et al. (2009) who

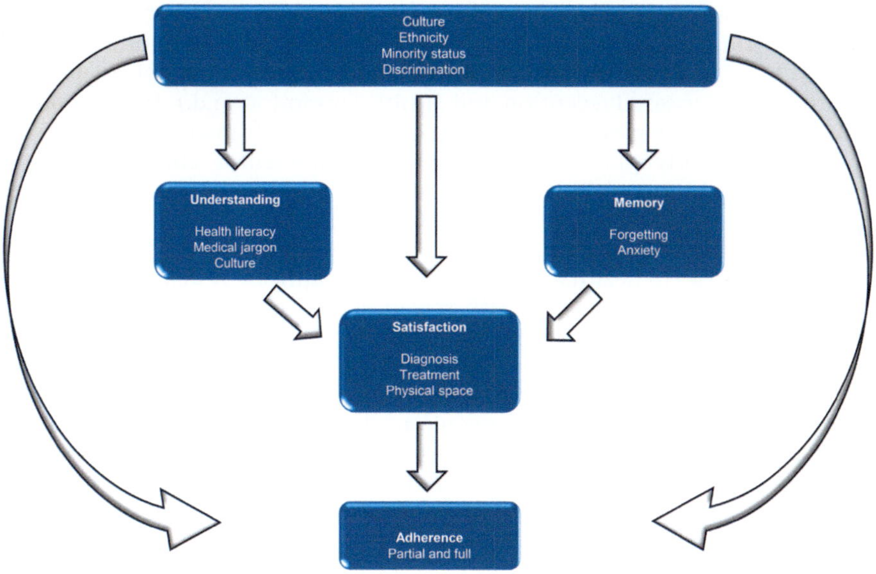

Figure 6.1
Socio-cultural-cognitive model of adherence

Source: Author, based on Ley (1986)

asked patients to point to various parts of the abdomen, around 38.4% were able to locate the stomach, 52.9% knew where the liver was, but only 31.4% could locate their lungs. There are anecdotal examples of medical jokes in which doctors have asked patients questions and received puzzling responses. When enquiring about any family history of heart problems, a doctor asked, 'Is there a history of cardiac arrest in your family?', the patient responded by saying 'No doctor, we have never been in trouble with the police!' While this may seem somewhat amusing, the important aspect in this example is the assumption on the part of the doctor that the patient would understand the medical terminology for the heart having stopped is a 'cardiac arrest'. Being unaware what cardiac meant, the patient responded to the word they were familiar with – 'arrest', albeit in a different context! In another example, when asking about a new symptom of urine leakage, a nurse asked the patient, 'Have you ever been incontinent before?', the patient replies 'No we have never been abroad!'. Again, it is the use of medical terminology that caused the misunderstanding, instead of using 'incontinent', a simpler non-medical term, such as 'leaked' would have been more appropriate. Patients may fear ridicule or embarrassment if they admit to being uncertain or confused about what a healthcare professional is asking, thus they may pretend to understand what has been said.

Understanding and health literacy

Despite being given instructions and/or advice about medication, treatment and/or lifestyle interventions, not all patients will be adherent. This can be due to a variety of factors that we will examine later in this chapter, but one very salient aspect of adherence is health literacy, which has been defined as "the degree to which individuals have the ability to find, understand, and use information and services to inform health-related decisions and actions for themselves and others" (Office of Disease Prevention and Health Promotion, n.d.). Health literacy can be influenced by past experience, educational level, ethnicity, culture, sexual and gender identity and disability. People have different levels and degrees of health literacy and poor health literacy has been associated with poor health outcomes (Parker, 2000). Nutbeam (2000) identified three levels of health literacy, the first level is **functional**, which involves the provision of basic health education on risks to health and how to use the healthcare system. It encourages adherence to medical advice, health screening and uptake of vaccinations. It does not involve communication, build personal skills or support independence in terms of reducing health risky behaviours or spontaneous uptake in health enhancing behaviours. The second level is concerned with **interactive health literacy**, which is about helping people to develop the skills and confidence to act on health advice, to ask questions during health consultations/appointments, so that they can engage in health decision-making, improve motivation, display independence and promote the uptake of healthy habits. The third level is **critical health literacy**, which focuses on the development of thinking and the skills required to take both personal and collective action to improve health. It involves understanding social, economic and environmental factors that affect health. For example, questioning health polices, such as the age at which screening for cervical or prostate cancers commences, and challenging governments about industrial practices that may have detrimental impacts on health, such as traffic pollution and air quality. Increasing an individual's health literacy can enhance their ability to have better control over health, which can lead to improved health outcomes.

The definition of health literacy provided by the Office of Disease Prevention and Health Promotion emphasised the individual's role in finding, understanding and using health information. However, it is incumbent on organisations, governments, healthcare systems and healthcare professions to ensure that the information they provide is understandable and presented in a range of formats to suit people's needs. A survey of 64 different health information sources in England that covered disease prevention, managing illness, health promotion, personal and public safety and the location and types of healthcare facilities found that much of the information was too complicated for a substantial proportion of the public to understand (Rowlands et al., 2015). This survey also highlighted that people who had low levels of health literacy were more likely to be from ethnic minorities and of low socioeconomic status. In the US, the National Heath Literacy survey conducted in 2003 showed similar findings. African American, Hispanic, American Indian and Alaskan Native adults had lower levels of health literacy compared to their White counterparts (Kutner et al., 2006). A systematic review of studies that assessed health literacy across 17 European countries found that between 33% and 50% of the population had difficulties in understanding health-related information (Baccolini et al., 2021). There is a common misconception that poor health literacy is always synonymous with low educational attainment, while there are some links between the two, many adults struggle to comprehend healthcare instructions, printed materials, healthcare communications, along with processes and policies to access the healthcare they require (Baccolini et al., 2021). When faced with an unfamiliar health-related situation (e.g. an acute disease or healthcare setting) or when interacting with healthcare professionals, even people who have high levels of health literacy may struggle to obtain and understand information to assist in healthcare decision-making (Berry et al., 2017).

Low health literacy is associated with poor health outcomes (Berkman et al., 2004) and a reduced likelihood of engaging in health enhancing behaviours that are known to prevent disease (Berkman et al., 2011). People with low health literacy tend to experience difficulty in managing chronic diseases (Dewalt et al., 2004) and are more likely to die prematurely (Rowlands et al., 2015). Even though health literacy is an important factor that can impact adherence and quality of life, it is something that healthcare professionals give little consideration to (Lambert et al., 2015). To help healthcare professionals improve written information and communication for patients in the UK, Health Education England, Public Health England, NHS England, & Community Health and Learning Foundation (2023) published a health literacy toolkit that links age and typical general literacy with different levels of complexity of health information. This includes advice on suitability of written, numerical and spoken information and suggests that healthcare professionals should make use of simple language, often referred to as plain English. Interventions to enhance health literacy have focused on adjusting communication through using pictograms (Sheridan et al., 2011), using the teach-back method (Ha Dinh et al., 2016) in which the patient is asked to reiterate in their own words, the information that has been provided by a healthcare professional and animations have also been used (Visscher et al., 2018).

How is health literacy measured?

There are over 150 scales available that purport to measure health literacy, making direct comparisons across studies difficult and there is no universal agreement as to which scale is the best (Nguyen et al., 2017). Scales include questions that measure aspects of understanding, reading, numeracy and pronunciation of medical words, with some only measuring one of these aspects (Altin et al., 2014). Using a single scale to assess an individual's health literacy can be misleading, for example, the Rapid Estimate of Adult Literacy in Medicine Scale (REALMS; Murphy et al., 1993) consists of 66 common medical and lay words to describe body parts and diseases. The individual is asked to read and pronounce these words; however, this scale just provides an indication of reading ability, rather than assessing health literacy per se. To achieve a comprehensive assessment of health literacy, the use of a **multidimensional scale** may be more appropriate. One such scale is the Health Literacy Questionnaire (HLQ; Osborne et al., 2013), which can be used to assess individual and population health literacy abilities, along with experiences with healthcare professionals and services. The HLQ consists of 44 questions that tap into nine domains (Figure 6.2), and these show areas in which people have health literacy strengths and weaknesses. Unlike other health literacy scales, the HLQ permits assessments to be made for each domain in order that health information can be tailored to meet specific needs and populations (Osborne et al., 2013).

Culture and health literacy

It is not clear the extent to which culture may exert an influence on health literacy, as measurement issues create problems in making meaningful comparisons across studies. In a systematic review of studies that had been conducted across Latin American and Caribbean countries, de Jesus et al. (2024) found that

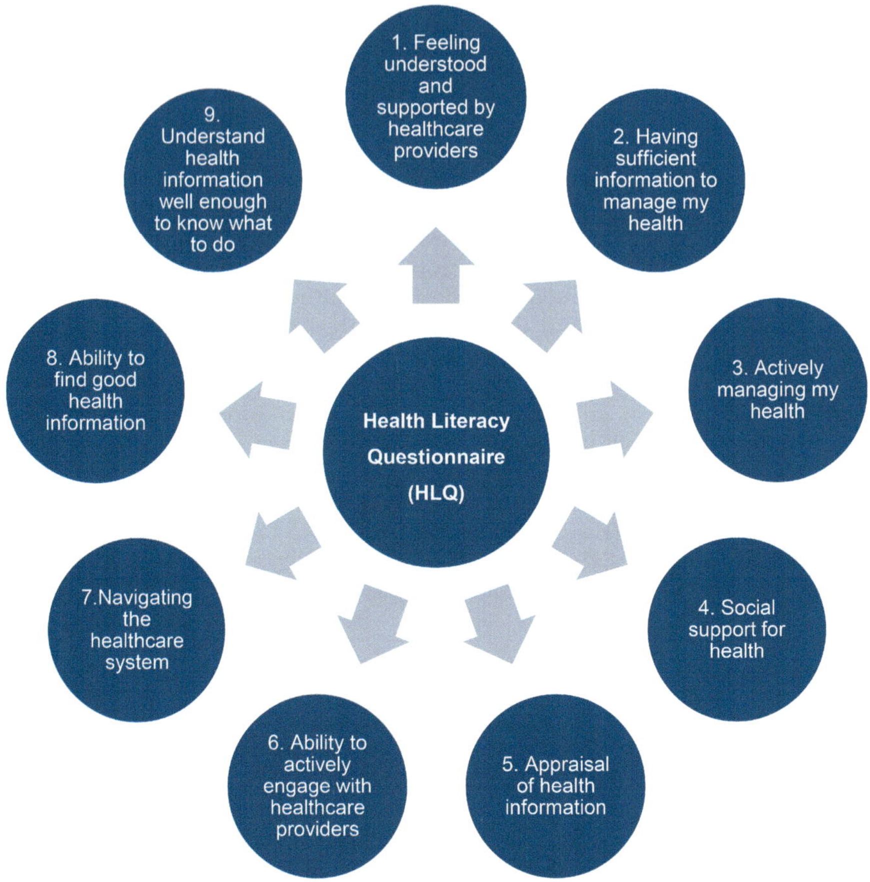

Figure 6.2
The nine domains of the Health Literacy Questionnaire (HLQ)

Source: Author, based on Osborne et al. (2013)

nearly 50% of participants had low levels of health literacy. However, just under 40% of the 22 measures used to assess health literacy had been validated in the languages of the countries where the studies had been conducted. Similar findings were reported by Wikkeling-Scott et al. (2019) in a review of health literacy across the Eastern Mediterranean region of Europe. These researchers concluded that measures developed in English-speaking countries and translated for use in other countries may not fully consider the linguistic nuances and culture of the regions in which they have been applied. When a researcher decides to use a scale that has been developed and validated in another language, they translate or back translate the content. **Back translation** refers to the process of one person translating a scale from the original language (e.g. English) into the target language (e.g. Arabic) and a second person translating the scale back into the original language (English), without looking at the original text. The original and back translated versions are compared to identify any discrepancies or differences in meaning that may be due to errors in translation or minor cultural nuances of language. While this process does permit adjustments to language, it does not consider cultural aspects of health, religion and subtle meanings in wording changes and tenses. Al Maqbali et al. (2020) provided an example of how linguistic back translation of a scale to measure health-related quality of life in people living with cancer (the Functional Assessment of Chronic Illness Therapy; FACIT) was insufficient to deal with subtle meanings that were culturally bound. The FACIT was originally developed for Western populations, but it has been successfully validated in many other languages. When the scale was used with Arabic patients in Oman, one item that referred to how satisfied people were with how they were coping with their illness produced inconsistent results. Al Maqbali et al. (2020) explained that in Islamic culture, illness is viewed as God's will, thus satisfaction with one's own coping of illness had no relevance to these patients, as according to God, illness was something they should be accepting of. Thus, when adapting health measurement tools for cross-cultural use, a direct linguistic translation is not enough, the cultural context must be considered to ensure concepts are meaningful. This includes ensuring that questionnaire items measure what they are supposed to and that items cover all aspects of the concept and are relevant to the target population. This process should include item assessment by experts and people from the target population (Osborne et al., 2022; Terwee et al., 2007).

The Australian Commission on Safety and Quality in Health Care (ACSQHE, 2015) reported that information across several countries (Australia, Canada, New Zealand and North America) indicated substantial differences in health literacy between Indigenous and non-Indigenous populations. Most information on health literacy is collected through survey methods using scales based on Western thinking about health literacy. In addition, these scales are designed for individual completion, but within Indigenous cultures, health decision-making is a shared activity. Hence, there is a need to think about ways of measuring health literacy that includes family members, the community and/or the village. Despite there being a plethora of scales to measure health literacy, there are some populations and communities for which there is no culturally appropriate health literacy scale; in such cases, it may be necessary to collect data through alternative means, such as interviews and/or group discussions. Rheault et al. (2021) conducted a mixed methods study in Australia to assess what information Aboriginal and Torres Strait Islander Peoples had received on their diagnosis, treatment, education, self-management of chronic illnesses and assessed their health literacy. Cultural safety and relevance of the study were enabled through partnership working with community Elders and Aboriginal Health workers, with the latter helping with data collection. Quantitative data were collected using the HLQ (Osborne et al., 2013), with questions read to participants to avoid embarrassing those who had low literacy abilities. Qualitative data were collected using semi-structured interviews, which were culturally adapted to use Aboriginal ways of exchanging and acquiring knowledge, based on oral storytelling, known as yarning. This is like interviewing, in that it helps to facilitate an exchange of information and stories, but without the imposition of Western semi-structured interview techniques that often interrupt with prompts to seek clarification or elicit further information (Lin et al., 2016). While it is disrespectful to interrupt the individual who is yarning, it can make it difficult to keep from straying off the topic being discussed. To address this, Bessarab and Ng'andu (2010) advise using different types of yarning for specific purposes during the research process. 'Social yarning' is an informal general discussion that can be used before 'research yarning', the latter is more focused on the topic under investigation. Findings from the Rheault et al. (2021)

study showed that participants had low health literacy scores across all nine domains of the HLQ. Participants who were below 55 years, female and had more years of education tended to have the highest health literacy. Qualitative data showed that participants had a fatal acceptance of developing a chronic disease and believed there was no way of preventing it or making it better. Every participant in the study had experiences of health professionals who had used medical terminology and some participants had received written health information, which was too difficult to understand, resulting in negative consequences for adhering to health advice. Participants admitted that feelings of embarrassment prevented them from asking for explanations. A salient theme centred on how healthcare professionals could help address Indigenous People's healthcare needs, along with the power imbalance between the healthcare professional and the patient. The use of yarning helped supplement and extend information obtained from the HLQ. It highlighted that patients required help to develop their health literacy skills but placed the onus on healthcare professionals to ensure that the information they provided was jargon free and communicated in a clear, respectful and culturally safe way. However, Rheault et al. (2021) stated that HLQ results should be interpreted with caution, as this particular outcome measure had not been previously validated for use within this population.

Based on a review of literature, MacAskill et al. (2022) also reported that limited information existed on Aboriginal and Torres Strait Islander Peoples' health literacy and that there were no validated outcome measures that were deemed culturally sensitive for this population. Rather than impose Western psychometric methods by using health literacy scales validated in White non-Indigenous populations, MacAskill et al. proposed that within general practice, doctors could explore health literacy by asking a few short questions in a non-judgemental yarning manner. For example, enquiring how confident the patient felt about filling in medical forms and how often they needed help in reading instructions or information from the doctor or pharmacy about health problems/medications. When using culturally specific approaches to access information on health literacy from Indigenous Peoples, there is a need to remember that even within the same country, there are variations in world views, traditions, language, dialects and beliefs (Vass et al., 2011). Most studies into the health literacy of Indigenous Peoples are situated in Western knowledge and ways of knowing, ignoring the importance of how culture, language and Indigenous knowledge are integrated and conceptualised with holistic health (Boot & Lowell, 2019). These authors analysed a range of policy and practice documents about health literacy from Australia, Canada and New Zealand and found that while there was recognition of the importance of Indigenous health knowledge, its promotion and guidance in healthcare professional training were limited.

Health literacy and gender identity

A plethora of research shows that LGBTQI+ (lesbian, gay, bisexual, transgender, queer plus) populations have poorer health outcomes than their cisgender and heterosexual counterparts; however, relatively little research has been conducted into the health literacy of LGBTQI+ populations. Eliason et al. (2017) developed a health literacy scale consisting of 20 items, which included 10 general questions about health literacy and 10 that were specific to lesbian, gay and bisexual (LGB) information and skills. Results indicated that participants who shared their sexual orientation with healthcare providers had higher health literacy and better health compared to those who felt unable to disclose this information. This was a pilot study and the authors acknowledged the need to conduct larger studies on more diverse populations. Transgender people often experience more healthcare professional stigma and discrimination compared to their cisgender counterparts (Aparicio-García et al., 2018). This is compounded by health professionals' lack of knowledge about **trans-specific care**, which can have negative health consequences, as transgender people may avoid seeking medical help due to fear of mistreatment (Teti et al., 2021). To increase their own health literacy and engage in health decision-making, many transgender people have resorted to searching the internet and joining transgender online communities where people can share health-related information (Pho et al., 2022).

Health literacy and learning disabilities

People with learning disabilities are at a greater risk of developing obesity, type 2 diabetes (T2DM) and cardiovascular disease (CVD) (White et al., 2024), they also exhibit these diseases earlier in life than the general population. Reduced communication and literacy skills can be barriers to developing sufficient health literacy to enable use of health information about unhealthy lifestyle habits, such as poor nutrition, low physical activity and incorrect use of medication (Chinn & Homeyard, 2017). The extent of a learning disability may mean that not everyone will be able to access, understand and benefit from health information and assistance may be provided by learning disability nurses, support workers or general practitioners ([GPs], Marks & Sisirak, 2017). Training programmes using visual aids and game-like questions may help people with learning disabilities to self-manage their health (Feldman et al., 2016), but their development can be resource intensive and usually only suitable for people with mild disabilities. Nevertheless, these activities can help in the development of functional health literacy skills and increase short-term adherence to advice and treatment regimens. There is a need to go further to empower people with learning disabilities to become actively involved in the self-management of health behaviours by shifting power dynamics in decision-making actions (Chinn & Homeyard, 2017; Marks & Sisirak, 2017). Moreover, people with learning disabilities are often excluded from taking part in health-related research due to concerns about **lacking capacity to consent**, or assumptions about inability to understand study descriptions and complete outcome measures (Bishop et al., 2024; Brooks et al., 2025). However, the use of coproduction and participatory methods in research can help overcome these problems, enabling people with learning disabilities to be included in health-related research (Davison et al., 2022) to develop their interactive and critical health literacy skills.

BOX 6.2
CRITICAL THINKING

Health literacy can have consequences for adherence to medication and healthcare-related instructions. Consider how well you understand health information, for example if you were advised to eat a healthy diet, would you know what that meant? How and where do you obtain health information? How do you know if the source of health information is factual?

Memory and adherence

One of the most frequent reasons for not attending medical appointments, taking medication at the correct time, the correct dose and carrying out health-related instructions is, 'I forgot'. The amount, complexity and the way in which information is delivered during a medical appointment can impact a patient's recall. For some people, the ability to remember such information is like learning a new language and it has been estimated that only about 20% of the information conveyed during a medical appointment is retained (Kessels, 2003). Patients may feel anxious when they attend medical appointments, which can have negative impacts on their understanding and memory (Legg et al., 2015). Recent research with patients who were attending a 'fast track' diagnostic clinic for colorectal cancer found that patients with high levels of anxiety recalled less information than those with low levels of anxiety (Nguyen et al., 2019). Thus, it is incumbent upon healthcare professionals to supplement verbal information (or signed, for people who are deaf) provided during a medical appointment with written information (or audio recorded for people who are blind) that highlights the most salient details that they wish the patient to remember or attend to, as this can help adherence.

Satisfaction and adherence

When patients are involved with healthcare professionals in collaborative treatment planning and decision-making about their health, it engenders trust, builds a therapeutic alliance and improves adherence. Healthcare providers often assess patient satisfaction of their services through post-visit surveys, which can help to determine aspects of service provision that are valued and those that may need to be enhanced. Patient satisfaction can have direct implications for adherence to prescribed medication, healthcare advice and future appointment attendance (Barbosa et al., 2012). There are a multiplicity of patient and health professional characteristics that can exert an influence on satisfaction and adherence. Within the UK, patient satisfaction with the National Health Service (NHS) is routinely measured and in 2024, it had fallen to its lowest ever at 21% overall. Satisfaction with accident and emergency services was 19% and general practitioner (GP) services satisfaction was 31%. Lower satisfaction scores were mainly due to longer waiting times to get appointments and hospital care, but satisfaction with quality of care was much higher at 51% (Taylor et al., 2025).

We learned in Chapter 5 that when people have symptoms, they often try to identify a cause and this may lead to patient expectations about the need for symptoms to be explored and types of treatments to manage or control symptoms. Treatment, prescribed medication, diagnosis or lack of referral to a specialist service can have negative consequences on patient satisfaction and subsequent adherence. Patent satisfaction is generally higher when healthcare professionals are perceived as more caring, approachable, viewed as taking a collaborative approach by showing empathy (Keshtkar et al., 2024) and exhibiting effective communication skills (Allen et al., 2023). Providing sufficient information for patients to become involved in their own care and avoiding the use of medical jargon are rated by patients as being important (Jahng et al., 2005). However, not being able to access disease- and medication-related information in a patient's own language can impact health literacy and satisfaction, especially when professional interpreters are not available and patients have to rely on family or friends to translate personal healthcare information (Alhomoud et al., 2015). In addition, the physical (cleanliness of and comfort of rooms and waiting areas, accessibility, signage and seating and privacy) and organisational aspects (continuity of care, ease of making appointments, waiting times and coordination with other services and/or departments) can also impact patient satisfaction (Keshtkar et al., 2024).

Assessing adherence

Medication

Estimating adherence to medication is fraught with difficulty, as figures vary according to the type of medication, the actual disease, whether the disease is acute or chronic and the costs of medication. How adherence is defined is important too, for example, total adherence means the full prescribed dose is taken, at the prescribed time and interval, along with instructions regarding the temporal relationship with food. Quite often healthcare professionals overestimate patient adherence (Miller et al., 2002) and attribute nonadherence as being the fault of the patient, but there are multiple interacting factors that can contribute to medication nonadherence.

Assessing adherence to medication

The WHO (2003) estimated that adherence to treatment for chronic diseases was only about 50% and that improving adherence could have substantial health benefits compared to trying to improve treatments themselves (Anghel et al., 2019). One of the problems facing healthcare practitioners and researchers alike is how to measure adherence. Ways of measuring adherence have included direct, indirect, subjective and objective methods. There is no 'gold standard' method of measuring adherence to medication, but one of the most obvious ways to measure adherence to medication is to ask the patient if they have been taking their medication. However, the way in which the question is phrased can influence the answer. A direct question may be perceived as challenging and the patient may not want to admit to nonadherence. Furthermore, the patient may have partially adhered, in that the medication was taken, but a lower or high dose or not taken at the correct time interval. Instead of asking 'Have you been taking your medication?', a less confrontational and more acceptable way could be to invite explanation and discussion. For example, 'Some patients have difficulty in taking this medication, how have you been managing?' This is less challenging and permits the patient to disclose any difficulties they may have experienced or reasons for deviating from the prescribed instructions. It is also important to note that adherence to medication covers taking the dose at specific times of the day, with food or before food, or avoidance of specific foods, or not drinking alcohol, as these may interact with medication.

Other ways to measure medication adherence include whether the person has sought a repeat prescription and/or counting the number of remaining tablets to determine how much of a medication has been taken. However, these two methods may not provide a good indication of adherence, as requesting a repeat prescription does not mean that the person has taken the medication, it just means they have asked for more! Likewise with tablet counts, we know how many tablets have been taken out of the supply, but we do not know if the person has ingested those tablets, thrown them out or given them to someone else. A reduction in a person's symptoms may be an indicator that they have adhered to their medication, but some symptoms will respond to lifestyle changes and resolve over time without the need for medication. Objective measures such as blood and urine tests may provide an indication of whether certain medications have been taken. These can be of use for specific conditions, but a range of factors can affect such tests, such as individual differences in how well people metabolise medication, the speed at which this happens, the impact of diet, physical activity, along with other medications and supplements. There is general agreement that measurement of adherence is fraught with difficulties and due to the variety of diseases, populations, healthcare services and ways in which adherence is defined and measured, assessing results across studies is fraught with difficulty (Nguyen et al., 2014).

Barriers to medication adherence

The WHO proposed a Multidimensional Adherence Model (MAM) that outlines multiple factors that may impact medication adherence (see Figure 6.3), which include patient, socioeconomic treatment, condition (disease) and healthcare system issues (WHO, 2003). The MAM is viewed as being a holistic model, as it addresses many of the intersecting biopsychosocial factors that impact medication adherence. In explaining the model, the WHO (2003) outlined how people in low-income countries may, due to socioeconomic factors, face stark choices between the costs of medication and the needs of their families. Even for patients in high-income countries, the costs of healthcare and medications can have adverse impacts on adherence (Piette et al., 2011). Australian Aboriginal and Torres Strait Islander peoples have highlighted that making medications more affordable and accessible, especially for people of lower socioeconomic status, could help to improve adherence (Davidson et al., 2010). Something that was echoed by Reese et al. (2025) when investigating Indigenous women's perceptions, beliefs and experiences related to medication. These researchers found that the financial constraints imposed by medication costs meant family members tried to make medication last longer by taking **partial doses**, spreading the prescribed amount for one day, over several days. The women suggested that doctors should factor in the expense of medications before prescribing them.

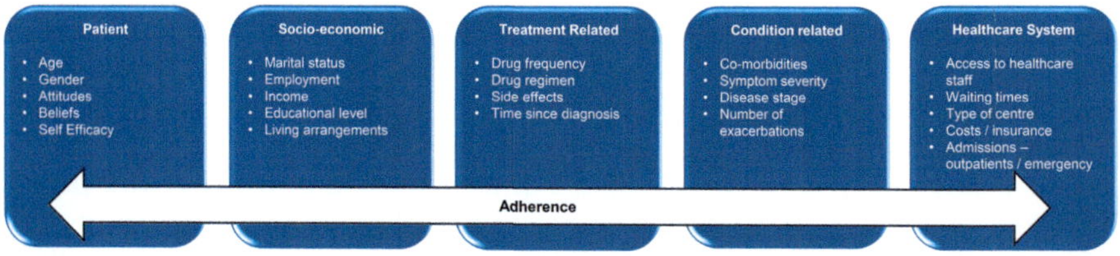

Figure 6.3
The WHO Multidimensional Adherence Model of Medication

Source: Author based on the WHO (2003)

In assessing the barriers and facilitators to medication adherence across a range of chronic disease studies (cancer, diabetes, asthma, human immunodeficiency virus/acquired immunodeficiency syndrome (HIV/AIDS), hypertension and epilepsy), Konstantinou et al. (2020) reported that nonmodifiable intersectional factors, such as low income, educational level, poor social support, living in rural locations and being under 30 years old, had negative impacts on adherence. Similar findings have been reported when attempting to investigate adherence to antidiabetic medication and belonging to a minority ethnic group (non-Whites in the US and non-Europeans in New Zealand). Results summarised within a systematic review showed that the intersections of income, health literacy and educational level also had implications for adherence within these populations (Studer et al., 2023).

Ethnicity, culture and adherence to medication

There are cross-cultural differences in the perceived benefits and harms associated with Western medications, especially long-term use, with traditional (non-Western) treatments being seen as preferable (Asiri et al., 2023). Within the UK, Alhomoud et al. (2015) reported that patients from South Asian and Middle Eastern origin were persuaded by relatives to avoid taking prescribed medications due to perceived harms outweighing any health benefits. Not receiving sufficient information about medication side effects and drug interactions that may be caused by **polypharmacy** (use of multiple medications by one person) was a concern for Indigenous women in the US. In addition, these women were worried about becoming addicted to pain medications and preferred to use traditional medicines over antibiotics, as the latter were viewed as treating symptoms rather than the underlying cause of a disease (Reese et al., 2025). A meta-synthesis of diabetes and cardiovascular medication adherence in people of South Asian origin found that patients who held positive beliefs about traditional medicines also had concerns about the toxicity of Western prescribed medications, which functioned as a barrier to adherence (Kumar et al., 2016). Levesque et al. (2024) explored adherence to medication in Indigenous patients, they found that nonadherence increased when patients felt that their health problems had not been thoroughly investigated and they had not received clear explanations of their medical condition or how the medication would help.

From a cultural perspective, adherence to diabetes medication can be affected by the stigma of being diagnosed with the condition, as some South Asian patients do not even tell their families about their diagnosis and treatment. South Asian patients in the UK have reported that a main barrier to controlling blood glucose comes from within their own communities, especially during family and community gatherings when the cultural etiquette involves eating sweet treats. Singh et al. (2012) found that the stigma of having diabetes was greater for young women of South Asian descent who were unmarried, as culturally, the disease was linked with having a physical weakness, which could have adverse consequences for marriage prospects. To avoid social stigma, many patients complied with the community norm of eating foods high in sugar. Family members often reinforce the stigma of diabetes by urging the individual not to divulge their diagnosis and some patients and family members were unaware of the long-term consequences of poorly controlled diabetes. In the same study, White patients also found dietary management was the most challenging aspect of diabetes, followed by the inconvenience of injecting insulin. White patients did not convey feelings of stigma or refrained from telling others about their condition; however, they did have concerns about injecting insulin, due to the others' stereotypic notions that injecting was associated with the use of illicit drugs.

Religious beliefs and adherence to medication

Religious beliefs can exert a strong influence on adherence to medication. Muslims are obligated to fast (refrain from food, drinks and medication) from sunrise to sunset during the holy month of **Ramadan**. People who have medical conditions, such as type 1 diabetes and solid organ transplants, are exempt from fasting during this time. Despite receiving advice from their doctor to avoid fasting, many patients disregard this advice to fulfil their religious obligations (Abolaban & Al-Moujahed, 2017). In exploring patient medication behaviours in South Asian and Middle Eastern Muslims living in the UK, Alhomoud et al. (2015) found that during Ramadan, many patients altered their medication regimen without consulting their doctors or pharmacists and believed that the temporary pause in medication, changing the dose or timing of doses would not be harmful to their health. Thousands of Muslims make the religious pilgrimage to Mecca for the Hajj every year, during this time, many people intentionally stop taking medications without health professional advice. Some Muslims believe that adhering to medication during this time is unnecessary, they prefer to drink the sacred Zamzam water, which originates from the ground underneath the Grand Mosque in Mecca, believing that this will not only keep their symptoms under control but also help to promote good overall health (Alhomoud et al., 2015). From these examples, it is clear that healthcare professionals must try to understand the spiritual needs of patients during Ramadan and the Hajj and provide considered and culturally sensitive advice to assist patients to fast safely. It has been suggested that any patient who has a medical condition that could be exacerbated by fasting, should be offered a pre-fasting assessment to discuss health concerns. This is especially salient for people with type 1 diabetes so that they are aware of and understand the warning signs of high and low blood glucose (Hassanein et al., 2017; Jahng et al., 2005).

Evidence also shows that religion and/or spiritual beliefs can increase adherence to medication in some chronic diseases. Jamil et al. (2022) explored health beliefs and medication adherence in South Asian immigrants in the US who had been prescribed medication for cardiovascular disease and T2DM. Patients who held religious or spiritual beliefs felt that they had a duty to take care of their health and this acted as a motivator to adhere to medication. These researchers also found that adhering to medication was associated with having a collaborative relationship with their healthcare professionals and support from family members.

BOX 6.3
CRITICAL THINKING

We know that adhering to health instructions and information is important. What personal, social, cultural and economic factors make it easier or harder to adhere to health recommendations?

Adherence to medication and chronic disease

There is limited research into adherence to medication for chronic diseases in LGBTQI+ populations, with the focus being on the human immunodeficiency virus (HIV) treatment for people who are HIV positive and preventative medications for people who are HIV negative. HIV affects the immune system, it cannot be cured, but it can be managed with **antiretroviral therapy** (ART) medications. Treatment for HIV can be compromised by poor adherence on the part of the patient and may involve a range of medication regimes that have varying side effects, nonadherence with ART can be poor, leading to excesses in morbidity and morality (Tadese et al., 2024). A range of factors can impact on adherence to ART, people who are employed, have higher incomes and educational levels, tend to have better adherence to ART, than people of lower socioeconomic status (Peltzer & Pengpid, 2013). Within the US, many African Americans have lower adherence rates to ART than other ethnic groups (Simoni et al., 2012). It has been postulated that this may be due, in part, to African American beliefs about HIV being a genetically engineered virus specifically targeted at poor African Americans, who are then used as 'guinea-pigs' to test out new ART medications (Bogart et al., 2010). In addition, many African Americans have a distrust of healthcare professionals due to experiences of paternalist care, microaggressions and discrimination, all of which can have negative consequences for medication adherence (Saha et al., 2011). To assess adherence barriers to ART in South Africa, Kagee and Delport (2010) interviewed patient advocates who supported patients with HIV. They found multifactorial reasons for nonadherence to ART, which included side effects of the medication, food insecurity (which led to problems taking medication on an empty stomach), transport issues to get to medical clinics, overcrowding and lack of confidentiality at clinics and judgemental attitudes from healthcare professionals. In addition, there were individual beliefs about HIV being God's will and it would be going against God's will to take medication to try to control or cure the disease, with those who received spiritual healing being less likely to adhere to medication. Medications to prevent HIV are known as **Pre-Exposure Prophylaxis** (PrEP). While PrEP can reduce the chance of getting HIV by around 99%, a scoping review found that transgender women's willingness to take PrEP was around 80%, but actual adherence was 35.4%. Barriers to PrEP included stigma, financial costs, medical mistrust and substance misuse (Teng et al., 2023).

When exploring LGBTQI+ research on medication adherence, some degree of caution may be required due to the terminology used. In a review of 937 studies, Rebić et al. (2023) found that the terms 'gender' and 'sex' were used interchangeably in 25% of studies. Furthermore, in 55% to 64% of studies, authors switched between terminology used to denote gender - 'men/women' and biological sex - 'male/female'. Such practices may mask intersectional health inequities and reporting of health outcomes for LGBTQI+ populations.

Healthcare system issues and adherence

People from LGBTQI+ groups are at greater risk of cardiovascular diseases, cancer and respiratory diseases than their cisgender and heterosexual counterparts (Fredriksen-Goldsen et al., 2017; Lick et al., 2013), which is thought to be due to minority stress. Many LGBTQI+ individuals are subjected to discrimination and harassment not just from the public, they often encounter institutional healthcare discrimination, which can be compounded by a lack of health professional competence to address the specific needs of this population (Haviland et al., 2020; Milner & McNally, 2020). In the US, a 2023 survey revealed that LGBTQI+ patients were twice as likely to experience negative interactions with healthcare providers compared to cisgender and heterosexual patients and this was more marked for Black and Hispanic adults, those on low incomes and younger adults (Montero et al., 2024). Many people from LGBTQI+ communities avoid seeking help for health problems, ignore cancer screening invitations, resort to concealing their gender and sexual identities when accessing healthcare (Layland et al., 2020; Saunders et al., 2021) and avoid repeat appointments, all of which can have negative impact on adherence to medication (Brooks et al., 2025; Mitzel et al., 2015). In the US, discrimination and stigmatising health barriers are even worse for LGBTQI+ people who come from ethnic minority groups, as they must overcome the intersection of multiple minority identities (Layland et al., 2020). Since January 2025, the rights of LGBTQI+ individuals in the US have been eradicated due to polices implemented by President Trump's administration. This has created further barriers to healthcare services, increased structural discrimination and abolishing current and future funding for health disparity research and care for LGBTQI+ populations (Cahill, 2025).

Noninclusive research practices and adherence

In 2023, the WHO estimated that one in six people across the globe were living with some type of disability and many require medication to manage their symptoms. People with disabilities, such as spinal cord injuries, multiple sclerosis, arthritis and strokes, may need to take multiple medications (Frahm et al., 2019; Gomides et al., 2021; Ostwald et al., 2006). Despite the number of people living with disabilities who are taking multiple medications (polypharmacy), there have been relatively few studies conducted on disability and adherence to medications, which may be due to disability being considered an exclusion criterion in many research studies. A systematic review of interventional studies on how to enhance medication adherence in chronic conditions (CVD, HIV/AIDS, hypertension, diabetes and respiratory disorders) found that even though women, older people and ethnic minorities face a greater prevalence of disability, they tended to be excluded from research studies (Nieuwlaat et al., 2014). This led Schwartz and Unni (2021) to re-explore the exclusion criteria of studies that Nieuwlaat et al. (2014) had included in their systematic review. Schwartz and Unni found that 34% of studies had excluded people because they had hearing, physical and/or cognitive disabilities. Such findings highlight the need for research to be more inclusive to represent the needs of people with disabilities, as they are an underrepresented population who may have specific needs to help improve their medication adherence and symptom control.

How to improve adherence to medication

Most of us will be familiar with non-intentional adherence, this is when an individual simply forgets to take their medication, to do exercises, misses a treatment appointment because they forgot, in fact the most cited reason for nonadherence is 'I forgot'. For medication, this can be overcome by using tablet boxes, with medication dispensed daily in a box for each day and compartments for morning, afternoon, evening and bedtime. Doing this can help an individual to check that they have taken the correct medication each day at the appropriate time. It is possible that an individual will forget to use their medication box, one strategy for overcoming this is to keep the box in the kitchen, near the kettle or the sink as a reminder, or to enable a mobile phone or smart speaker reminder.

In the past, it was thought that a person's health beliefs about the seriousness of an illness and the ensuing consequences would have an impact on medication adherence, that is, the more serious the illness the better the adherence. This does not seem to be the case, as people with life-threatening or eye conditions that can lead to blindness are no more likely to adhere to medication than those who take medication for non-life-threatening conditions. To try and explain how healthcare practitioners can help patients adhere to medication, Unni and Bae (2022) proposed the Hierarchical Model for Medication Adherence (HMMA, Figure 6.4). This suggests that for a person to adhere to medication, they need sufficient health literacy, appropriate beliefs about illness, belief about medication and medication self-efficacy.

When people have a good level of health literacy, it means that they understand their illness, their medication and the reasons for taking it, along with implications of nonadherence. The HMMA suggests that adherence is affected by health literacy, illness beliefs about the disease severity and how susceptible an individual believes they are to symptoms worsening. However, as we will see in Chapter 7, disease severity is not good a good predictor of engaging in health behaviours, even when coupled with cues to action, such as media campaigns and information leaflets. If the individual is knowledgeable about the benefits and any side effects of medication, their adherence decisions will depend on weighing the pros and cons of taking the medication. Beliefs about medication can impact adherence, if a medication is viewed as helping to control symptoms, reduce disease risks and there are very few or quite manageable side effects, the likelihood of

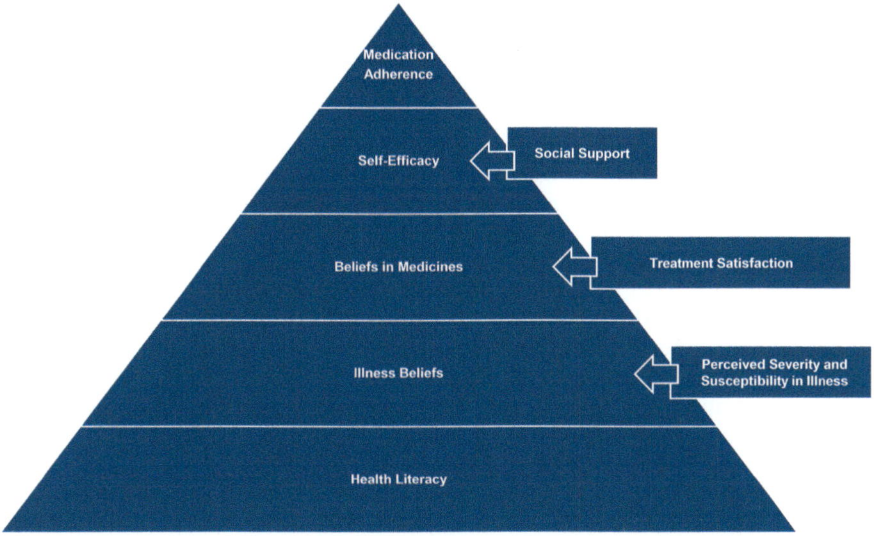

Figure 6.4
The Hierarchical Model for Medication Adherence (HMMA)

Source: Unni and Bae (2022)

adhering to medication may increase. There may be a need for help from others, with family or carer reminders to take medication and/or instrumental support, whereby someone orders, collects and delivers medication to community dwelling patients. The final aspect of this model is self-efficacy, which is concerned with an individual's confidence that they can take the medication as prescribed. People who have higher levels of medication self-efficacy generally display higher medication adherence. Unni and Bae (2022) believe that to assist patients with medication adherence, all the factors within their model must be in place.

Given that patients are the main stakeholders in the receipt of healthcare, it is imperative to ensure that patient needs are considered when medication is being prescribed. For patients to adhere to medication, they need to have some understanding of the health condition, why medication is being prescribed and how to take it. Thus, it is incumbent upon healthcare professionals to provide tailored health literacy advice that includes consideration of educational level, culture, polypharmacy, any food or drink restrictions associated with specific medications and medication side effects. In some healthcare services, the costs of medication may need to be considered and discussed with patients, as financial factors can be a barrier to adherence (Aremu et al., 2022).

Reasons for nonattendance at medical appointments

The cost to the health service for nonattendance at GP appointments in England in 2019 was around £216 million (Parsons et al., 2023). A systematic review of missed GP appointments across five countries (Australia, Canada, Malaysia, UK and US) found that on average, patients missed 15.2% of appointments, due to forgetting, the weather, transport problems, family, childcare and work commitments. Analysis of demographic factors showed those most likely to miss appointments were under 21 years old and from lower socioeconomic groups (Ellis et al., 2017; Parsons et al., 2021). This was confirmed by Alturbag (2024) who found that across a range of hospital appointment types and countries, older patients and those with higher levels of education were less likely to miss medical appointments.

Apart from having a financial impact, missed appointments can mean that other patients are waiting longer to see a healthcare professional and this may contribute to delayed diagnoses, treatment and needless suffering. For patients who must be seen in person, transport can be a barrier to attending medical appointments, especially for the elderly, patients with disabilities or people living in rural areas with poor transport links. GP working practices across the UK have changed since the COVID-19 pandemic, with more patients being offered online and telephone appointments. This has helped reduce missed appointments (Digital NHS, 2019), but it may act as a barrier for people with hearing impairments and those from lower socioeconomic groups who may not be able to access online appointments due to lack of internet access (Bryce et al., 2021).

Nonattendance at medical appointments and cultural factors

Research shows that nonattendance at medical appointments can also be influenced by cultural and geographical issues, which is especially true for Indigenous

Peoples (Copeland et al., 2017; Davy et al., 2016). Indigenous Australians are three times less likely to turn up for scheduled medical appointments compared to their non-Indigenous counterparts (Nancarrow et al., 2014). To get a fuller understanding of the reasons for nonattendance, researchers tried using structured telephone surveys; however, this does not always work for Indigenous Australian patients (Copeland et al., 2017), due to telephone and mobile phone signal problems related to geographical remoteness. More importantly, direct questioning about nonattendance is culturally inappropriate and interpreted as apportioning blame. To overcome these twin problems, Copeland et al. (2017) conducted interviews with patients who had attended for ophthalmology appointments but had missed a previous appointment. They found that the three most common reasons for nonattendance were appointments being scheduled at short notice and having other commitments (39%), transport problems (19%) and having forgotten about the appointment (14%). The short notice in scheduling appointments was a deliberate attempt by staff to increase attendance, as previous experiences had shown that appointments made more than a week in advance were unlikely to be attended. To combat the logistics of patients travelling to clinics, local staff who knew where people lived provided transport to clinics, forgetfulness was addressed using several types of appointment reminders, including postal mail, e-mail, telephone, in person and hand-delivered reminders, with all patients receiving more than one type of reminder. The researchers concluded that this patient-centred approach was successful due to the time and investment of staff who understood the specific barriers to attendance for this population.

Within Canada, around 60% of the Indigenous population live in rural or remote areas (Organisation for Economic Cooperation and Development, 2020), the remoteness of such communities may impact adherence to medications due to difficulties in reaching pharmacies (Orr, 2011). In addition, Mandal and Phillips (2022) pointed out that the difficulty in retaining healthcare professionals in rural locations and high staff turnover may contribute to understaffing, a lack of trust, continuity of care and cultural competence, all of which may adversely impact adherence.

While there may be some similarity in reasons for nonattendance between Indigenous and non-Indigenous populations (e.g. forgetting about the appointment and transport issues), negative healthcare experiences, such as discrimination, racism and unmet needs, are salient factors for Indigenous patients not attending medical appointments (Harris et al., 2019). Health professionals may unconsciously relay biased attitudes towards Indigenous patients through the use of stereotypic descriptors by using labels, such as 'non-compliers' or 'drug seekers'. Indigenous patients may present to healthcare services later in a disease trajectory, with higher disease burdens, and healthcare professionals may view these patients through a biased lens as less worthy of care and less capable of looking after their own health (Turpel-Lafond, 2020). Across the Western and colonialised world, healthcare provision tends to be delivered within a Western biomedical framework, which emphasises individual responsibility, such an approach ignores the understanding and importance of harmony with the land and spirituality that are central aspects of Indigenous holistic health. This discord helps maintain a power imbalance between healthcare professions and Indigenous peoples that can impact adherence. Poor doctor – patient communication, along with a lack of continuity of care can have negative consequences for adherence (Orr, 2011). Recognising the needs of and listening to the wishes of Indigenous patients, including being open and accepting the use of traditional healing, can have positive impacts on patient empowerment, which can facilitate adherence (Ratner et al., 2017).

To combat nonattendance at medical appointments, healthcare services are resorting to sending text and e-mail reminders or phoning up patients to confirm that they intend to come to the appointment. However, research by Alhamad (2013) indicated that some missed appointments could be explained by patients having received notifications too late for them to attend. Within the UK, non-emergency access to hospital consultants, treatment and tests usually involves making an appointment with a GP, who then refers the patient to a hospital. This can be a lengthy process and there is a correlation between the length of time to get an appointment and nonattendance, which may be due to symptoms having been resolved, reduced or patients having sought privately funded treatment but not cancelling their NHS appointment.

Some studies report gender differences in missed medical appointments. In a systematic review, Alturbag (2024) reported on studies conducted in Australia, Demark, the UK and Singapore; they found that women were more likely to attend appointments compared to men. Previous research has suggested that men are less inclined to attend for treatment and screening because they often try to self-manage medical problems (Niño de Guzmán Quispe et al., 2021), but this is not a universal finding. Transport issues related to cultural factors were the main reason for women being more likely to miss appointments than men in Saudi Arabia (Alturbag, 2024). Prior to 2018, women in Saudi Arabia were not permitted to drive cars and even today, cultural prohibitions about unaccompanied women using public transport remain.

Within Oman, Alawadhi et al. (2022) found that forgetting about a medical appointment was one of the main reasons for women's nonattendance, which occurred even if text message reminders had been sent. These researchers explained that when women attend hospital appointments, they are usually accompanied by a man (family member) who acts as a chaperone and registers the woman's attendance. Any follow-up appointments are sent to the chaperone's mobile number, rather than to the woman, who may not have been informed of subsequent appointments. Even if attending an appointment on their own, for cultural reasons, women in Oman will not provide their personal mobile telephone number, especially as patient check-in staff are more likely to be men.

There are many intersecting factors that impact adherence, which include personal, health system, income, education, religion, ethnicity, culture, gender and sexual orientation. It is apparent that training in cultural competence may help healthcare professionals to understand patient needs and beliefs about illness, culture backgrounds and religious beliefs, along with preferences around the use of traditional health practices. Training may also help health professionals to reflect on their own unconscious biases, especially when interacting with patients from marginalised and minority groups.

Chapter Summary

Define the concept of adherence in healthcare contexts

Adherence involves active engagement in making healthy lifestyle choices, treatment-related decisions and attendance at health-related appointments. Adherence can be partial, meaning that not all instructions and advice have been followed. Adherence can be influenced by a range of cognitive, social and cultural factors.

Describe the socio-cultural-cognitive model of adherence that goes beyond understanding, memory and satisfaction when considering factors that influence adherence

Ley's (1986) conceptualisation of adherence provides explanations of why people do not adhere to medication, treatment or advice that includes understanding, satisfaction and memory, but fails to consider cultural beliefs, ethnicity, minority status associated with gender identity, sexual orientation and disability and past discriminatory experience.

Explain the concept of health literacy and discuss how it influences patient adherence and health outcomes

Health literacy is concerned with an individual's ability to locate, understand and make use of health information and how to use services. Nutbeam (2000) identified three levels of health literacy, which are functional, interactive and critical. Low health literacy is associated with poorer adherence and health outcomes, which can be related to lower educational levels, culture and health beliefs.

Identify methods used to measure health literacy and why they may not be applicable to everyone

There are over 150 scales that measure health literacy, but they vary in the degree to which they tap into the multidimensional nature of health literacy, with some only providing an indication of being able to read and pronounce words. A multidimensional scale can be more appropriate in assessing health literacy, but the scale used needs to be culturally appropriate for the population for whom it is used. For example, health literacy scales are usually based on Western conceptualisations of health and ignore the holistic nature of Indigenous health, thereby ignoring important cultural aspects of health and disease in these populations.

Explain how culture, ethnicity and intersectionality can shape adherence

Culture shapes beliefs about illness, health, medications and health behaviours, which can be further influenced by religious beliefs. Previous discriminatory healthcare experiences due to ethnicity, gender identity, sexual orientation and disability can intersect, impacting trust in healthcare professionals, which can have detrimental impacts on adherence.

Outline the key components of the World Health Organization's Multidimensional Adherence Model

This model identifies five components that can interact to influence adherence to medication. Patient factors include demographic characteristics, attitudes and health literacy. Socioeconomic factors, such as marital status, employment, income and education levels, can have impacts on health literacy and affordability of medications. Treatment-related factors are connected to treatment complexity, as well as side effects and duration of medication. Condition-related factors are concerned with the chronicity of the disease, how severe symptoms are and more so if the person has other diseases. Healthcare-related factors can include the patient/healthcare professional relationships and being able to access care and waiting times.

Describe strategies to improve medication adherence, included in the hierarchical model of adherence

Adherence to medication can be enhanced through better health literacy, addressing illness beliefs about the medication and improving social support from others. The latter can include reminders to take medication, ordering and collecting medication on behalf of an individual. The importance of a person believing that they can take the medication as prescribed, that is self-efficacy, is the final aspect in this model.

Explain how culture, ethnicity and intersectionality can shape nonadherence at medical appointments

Often, the key reason for nonattendance is 'I forgot'; however, other factors such as the weather, transport problems, caring responsibility and socioeconomic status can impact attendance. Living in a rural location and time from receipt of appointment to the appointment date can also affect decisions to attend medical appointment. Factors such as ethnicity and gender can present as intersectional barriers to using public transport and being able to attend appointments without a chaperone in some cultures.

Keywords

Immunosuppressive: Medication that reduces or suppresses the immune response, usually used to prevent rejection of transplanted organs.

Adherence: Involves active engagement in making healthy lifestyle choices, treatment-related decisions and attendance at health-related appointments.

Intentional nonadherence: Making an active decision not to adhere to medical advice, treatment or attend appointments. Intentional nonadherence can also be partial.

Unintentional nonadherence: Usually related to forgetting to take medication or attend appointments or not understanding the health advice or instructions provided by a healthcare professional.

Functional health literacy: Being able to read, understand and use health information to make health decisions about taking medication or attending appointments.

Interactive health literacy: The ability to actively engage in conversations and decision-making with healthcare professionals, asking questions and applying health information to daily living.

Critical health literacy: To critically analyse health information, evaluate relevance of the information and engage in critical thinking about healthcare policies and advocate for change.
Multidimensional scale: A scale that measures more than one aspect of the topic being assessed.
Back translation: Text is translated from the original language into the target language by one person and translated back into the original language by another person.
Trans-specific care: Healthcare that is tailored to suit the needs of transgender people.
Lacking ability to consent: When an individual cannot understand information to make informed decisions about their own healthcare due to learning disability, age, severe mental health problems or other conditions and problems that impact cognitive ability.
Partial doses: Not taking the full dose of a prescribed medication.
Polypharmacy: The use of multiple medications at the same time.
Ramadan: A month of fasting from dawn to sunset that occurs annually in the Muslim faith.
Antiretroviral therapy: Medication prescribed for an individual who has HIV, to suppress the immune system and prevent the development of AIDS.
Pre-Exposure Prophylaxis: A preventative medication taken by people who are HIV negative to reduce the risk of contracting HIV.
Stereotypic descriptors: Words or phrases that are used to generalise beliefs to all people within certain groups, usually based on ethnicity, religion, socioeconomic status, disability, gender identity and sexual orientation.

Key Readings

Alturbag, M. (2024). Factors and reasons associated with appointment non-attendance in hospitals: A narrative review. *Cureus*, *16*(4): e58594. https://doi.org/10.7759/cureus.58594

Aremu, T. O., Oluwole, O. E., Adeyinka, K. O., & Schommer, J. C. (2022). Medication adherence and compliance: Recipe for improving patient outcomes. *Pharmacy*, *10*(5), 106. https://doi.org/10.3390/pharmacy10050106

Dale, S. K., Bogart, L. M., Wagner, G. J., Galvan, F. H., & Klein, D. J. (2016). Medical mistrust is related to lower longitudinal medication adherence among African-American males with HIV. *Journal of Health Psychology*, *21*(7), 1311–1321. https://doi.org/10.1177/1359105314551950

These reflective questions are designed to encourage you to think about the material presented in this chapter:

1. Outline what is meant by adherence and explain factors that may influence adherence across different population groups.
2. What is health literacy and why is it important for adherence?
3. How can culture affect whether people attend medical appointments?

References

Abolaban, H., & Al-Moujahed, A. (2017). Muslim patients in Ramadan: A review for primary care physicians. *Avicenna Journal of Medicine, 7*(3), 81–87. https://doi.org/10.4103/ajm.AJM_76_17

Alawadhi, A., Palin, V., & van Staa, T. (2022). Investigating the reasons for missing an outpatient appointment in Royal Hospital, Sultanate of Oman: Perspectives of patients and medical staff in a survey. *Health Science Reports, 5*, e470. https://doi.org/10.1002/hsr2.470

Alhamad, Z. M. (2013). Reasons for missing appointments in general clinics of primary health care center in Riyadh Military Hospital, Saudi Arabia. *International Journal of Medicine Science and Public Health, 2*, 258–67. https://doi.org/10.5455/ijmsph.2013.2.256-265

Alhomoud, F., Dhillon, S., Aslanpour, Z., & Smith, F. (2015). South Asian and Middle Eastern patients' perspectives on medicine-related problems in the United Kingdom. *International Journal of Clinical Pharmacy, 37*(4), 607–615. https://doi.org/10.1007/s11096-015-0103-6

Allen, K. A., Charpentier, V., Hendrickson, M. A., Kessler, M., Gotlieb, R., Marmet, J., Hause, E., Praska, C., Lunos, S., & Pitt, M. B. (2023). Jargon be gone - Patient preference in doctor communication. *Journal of Patient Experience, 10*, 23743735231158942. https://doi.org/10.1177/23743735231158942

Al Maqbali, M., Hughes, C., Gracey, J., Rankin, J., Hacker, E., & Dunwoody, L. (2020). Psychometric properties of the Arabic version of the functional assessment of chronic illnesses therapy-fatigue in Arabic cancer patients. *Journal of Pain and Symptom Management, 59*(1), 130–138.e2. https://doi.org/10.1016/j.jpainsymman.2019.10.008

Altin, S. V., Finke, I., Kautz-Freimuth, S., & Stock, S. (2014). The evolution of health literacy assessment tools: A systematic review. *BMC Public Health, 14*, 1207. https://doi.org/10.1186/1471-2458-14-1207

Alturbag, M. (2024). Factors and reasons associated with appointment non-attendance in hospitals: A narrative review. *Cureus 16*(4): e58594. https://doi.org/10.7759/cureus.58594

Anghel, L. A., Farcas, A. M., & Oprean, R. N. (2019). An overview of the common methods used to measure treatment adherence. *Medicine and Pharmacy Reports, 92*(2), 117–122. https://doi.org/10.15386/mpr-1201

Aparicio-García, M. E., Díaz-Ramiro, E. M., Rubio-Valdehita, S., López-Núñez, M. I., & García-Nieto, I. (2018). Health and well-being of cisgender, transgender and non-binary young people. *International Journal of Environmental Research and Public Health, 15*(10), 2133. https://doi.org/10.3390/ijerph15102133

Aremu, T. O., Oluwole, O. E., Adeyinka, K. O., & Schommer, J. C. (2022). Medication adherence and compliance: Recipe for improving patient outcomes. *Pharmacy, 10*(5), 106. https://doi.org/10.3390/pharmacy10050106

Asiri, R., Robinson-Barella, A., Iqbal, A., Todd, A., & Husband, A. (2023). Understanding the influence of ethnicity on adherence to antidiabetic medication: Meta-ethnography and systematic review. *PloS One, 18*(10), e0292581. https://doi.org/10.1371/journal.pone.0292581

Australian Commission on Safety and Quality in Health Care (2015). *Health literacy: Taking action to improve safety and quality*. Australian Commission on Safety and Quality in Health Care. https://www.safetyandquality.gov.au/publications-and-resources/resource-library/health-literacy-taking-action-improve-safety-and-quality

Baccolini, V., Rosso, A., Di Paolo, C., Isonne, C., Salerno, C., Miglara, C., Prencipe, G. P., Massimi, A., Marzuillo, C., De vito, C., Villari, P., & Romano, F. (2021). What is the prevalence of low health literacy in European Union member states? A systematic review and meta-analysis. *Journal of General Internal Medicine, 26*, 753–761. https://doi.org/10.1007/s11606-020-06407-8

Barbosa, C. D., Balp, M. M., Kulich, K., Germain, N., & Rofail, D. (2012). A literature review to explore the link between treatment satisfaction and adherence, compliance, and persistence. *Patient Preference and Adherence, 6*, 39–48. https://doi.org/10.2147/PPA.S24752

Berkman, N. D., Dewalt, D. A., Pignone, M. P., Sheridan, S. L., Lohr, K. N., Lux, L., Sutton, S. F., Swinson, T., & Bonito, A. J. (2004). Literacy and health outcomes. *Evidence Report/Technology Assessment, 87*, 1–8.

Berkman, N., Sheridan, S., Donahue, K., Halpern, D., & Crotty, K. (2011). Low health literacy and health outcomes: An updated systematic review. *Annals of Internal Medicine, 15*(2), 97–107. https://doi.org/10.7326/0003-4819-155-2-201107190-00005

Berry, L. L., Danaher, T. S., Beckham, D., Awdish, R. L. A., & Mate, K. S. (2017). When patients and their families feel like hostages to health care. *Mayo Clinic Proceedings, 92*(9), 1373–1381. https://doi.org/10.1016/j.mayocp.2017.05.015

Bessarab, D., & Ng'andu, B. (2010). Yarning about yarning as a legitimate method in Indigenous research. *International Journal of Critical Indigenous Studies, 3*(1), 37–50. https://doi.org/10.5204/ijcis.v3i1.57

Bishop, R., Laugharne, R., Shaw, N., Russell, A. M., Goodley, D., Banerjee, S., Clack, E., Shankar, R.; SpeakUp, CHAMPS (2024). The inclusion of adults with intellectual disabilities in health research - Challenges, barriers and opportunities: A mixed-method study among stakeholders in England. *Journal of Intellectual Disability Research, 68*(2), 140–149. https://doi.org/10.1111/jir.13097

Bogart, L. M., Wagner, G., Galvan, F. H., & Banks, D. (2010). Conspiracy beliefs about HIV are related to antiretroviral treatment nonadherence among African American men with HIV. *Journal of Acquired Immune Deficiency Syndromes, 53*(5), 648–655. https://doi.org/10.1097/QAI.0b013e3181c57dbc

Boot, G. R., & Lowell, A. (2019). Acknowledging and promoting Indigenous knowledges, paradigms, and practices within health literacy-related policy and practice documents across Australia, Canada, and New Zealand. *The International Indigenous Policy Journal, 10*(3). https://ir.lib.uwo.ca/iipj/vol10/iss3/2

Brooks, B. D., Job, S. A., Kaniuka, A. R., Kolb, R., Unda Charvel, P., & Araújo, F. (2025). Healthcare discrimination and treatment adherence among sexual and gender minority individuals living with chronic illness: The mediating effects of anticipated discrimination and depressive symptoms. *Psychology & Health, 40*(2), 304–320. https://doi.org/10.1080/08870446.2023.2220008

Bryce, C., O'Connell, M. D., Dale, J., Underwood, M., & Atherton, H. (2021). Online and telephone access to general practice: A cross-sectional patient survey. *BJGP Open, 5*(4). https://doi.org/10.3399/BJGPO.2020.0179

Cahill, S. R. (2025). A severe dismantling of LGBTQI+ health equity and equality: Impact of new U.S. policies on the global response to HIV. *Journal of the International AIDS Society, 28*(5), e26485. https://doi.org/10.1002/jia2.26485

Chinn, D., & Homeyard, C. (2017). Easy read and accessible information for people with intellectual disabilities: Is it worth it? A meta-narrative literature review. *Health Expectations, 20*(6), 1189–1200. https://doi.org/10.1111/hex.12520

Copeland, S., Muir, J., & Turner, A. (2017). Understanding Indigenous patient attendance: A qualitative study. *Australian Journal of Rural Health, 25*, 268–274. https://doi.org/10.1111/ajr.12348

Davidson, P. M., Abbott, P., Davison, J., & DiGiacomo, M. (2010). Improving medication uptake in Aboriginal and Torres Strait islander Peoples. *Heart Lung and Circulation, 19*(5–6), 372–377. https://doi.org/10.1016/j.hlc.2010.01.010

Davison, J., Maguire, S., McLaughlin, M., & Simms, V. (2022). Involving adolescents with intellectual disability in the adaptation of self-reported subjective well-being measures: Participatory research and methodological considerations. *Journal of Intellectual Disability Research, 66*(7), 628–641. https://doi.org/10.1111/jir.12936

Davy, C., Harfield, S., McArthur, A., Munn, Z., & Brown, A. (2016). Access to primary health care services for Indigenous peoples: A framework synthesis. *International Journal for Equity in Health, 15*, 163. https://doi.org/10.1186/s12939-016-0450-5

de Jesus, P. R., Bianchini, B., Ziegelmann, P. K., & Dal Pizzol, T. D. S. (2024). The low health literacy in Latin America and the Caribbean: A systematic review and meta-analysis. *BMC Public Health, 24*, 1478. https://doi.org/10.1186/s12889-024-18972-2

Dewalt, D. A., Berkman, N. D., Sheridan, S., Lohr, K. N., & Pignone, M. P. (2004). Literacy and health outcomes: A systematic review of the literature. *Journal of General Internal Medicine, 19*(12), 1228–1239. https://doi.org/10.1111/j.1525-1497.2004.40153.x

Digital NHS (2019). *Appointments in general practice November 2019*. https://digital.nhs.uk/data-and-information/publications/statistical/appointments-in-general-practice/november-2019

Eliason, M. J., Robinson, P., & Balsam, K. (2017). Development of an LGB-specific health literacy scale. *Health Communication, 33*(12), 1531–1538. https://doi.org/10.1080/10410236.2017.1372052

Ellis, D. A., McQueenie, R., McConnachie, A., Wilson, P., & Williamson, A. E. (2017). Demographic and practice factors predicting repeated non-attendance in primary care: A national retrospective cohort analysis. *The Lancet. Public Health, 2*(12), e551–e559. https://doi.org/10.1016/S2468-2667(17)30217-7

Feldman, M. A., Owen, F., Andrews, A. E., Tahir, M., Barber, R., & Griffiths, D. (2016). Randomized control trial of the 3Rs health knowledge training program for persons with intellectual disabilities. *Journal of Applied Research in Intellectual Disabilities, 29*(3), 278–288. https://doi.org/10.1111/jar.12186

Foley, L., Larkin, J., Lombard-Vance, R., Murphy, A. W., Hynes, L., Galvin, E., & Molloy, G. J. (2021). Prevalence and predictors of medication non-adherence among people living with multimorbidity: A systematic review and meta-analysis. *BMJ Open, 11*(9), e044987. https://doi.org/10.1136/bmjopen-2020-044987

Frahm, N., Hecker, M., & Zettl, U. K. (2019). Multi-drug use among patients with multiple sclerosis: A cross-sectional study of associations to clinicodemographic factors. *Scientific Reports, 9*(1), 3743. https://doi.org/10.1038/s41598-019-40283-5

Fredriksen-Goldsen, K. I., Kim, H. J., Shui, C., & Bryan, A. E. (2017). Chronic health conditions and key health indicators among lesbian, gay, and bisexual older US adults, 2013–2014. *American Journal of Public Health, 107*(8), 1332–1338. https://doi.org/10.2105/AJPH.2017.303922

Gandolfini, I., Palmisano, A., Fiaccadori, E., Cravedi, P., & Maggiore, U. (2022). Detecting, preventing and treating non-adherence to immunosuppression after kidney transplantation. *Clinical Kidney Journal, 15*(7), 1253–1274. https://doi.org/10.1093/ckj/sfac017

Gomides, A. P. M., Albuquerque, C. P., Santos, A. B. V., Amorim, R. B. C., Bértolo, M. B., Júnior, P. L., Santos, I. A., Giorgi, R. D., Sacilotto, N. C., Radominski, S. C., Borghi, F. M., Guimarães, M. F. B. R., Pinto, M. R. C., Resende, G. G., Bonfiglioli, K. R., Carriço, H., Sauma, M. F. L. C., Sauma, M. L., Medeiros, J. B., Pereira, I. A., & Pinheiro, G. R. C. (2021). High levels of polypharmacy in rheumatoid arthritis - a challenge not covered by current management recommendations: Data from a large real-life study. *Journal of Pharmacy Practice, 34*(3), 365–371. https://doi.org/10.1177/0897190019869158

Ha Dinh, T. T., Bonner, A., Clark, R., Ramsbotham, J., & Hines, S. (2016). The effectiveness of the teach-back method on adherence and self-management in health education for people with chronic disease: A systematic review. *JBI Database of Systematic Reviews and Implementation Reports, 14*(1), 210–247. https://doi.org/10.11124/jbisrir-2016-2296

Harris, R. B., Cormack, D. M., & Stanley, J. (2019). Experience of racism and associations with unmet need and healthcare satisfaction: The 2011/12 adult New Zealand health survey. *Australian and New Zealand Journal of Public Health, 43*(1), 75–80. https://doi.org/10.1111/1753-6405.12835

Hassanein, M., Al-Arouj, M., Hamdy, O., Bebakar, W. M. W., Jabbar, A., Al-Madani, A., Hanif, W., Lessan, N., Basit, A., Tayeb, K., Omar, M., Abdallah, K., Al Twaim, A., Buyukbese, M. A., El-Sayed, A. A., Ben-Nakhi, A. & International Diabetes Federation, in collaboration with the Diabetes and Ramadan International Alliance (2017). Diabetes and Ramadan: Practical guidelines. *Diabetes Research and Clinical Practice, 126*, 303–316. https://doi.org/10.1016/j.diabres.2017.03.003

Haviland, K. S., Swette, S., Kelechi, T., & Mueller, M. (2020). Barriers and facilitators to cancer screening among LGBTQ individuals with cancer. *Oncology Nursing Forum, 47*(1), 44–55. https://doi.org/10.1188/20.ONF.44-55

Health Education England, Public Health England, NHS England, & Community Health and Learning Foundation. (2023). *Health literacy toolkit* (2nd ed.). NHS England Knowledge and Library Services. Retrieved July 29, 2025, from https://library.nhs.uk/health-literacy/

Jahng, K. H., Martin, L. R., Golin, C. E., & DiMatteo, M. R. (2005). Preferences for medical collaboration: Patient-physician congruence and patient outcomes. *Patient Education and Counseling, 57*(3), 308–314. https://doi.org/10.1016/j.pec.2004.08.006

Jamil, A., Jonkman, L. J., Miller, M., Jennings, L., & Connor, S. E. (2022). Medication adherence and health beliefs among South Asian immigrants with diabetes in the United States: A qualitative study. *Journal of the American College of Clinical Pharmacology, 5*(8), 829–836. https://doi.org/10.1002/jac5.1668

Kagee, A., & Delport, T. (2010). Barriers to adherence to antiretroviral treatment: The perspectives of patient advocates. *Journal of Health Psychology, 15*(7), 1001–1011. https://doi.org/10.1177/1359105310378180

Keshtkar, L., Madigan, C. D., Ward, A., Ahmed, S., Tanna, V., Rahman, I., Bostock, J., Nockels, K., Wang, W., Gillies, C. L., & Howick, J. (2024). The effect of practitioner empathy on patient satisfaction: A systematic review of randomized trials. *Annals of Internal Medicine, 177*(2), 196–209. https://doi.org/10.7326/M23-2168

Kessels, R. P. (2003). Patients' memory for medical information. *Journal of the Royal Society of Medicine, 96*(5), 219–222. https://doi.org/10.1177/014107680309600504

Konstantinou, P., Kassianos, A. P., Georgiou, G., Panayides, A., Papageorgiou, A., Almas, I., Wozniak, G., & Karekla, M. (2020). Barriers, facilitators, and interventions for medication adherence across chronic conditions with the highest non-adherence rates: A scoping review with recommendations for intervention development. *Translational Behavioral Medicine, 10*(6), 1390–1398. https://doi.org/10.1093/tbm/ibaa118

Kumar, K., Greenfield, S., Raza, K., Gill, P., & Stack, R. (2016). Understanding adherence-related beliefs about medicine amongst patients of South Asian origin with diabetes and cardiovascular disease patients: A qualitative synthesis. *BMC Endocrine Disorders, 16*(1), 24. https://doi.org/10.1186/s12902-016-0103-0

Kutner, M., Greenberg, E., Jin, Y., & Paulsen, C. (2006). *The health literacy of America's adults: Results from the 2003 national assessment of adult literacy*. National Center for Education Statistics. https://nces.ed.gov/pubsearch/pubsinfo.asp?pubid=2006483

Lambert, K., Mullan, J., Mansfield, K., & Lonergan, M. (2015). A cross-sectional comparison of health literacy deficits among patients with chronic kidney disease. *Journal of Health Communication, 20*(2), 16–23. https://doi.org/10.1080/10810730.2015.1080329

Layland, E. K., Carter, J. A., Perry, N. S., Cienfuegos-Szalay, J., Nelson, K. M., Bonner, C. P., & Rendina, H. J. (2020). A systematic review of stigma in sexual and gender minority health interventions. *Translational Behavioral Medicine, 10*(5), 1200–1210. https://doi.org/10.1093/tbm/ibz200

Legg, A. M., Andrews, S. E., Huynh, H., Ghane, A., Tabuenca, A., & Sweeny, K. (2015). Patients' anxiety and hope: Predictors and adherence intentions in an acute care context. *Health Expectations, 18*(6), 3034–3043. https://doi.org/10.1111/hex.12288

Levesque, A., Verde, M., Li, H. Z., Yu, B., & Chen, X. (2024). Factors influencing medical adherence among First Nations patients of European ancestry: Data from Canada. *SSM Qualitative Research in Health, 5*, 100424. https://doi.org/10.1016/j.ssmqr.2024.100424

Ley, P. (1986). Cognitive variables and noncompliance. *Journal of Compliance in Health Care, 1*(2), 171–188.

Lick, D. J., Durso, L. E., & Johnson, K. L. (2013). Minority stress and physical health among sexual minorities. *Perspectives on Psychological Science, 8*(5), 521–548. https://doi.org/10.1177/1745691613497965

Lin, I., Green, C., & Bessarab, D. (2016). 'Yarn with me': Applying clinical yarning to improve clinician–patient communication in Aboriginal health care. *Australian Journal of Primary Health, 22*(5), 377–382. https://doi.org/10.1071/PY16051

MacAskill, W., Rolleston, R. M., Brumpton, K., & Pinidiyapathiage, J. (2022). Assessing the health literacy of Aboriginal and Torres Strait Islander peoples presenting to general practice. *Australian Journal of General Practice, 51*(8), 621–625. https://doi.org/10.31128/AJGP-07-21-6100

Mandal, A., & Phillips, S. (2022). To stay or not to stay: The role of sense of belonging in the retention of physicians in rural areas. *International Journal of Circumpolar Health, 81*(1), 2076977. https://doi.org/10.1080/22423982.2022.2076977

Marks, B., & Sisirak, J. (2017). Nurse practitioners promoting physical activity: People with intellectual and developmental disabilities. *The Journal for Nurse Practitioners, 13*(1), 1–5. https://doi.org/10.1016/j.nurpra.2016.10.023

Miller, L. G., Liu, H., Hays, R. D., Golin, C. E., Beck, C. K., Asch, S. M., Ma, Y., Kaplan, A. H., & Wenger, N. S. (2002). How well do clinicians estimate patients' adherence to combination antiretroviral therapy? *Journal of General Internal Medicine, 17*(1), 1–11. https://doi.org/10.1046/j.1525-1497.2002.09004.x

Milner, G. E., & McNally, R. J. (2020). Nonadherence to breast and cervical cancer screening among sexual minority women: Do stigma-related psychological barriers play a role? *Health Psychology, 39*(10), 891–899. https://doi.org/10.1037/hea0000887

Mitzel, L. D., Vanable, P. A., Brown, J. L., Bostwick, R. A., Sweeney, S. M., & Carey, M. P. (2015). Depressive symptoms mediate the effect of HIV-related stigmatization on medication adherence among HIV-infected men who have sex with men. *AIDS and Behavior, 19*(8), 1454–1459. https://doi.org/10.1007/s10461-015-1038-6

Montero, A., Hamel, L., Artiga, S., & Dawson, L. (2024). *LGBT adults' experiences with discrimination and health care disparities: Findings from the KFF survey of racism, discrimination, and health*. KFF. https://www.kff.org/report-section/lgbt-adults-experiences-with-discrimination-and-health-care-disparities-findings/

Murphy, P. W., Davis, T. C., Long, S. W., Jackson, R. H., & Decker, B. C. (1993). Rapid Estimate of Adult Literacy in Medicine (REALM): A quick reading test for patients. *Journal of Reading, 37*, 124–130. https://www.jstor.org/stable/40033408

Nancarrow, S. A., Bradbury, J., & Avila, C. (2014). Factors associated with non-attendance in a general practice super clinic population in regional Australia: A retrospective cohort study. *The Australasian Medical Journal, 7*, 323–333. https://doi.org/10.4066/AMJ.2014.2098

Nguyen, T. M., La Caze, A., & Cottrell, N. (2014). What are validated self-report adherence scales really measuring?: A systematic review. *British Journal of Clinical Pharmacology, 77*(3), 427–445. https://doi.org/10.1111/bcp.12194

Nguyen, T. H., Paasche-Orlow, M. K., & McCormack, L. A. (2017). The state of the science of health literacy measurement. *Information Services & Use, 37*, 189–203. https://doi.org/10.3233/ISU-170827

Nguyen, M. H., Smets, E. M. A., Bol, N., Bronner, M. B., Tytgat, K. M. A. J., Loos, E. F., & van Weert, J. C. M. (2019). Fear and forget: How anxiety impacts information recall in newly diagnosed cancer patients visiting a fast-track clinic. *Acta Oncologica, 58*(2), 182–188. https://doi.org/10.1080/0284186X.2018.1512156

Nieuwlaat, R., Wilczynski, N., Navarro, T., Hobson, N., Jeffery, R., Keepanasseril, A., Agoritsas, T., Mistry, N., Iorio, A., Jack, S., Sivaramalingam, B., Iserman, E., Mustafa, R. A., Jedraszewski, D., Cotoi, C., & Haynes, R. B. (2014). Interventions for enhancing medication adherence. *The Cochrane Database of Systematic Reviews, 2014*(11), CD000011. https://doi.org/10.1002/14651858.CD000011.pub4

Niño de Guzmán Quispe, E., Martínez García, L., Orrego Villagrán, C., Heijmans, M., Sunol, R., Fraile-Navarro, D., Pérez-Bracchiglione, J., Ninov, L., Salas-Gama, K., Viteri García, A., & Alonso-Coello, P. (2021). The perspectives of patients with chronic diseases and their caregivers on self-management interventions: A scoping review of reviews. *The Patient, 14*(6), 719–740. https://doi.org/10.1007/s40271-021-00514-2

Nutbeam, D. (2000). Health literacy as a public health goal: A challenge for contemporary health education and communication strategies into the 21st century. *Health Promotion International, 15*, 259–267. http://doi.org/10.1093/heapro/15.3.259

Office of Disease Prevention and Health Promotion (n.d). *Health literacy – Healthy people 2030: Personal health literacy*. U.S. Department of Health and Human Services. https://odphp.health.gov/healthypeople/priority-areas/health-literacy-healthy-people-2030

Organisation for Economic Cooperation and Development. (2020). *Linking Indigenous communities with regional development in Canada*. https://www.oecd.org/en/publications/linking-indigenous-communities-with-regional-development-in-canada_fa0f60c6-en.html

Orr, P. (2011). Adherence to tuberculosis care in Canadian Aboriginal populations Part1: Definition, measurement, responsibility, barriers. *International Journal of Circumpolar Health, 70*(2), 113–127. https://doi.org/10.3402/ijch.v70i2.17809

Osborne, R. H., Batterham, R., Elsworth, G. R., Hawkins, M., & Buchbinder, R. (2013). The grounded theory, psychometric development and initial validation of the Health Literacy Questionnaire (HLQ). *BMC Public Health, 13*, 658. https://doi.org/10.1186/1471-2458-13-658

Osborne, R. H., Cheng, C. C., Nolte, S., Elmer, S., Besancon, S., Budhathoki, S. S., Debussche, X., Dias, S., Kolarčik, P., Loureiro, M. I., Maindal, H., Nascimento do O, D., Smith, J. A., Wahl, A., Elsworth, G. R., & Hawkins, M. (2022). Health literacy measurement: Embracing diversity in a strengths-based approach to promote health and equity, and avoid epistemic injustice. *BMJ Global Health, 7*(9), e009623. https://doi.org/10.1136/bmjgh-2022-009623

Ostwald, S. K., Wasserman, J., & Davis, S. (2006). Medications, comorbidities, and medical complications in stroke survivors: The CAReS study. *Rehabilitation 31*(1), 10–14. https://doi.org/10.1002/j.2048-7940.2006.tb00004.x

Parker, R. (2000). Health literacy: A challenge for American patients and their health care providers. *Health Promotion International, 15*(4), 277–283. https://doi.org/10.1093/heapro/15.4.277

Parsons, J., Bryce, C., & Atherton, H. (2021). Which patients miss appointments with general practice and the reasons why: A systematic review. *The British Journal of General Practice, 71*(707), e406–e412. https://doi.org/10.3399/BJGP.2020.1017

Parsons, J., Abel, G., Mounce, L. T., & Atherton, H. (2023). The changing face of missed appointments. *The British Journal of General Practice, 73*(728), 134–135. https://doi.org/10.3399/bjgp23X732249

Peltzer, K., & Pengpid, S. (2013). Socioeconomic factors in adherence to HIV therapy in low- and middle-income countries. *Journal of Health, Population, and Nutrition, 31*(2), 150–170. https://doi.org/10.3329/jhpn.v31i2.16379

Pho, A. T., Bakken, S., Lunn, M. R., Lubensky, M. E., Flentje, A., Dastur, Z., & Obedin-Maliver, J. (2022). Online health information seeking, health literacy, and human papillomavirus vaccination among transgender and gender-diverse people. *Journal of the American Medical Informatics Association, 29*(2), 285–295. https://doi.org/10.1093/jamia/ocab150

Piette, J. D., Beard, A., Rosland, A. M., & McHorney, C. A. (2011). Beliefs that influence cost-related medication non-adherence among the "haves" and "have nots" with chronic diseases. *Patient Preference and Adherence, 5*, 389–396. https://doi.org/10.2147/PPA.S23111

Ratner, N., Davis, E., Lhotka, L., Wille, S., & Walls, M. (2017). Patient-centered care, diabetes empowerment, and type 2 diabetes medication adherence among American Indian patients. *Clinical Diabetes, 35*(5), 281–285. https://doi.org/10.2337/cd17-0008

Rebić, N., Law, M. R., Cragg, J., Brotto, L. A., Ellis, U., Garg, R., Park, J. Y., & De Vera, M. A. (2023). What's sex and gender got to do with it? A scoping review of sex- and gender-based analysis in pharmacoepidemiologic studies of medication adherence. *Value in Health, 26*(9), 1413–1424. https://doi.org/10.1016/j.jval.2023.04.002

Reese, S. E., Liddell, J. L., & Mascarena, L. (2025). You just want to give me some medicine and be on my way: Preferences, beliefs, and experiences related to Western medication among members of a state-recognized tribe. *Journal of Holistic Nursing, 43*(2), 176–189. https://doi.org/10.1177/08980101231219357

Rheault, H., Coyer, F., & Bonner, A. (2021). Chronic disease health literacy in First Nations people: A mixed methods study. *Journal of Clinical Nursing, 30*, 2683–2695. https://doi.org/10.1111/jocn.15757

Rowlands, G., Protheroe, J., Winkley, J., Richardson, M., Seed, P. T., & Rudd, R. (2015). A mismatch between population health literacy and the complexity of health information: An observational study. *The British Journal of General Practice, 65*(635), e379–e386. https://doi.org/10.3399/bjgp15X685285

Saha, S., Sanders, D. S., Korthuis, P. T., Cohn, J. A., Sharp, V. L., Haidet, P., Moore, R. D., & Beach, M. C. (2011). The role of cultural distance between patient and provider in explaining racial/ethnic disparities in HIV care. *Patient Education and Counseling, 85*(3), e278–e284. https://doi.org/10.1016/j.pec.2011.01.012

Saunders, C. L., Massou, E., Waller, J., Meads, C., Marlow, L. A., & Usher-Smith, J. A. (2021). Cervical screening attendance and cervical cancer risk among women who have sex with women. *Journal of Medical Screening, 28*(3), 349–356. https://doi.org/10.1177/0969141320987271

Schwartz, J. K., & Unni, E. (2021). Inclusion of people with disabilities in research to improve medication adherence: A systematic review. *Patient Preference and Adherence, 15*, 1671–1677. https://doi.org/10.2147/PPA.S314135

Sheridan, S. L., Halpern, D. J., Viera, A. J., Berkman, N. D., Donahue, K. E., & Crotty, K. (2011). Interventions for individuals with low health literacy: A systematic review. *Journal of Health Communication, 16*(3), 30–54. https://doi.org/10.1080/10810730.2011.604391

Simoni, J. M., Huh, D., Wilson, I. B., Shen, J., Goggin, K., Reynolds, N. R., Remien, R. H., Rosen, M. I., Bangsberg, D. R., & Liu, H. (2012). Racial/ethnic disparities in ART adherence in the United States: Findings from the MACH14 study. *Journal of Acquired Immune Deficiency Syndromes, 60*(5), 466–472. https://doi.org/10.1097/QAI.0b013e31825db0bd

Singh, H., Cinnirella, M., & Bradley, C. (2012). Support systems for and barriers to diabetes management in South Asians and Whites in the UK: Qualitative study of patients' perspectives. *BMJ Open, 2*(6), e001459. https://doi.org/10.1136/bmjopen-2012-001459

Studer, C. M., Linder, M., & Pazzagli, L. (2023). A global systematic overview of socioeconomic factors associated with antidiabetic medication adherence in individuals with type 2 diabetes. *Journal of Health, Population, and Nutrition, 42*(1), 122. https://doi.org/10.1186/s41043-023-00459-2

Tadese, B. K., Hennessy, F., Salmon, P., Holbrook, T., & Prajapati, G. (2024). Adherence to antiretroviral therapy and its association with quality of life among people with HIV in the United States. *AIDS Care, 36*(12), 1869–1881. https://doi.org/10.1080/09540121.2024.2391439

Taylor, B., Lobont, C., Dayan, M., Merry, L., Jefferies, D., & Wellings, D. (2025). *Public satisfaction with the NHS and social care in 2024: Results from the British social attitudes survey*. The King's Fund & Nuffield Trust. National Centre for Social Research. Retrieved July 24, 2025, from https://www.kingsfund.org.uk/insight-and-analysis/reports/public-satisfaction-nhs-social-care-in-2024-bsa#satisfaction-with-the-nhs%C2%A0

Teng, F., Sha, Y., Fletcher, L. M., Welsch, M., Burns, P., & Tang, W. (2023). Barriers to uptake of PrEP across the continuum among transgender women: A global scoping review. *International Journal of STD & AIDS, 34*(5), 299–314. https://doi.org/10.1177/09564624231152781

Terwee, C. B., Bot, S. D., de Boer, M. R., van der Windt, D. A., Knol, D. L., Dekker, J., Bouter, L. M., & de Vet, H. C. (2007). Quality criteria were proposed for measurement properties of health status questionnaires. *Journal of Clinical Epidemiology, 60*(1), 34–42. https://doi.org/10.1016/j.jclinepi.2006.03.012

Teti, M., Kerr, S., Bauerband, L. A., Koegler, E., & Graves, R. (2021). A qualitative scoping review of transgender and gender non-conforming people's physical healthcare experiences and needs. *Frontiers in Public Health, 9*, 598455. https://doi.org/10.3389/fpubh.2021.598455

Turpel-Lafond, M. E. (2020). *In plain sight: Addressing Indigenous-specific racism and discrimination in B.C. health care*. https://engage.gov.bc.ca/app/uploads/sites/613/2020/11/In-Plain-Sight-Summary-Report.pdf

Unni, E., & Bae, S. (2022). Exploring a new theoretical model to explain the behavior of medication adherence. *Pharmacy, 10*(2), 43. https://doi.org/10.3390/pharmacy10020043

Vass, A., Mitchell, A., & Dhurrkay, Y. (2011). Health literacy and Australian Indigenous peoples: An analysis of the role of language and worldview. *Health Promotion Journal of Australia, 22*, 33–37. https://doi.org/10.1071/he11033

Visscher, B. B., Steunenberg, B., Heijmans, M., Hofstede, J. M., Devillé, W., van der Heide, I., & Rademakers, J. (2018). Evidence on the effectiveness of health literacy interventions in the EU: A systematic review. *BMC Public Health, 18*(1), 1414. https://doi.org/10.1186/s12889-018-6331-7

Weinman, J., Yusuf, G., Berks, R., Rayner, S., & Petrie, K. J. (2009). How accurate is patients' anatomical knowledge: A cross-sectional, questionnaire study of six patient groups and a general public sample. *BMC Family Practice, 10*, 43. https://doi.org/10.1186/1471-2296-10-43

Wikkeling-Scott, L. F., Ajja, R. J. Y., & Rikard, R. V. (2019). Health literacy research in the Eastern Mediterranean Region: An integrative review. *International Journal of Public Health, 64*, 523–533. https://doi.org/10.1007/s00038-018-01200-1

White, A., Sheehan, R., Ditzel, N., Ding, J., Roberts, C., Magill, N., Yu, M. K. L., Keagan-Bull, R., Chauhan, U., Tuffrey-Wijne, I., & Strydom, A. (2024). *Learning from lives and deaths – People with a learning disability and autistic people (LeDeR) report for 2023*. LeDeR Autism and Learning Disability Partnership, King's College London. https://www.kcl.ac.uk/ioppn/assets/pdfs/leder/leder-annual-report-2023.pdf

World Health Organization (2003). *Adherence to long-term therapies: Evidence for action*. Retrieved August 1, 2025, from https://iris.who.int/handle/10665/42682

World Health Organization (2023). *Ten facts about disability*. Retrieved August 1, 2025, from https://www.who.int/news-room/facts-in-pictures/detail/disabilities
World Health Organization (n.d.). *Health promotion: The mandate for health literacy*. Retrieved August 1, 2025, from https://www.who.int/teams/health-promotion/enhanced-wellbeing/ninth-global-conference/health-literacy

7 Health theories and models

Chapter contents

- Behaviour in the context of health psychology.
- Theories and models in health psychology.
- Early theories used to explain behaviours.
- Social cognitive models of health behaviour.
- Stage model of health behaviour.
- Behaviour prediction model of health.
- Multisystem model of health behaviour
- Indigenous models of health.
- Looking to the future.

Chapter objectives

After reading this chapter, you should be able to answer the following questions:

- Discuss how classical conditioning, operant conditioning and social learning theory may influence health behaviours.
- Outline the main components of the social cognitive models of health.
- Examine the stages and associated processes of change in the Transtheoretical Model.
- Discuss factors that influence behaviour intention in the Theory of Planned Behaviour.
- Outline the COM-B model and how it is related to intervention functions and policy categories in the Behaviour Change Wheel.
- Explain the Two-Eyed Seeing model and discuss why it is important to Indigenous health.
- Outline why the Medicine Wheel is of use when designing an intervention for Indigenous communities.
- Discuss how the He Pikinga Waiora model has been used as a guide to develop health interventions in New Zealand.

Behaviour in the context of health psychology

Actions or habits that improve overall health outcomes, such as physical activity, eating a healthy diet, getting sufficient sleep, engaging in stress management, disease preventative screening, vaccinations, health assessments, avoidance of harmful substances and maintaining social connections, are all viewed as **health**

DOI: 10.4324/9781003423157-7

enhancing behaviours. On the contrary, smoking, excessive alcohol consumption, eating an unhealthy diet, having a largely sedentary lifestyle and engaging in risky sexual behaviours, are all viewed as **health compromising behaviours**.

Theories and models in health psychology

Due to increased associations between lifestyle factors and disease, psychologists became interested in how to predict, explain and influence health enhancing and health risk behaviours. Kasl and Cobb (1966) viewed health behaviours as concerned with disease prevention or identifying disease before symptoms appeared, as in the case of cancer screening, focusing on the biomedical aspects of health behaviours. Whereas Conner and Norman (2015, p. 2) took a more holistic approach that considered health improvement, which was not tied to the notion of disease. Psychologists have developed numerous theories and models of health behaviour. Theories are systematic, they provide conceptual ideas, definitions and statements that can be used in a structured way to examine, predict and explain health behaviours (Glanz & Rimer, 2005). Models are a way of putting theories into action and a model can incorporate more than one theory. Theories and models use constructs or concepts that represent important variables (e.g. beliefs, attitudes, motivations, emotions, social norms, environmental and/or social influences); there are some overlaps between theories and models and the terms are often used interchangeably (Nilsen, 2015).

Theories and models have been used to predict and explain how individuals behave under specific circumstances. They are used to inform the development of interventions to promote behaviour change and need to be generalisable across different populations, social situations and environmental contexts (Skivington et al., 2021). The major theories and models used by health psychologists are based on Western conceptions of health that emphasise individual decision-making, which means that they may not directly transfer to cultures in which collective health decision-making is the norm.

Early theories used to explain behaviour

Classical conditioning

You may have heard of classical, operant conditioning and social learning theory; these types of learning propose that the likelihood of a behaviour occurring is dependent on the consequences associated with that behaviour. In **classical conditioning**, Pavlov (1927) showed that it was possible to teach a dog to salivate at the sound of a bell. Pavlov, who was a physiologist, conducted research into dogs' digestive systems; this research involved collecting saliva when the dogs were being fed. Salivation was a normal reflex that happened when the dogs smelt food, and it did not require any learning. Pavlov noticed that dogs salivated when they heard the footsteps of the person feeding them, as they had associated the sounds of footsteps with getting food. Pavlov wondered if it was possible to train a dog to salivate to another sound, such as a bell. The bell was a neutral stimulus, as the dogs had never heard it before, thus the bell had no meaning attached to it. Unsurprisingly, when Pavlov rang the bell the dogs did not respond. The bell was then paired with food (unconditioned stimulus) and the dogs salivated in response to

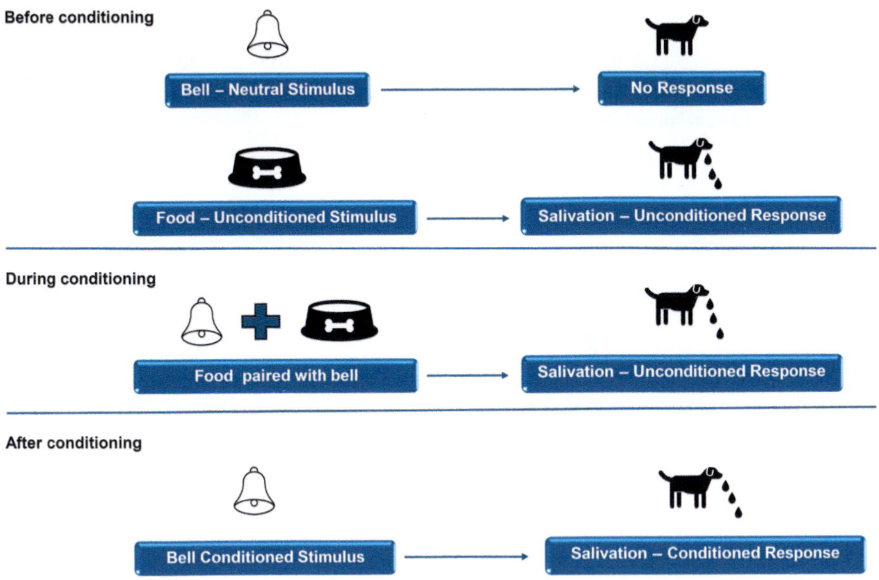

Figure 7.1
Classical conditioning in dogs

Source: Author

the food (unconditioned response). After several pairings of the food and bell, when Pavlov rang the bell, but presented no food, the dogs started to salivate. They had associated or learned the connection between food and the bell to the extent that the previously neutral bell had become a conditioned (learned) stimulus that produced salivation (conditioned response; see Figure 7.1). Pavlov went on to show how this type of learning could be generalised to different sounds, colours and objects. The important aspect of classical conditioning is that it involves reflexive behaviours that we have little control over, e.g. the fear response, salivation, the eye blink reflex, the vomit reflex, etc.

Behaviour therapy based on classical conditioning

Classical conditioning has been used to explain why in certain situations, patients can feel nauseated when they enter medical-type environments. Some chemotherapy drugs cause nausea and vomiting, this is despite the patient receiving drugs to prevent these symptoms. Patients may start to associate nausea and vomiting with some aspect of the hospital environment; this can include driving into the car park, sounds, smells and tastes of certain foods or drinks that were consumed during a hospital appointment (see Figure 7.2). Even after just one session of chemotherapy, up to one-third of patients report feelings of anticipatory nausea (Hickok et al., 2001; Stockhorst et al., 2006). Once this associative learning has occurred, it can be somewhat resistant to anti-nausea medication.

Anticipatory nausea may also be associated with anxiety about feeling sick due to the impending administration of chemotherapy; it may be helped by systematic desensitisation, which is a type of counterconditioning (Figueroa-Moseley et al., 2007). First, the patient is helped to make a hierarchical list of events that may

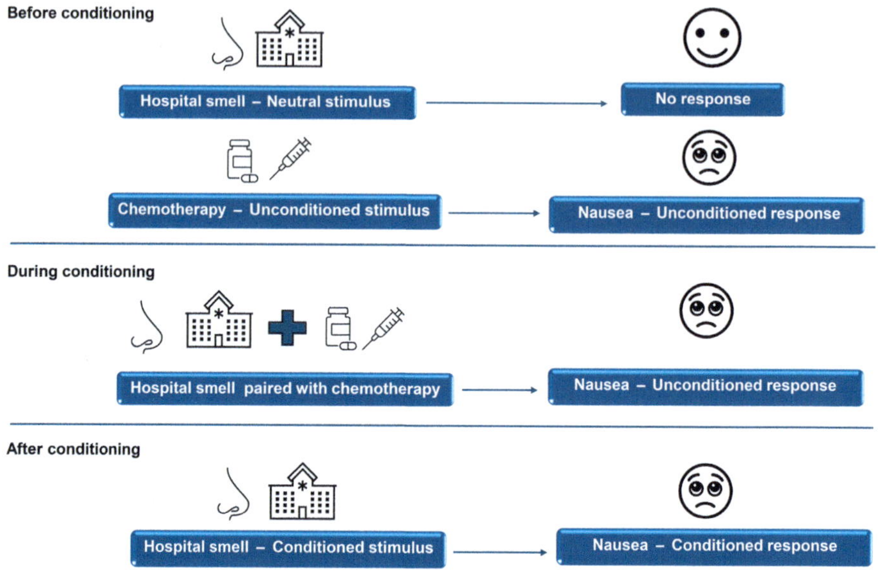

Figure 7.2
Classical conditioned nausea and smell of hospital

Source: Author

contribute to feeling anxious about nausea and sickness on the days they are having chemotherapy. This starts off with events that may cause mild anxiety about nausea, such as thoughts about going to the appointment, travelling to the hospital, seeing the hospital, smells associated with the car park, walking to the hospital doors and at the top of the hierarchy the specific hospital smell that induces nausea. Over several sessions, the patient is taught a progressive relaxation routine, when totally relaxed, they are asked to imagine getting ready to go to the hospital and gradually going through the hierarchy of activities associated with travelling to get their chemotherapy. If the patient starts to experience feelings of nausea when moving through the hierarchy, they are asked to indicate this and concentrate on relaxation. While systematic desensitisation is a useful adjunct in helping to treat anticipatory nausea, it is time consuming, as it usually requires one-to-one therapy, it takes around 10 sessions and may not be suitable for all patients (Hailey & White, 1983).

BOX 7.1
CRITICAL THINKING

An individual has an aversion to a specific drink, can you think how classical conditioning may be used to explain this?

How might classical conditioning be used to explain why an individual develops a fear of going to the dentist?

Operant conditioning

Operant conditioning is credited to Skinner (1953) whose early work with rats and later with pigeons illustrated how it was possible to condition (teach) voluntary behaviours (those which we have a choice over doing) using reinforcement (tangible rewards). Skinner was able to condition a pigeon to peck at a coloured disc (see Figure 7.3). As pigeons naturally engage in pecking behaviour, Skinner was able to gradually shape the pigeon's pecking behaviours using successive approximations. To manage this, the pigeon was placed in a special container, called a 'Skinner Box', which had a coloured disc on the wall. When the pigeon pecked the floor nearer to the disc, it received a food pellet, then it had to get closer to the disc before it received the food pellet, then it only got a pellet if it pecked the wall where the disc was placed and finally it only received a food pellet when the disc was pecked. Every time the pigeon pecked the disc, it was reinforced with food; this is an example of continuous reinforcement.

Skinner was able to change how often the pigeon was reinforced (received a food pellet) by using different schedules of reinforcement and these were based on time or the number of responses. A fixed interval (FI) meant that if the behaviour occurred within a set time period (e.g. 60 seconds) reinforcement was provided, which contrasted with varying the amount of time (variable interval; VI) the pigeon had to wait to get reinforced. If the pigeon was on a fixed ratio (FR) schedule, it had to peck at the disc a set number of times before getting reinforcement and on a variable ratio (VR) schedule, reinforcement was provided after a random number of responses. In VI and VR schedules, the reinforcer is provided at an average time or after an average number of responses respectively. For example, VI 5 means that on average, provided the behaviour occurs, the pigeon will be reinforced about every 5 minutes, but the time changes, the reinforcement could be delivered at the 3rd or 6th minute. For a VR 5, the pigeon gets reinforced, on average, after every 5th peck of the disc, but reinforcement will be received

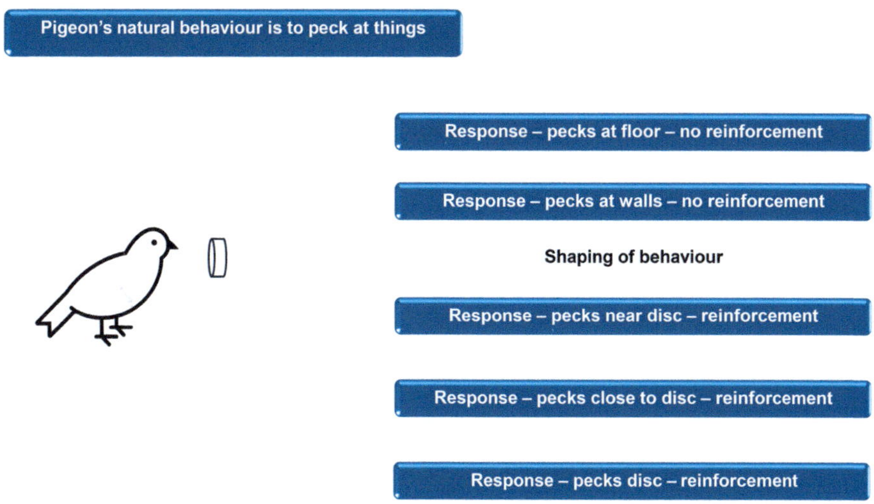

Figure 7.3
Operant conditioning of a pigeon

Source: Author

after an unpredictable number of target behaviours, e.g. it may happen on the 4th or 7th response. VI and VR schedules of reinforcement tend to result in higher response rates than fixed ones, with VR providing the greatest duration of responding, due to the unpredictability of reinforcement. In our everyday lives, we are exposed to various schedules of reinforcement, which can impact all types of behaviours, including health-related ones, such as the examples provided in Table 7.1.

The principles of operant conditioning are used in everyday life, take, for example, when we tell children if they are good, they will get some sweets or pocket money, hence their good behaviour is positively reinforced. The time interval between the target behaviour (being good) and reinforcement (sweets) must not be too long, especially for children, or the reinforcer (sweets) may not be associated with the target behaviour. Skinner distinguished between primary

Table 7.1 Schedule of reinforcement in health-related activities

Schedule	Behaviour	Reinforcer	Effect of no reinforcer
Continuous reinforcement received after every target behaviour.	Going out for a walk every day.	Chatting with friends when walking.	Friends go on holiday, no one to chat to, the individual may stop walking.
Fixed Interval (FI 7) Reinforcement received every 7 days (if the behaviour occurs).	Weekly weigh-in as part of a weight loss programme.	Receives praise for weight loss.	May eat less food and more healthily as weigh-in day approaches. Healthy food consumption may drop off after the reinforcer is received.
Variable Interval (VI 10) Reinforcement received at unpredictable time intervals, averaging every 10 days (if the behaviour occurs).	Takes medication daily and logs it in a health app, which is checked by a nurse:	Receives motivational praise from a nurse in the app at unpredictable time intervals. (e.g. day 9, day 10, day 8, day 12).	Reinforcement times are unpredictable. This can create moderately good adherence, as the patient does not know when adherence will be checked.
Fixed Ratio (FR 10) Reinforcement is received if the target behaviour happens on 10 occasions.	Individual commits to attending a physical activity programme for people who are recovering from a heart attack.	Receives a special tee-shirt after completion of 10 sessions.	Helps to promote physical activity through working to a milestone. Motivation may drop if no reinforcer is given and behaviour may become less consistent.
Variable Ratio (FR 12) Reinforcement given at after an unpredictable number of times exercises are completed, averaging 12th time (if the behaviour occurs).	Patient recovering from surgery is asked by a physiotherapist to undertake exercises and enter completion on an app.	Reinforced by motivational congratulatory app messages after an unpredictable number of times the exercises have been completed, e.g. 10th, 13th and 9th times.	Reinforcement for number of exercises completed is unpredictable, this can be motivational. Even if no app message is received, the unpredictability in receipt of previous congratulatory messages means the individual maintains steady engagement.

reinforcers that were necessary for survival, such as food, water, sleep, sex and secondary reinforcers, which had some value to the person, for example, sweets, praise, money, attention, etc. When a young child goes to a medical appointment or the dentist, they may be reinforced by receiving a sticker for being 'brave' or 'good'; however, Coxon et al. (2017) found that if children aged between four and eight years old were permitted to choose between 10 different reinforcers, comprised of stickers and small toys, none of the children selected the stickers. This does not indicate that stickers do not have reinforcing properties, rather that when faced with a choice, stickers were the least preferred, hence it may be necessary to assess the value of potential reinforcers before use.

BOX 7.2
CRITICAL THINKING

Do you engage in any health behaviours? What reinforces the likelihood of you repeating the behaviour? Can you identify the schedule of reinforcement that you receive?

It is also possible to increase behaviour through negative reinforcement, which involves the removal of something that is unpleasant. The behaviour of taking medication will be reinforced if it removes pain or troublesome symptoms (the unpleasant stimulus), thus making it more likely that an individual will take medication the next time they have a headache (assuming that there were no negative side effects of the medication or financial barriers to getting the medication). Other examples include putting on sunscreen to avoid getting sun burnt, taking insulin to avoid high blood glucose and using inhaled medication to keep lung conditions under control. If we look at the temporal (time) relationship between taking some medications, such as statins, used to reduce cholesterol in people with cardiovascular disease (CVD), the reinforcing properties of taking the medication are not only delayed, but they are not obvious to the patient, as assessment requires a blood test. This can have negative consequences for adherence (see Chapter 6), as the patient is not receiving any timely reinforcement for adhering to medication.

Often health behaviours are not quite as simple as the examples used above suggest. Going back to the use of sunscreen to prevent skin damage and painful sunburn. The application of sunscreen may be influenced by other factors, such as wanting to have a glowing 'healthy looking' suntan. While the unpleasant effects of too much sun may, in the short term, cause painful sunburn, some individuals view the aesthetic benefits of a suntan to be more important than the risk of developing skin cancer. This can be due to skin cancer taking many years to develop, making it easier for people to ignore the risks of getting sunburnt. In addition, other people can unintentionally reinforce unhealthy sun behaviours by telling a person that they look healthier with a suntan.

Unintentional reinforcement can also exert an influence on illness behaviours. An individual who has had a heart attack may feel anxious about adhering to a health professional's advice to engage in physical activity. Family members may also endorse the avoidance of physical activity through being oversolicitous, telling the individual to rest and provide more physical help than is required. This can reinforce sedentary behaviour beliefs about being disabled and the inability to care for oneself, thereby contributing to 'cardiac invalidism' (Bertoni et al., 2023; Itkowitz et al., 2003). While the principles of operant conditioning can be applied in different ways to help explain some health behaviours, social contexts, vicarious learning, that is, observation of others' behaviours and ensuing consequences can also exert an influence over a person's health behaviours.

Social Learning Theory

Bandura's **Social Learning Theory** (1977a) proposed that people not only learn from the consequences of their own behaviours (direct experiences), but they can also learn from observing others' behaviours, actions and the associated consequences. Bandura conducted many research studies about learning, the most famous was the Bobo doll study that examined if aggressive behaviour could be influenced by watching others. A group of children (the experimental group) watched an adult playing with an inflatable Bobo (clown) doll, the adult hit the doll, pushed it over and shouted at it. A second group of children saw an adult play non-aggressively (control group) with toys that included the Bobo doll. After this, the children were then permitted to play with the Bobo doll. Bandura et al. (1961) found that those who had watched an adult being aggressive towards the Bobo doll were more aggressive in their play than children in the control group. Bandura took this as evidence that children and, to a certain extent, adults, tend to model their behaviour on what they have observed in others, this is known as **vicarious learning**.

Social learning theory may help to explain some health behaviours; a teenager may start smoking after observing friends or family smoking cigarettes. Children may adopt the food habits of a parent, e.g. one parent may refuse to eat salad items referring to them as 'rabbit food', a child might imitate the behaviour and state that they do not like these foods, even though they have not tasted them. Seeing others being reinforced for health enhancing behaviours may increase the likelihood of that behaviour being adopted, e.g. someone on social media or a friend losing weight by following a 'new' diet may motivate others to do the same. However, social learning theory cannot explain all health behaviours, because we also make our own decisions, these can be based on our ability or inability to foresee the future consequences of actions and the impact of family and significant others.

Family, peers and role models

Family members, communities, adults, teachers, peers and other role models can be crucial to shaping a person's health behaviours, through information, support or social learning. The family is often cited as having a major impact on children in their formative years; this can be observed through child health behaviours, such as taking exercise, eating a healthy diet, along with hygiene practices such as brushing of teeth and hand washing. In early childhood, family members serve as the main role models for children, they help to shape their attitudes, beliefs and habits relating to health. For example, if a parent has a fear of the dentist, the child may also express such a fear without having ever visited the dentist. Peer groups and social networks can exert positive and negative influences on health behaviours, particularly during adolescence. Peer pressure can contribute to experimentation in health risky behaviours like smoking, vaping, drinking alcohol and experimenting with drugs. More importantly, peers and role models can influence the adoption of healthy behaviours, whereby athletes, teachers, community leaders, peers and mentors who promote healthy lifestyles can inspire others to do the same. Many health promotion campaigns make use of role models, for example, the UK celebrity chief Jamie Oliver led a campaign to promote healthier eating for children and the provision of more nutritious school meals. Cathy Freeman, an Olympic gold medallist (sprinter), helps to support the education and wellbeing of Indigenous children through the Cathy Freeman Foundation. The actor Angelina Jolie highlighted the role of genetic testing for the *BRCA* gene associated with some types of breast cancer. The tennis champion Serena Williams, through sharing life-threatening experiences when giving birth, helped to raise awareness of maternal health complications and racial disparities in healthcare.

BOX 7.3 CRITICAL THINKING

Health behaviours are shaped not only by knowledge, but by also what we observe others doing. How can health advertising use social influence, role models and observational learning to improve health outcomes?

Self-efficacy

The concept of **self-efficacy** (SE) refers to a person's belief in their own ability to accomplish a task or behaviour (an outcome; Bandura, 1977b). This usually depends on whether they think they have the knowledge and skills required to undertake the behaviour. SE can be increased or decreased by four efficacy expectations, these are mastery, vicarious learning (modelling), social persuasion and physiological responses. Take for example, a patient with chronic low back pain who has been referred to a physiotherapist, a series of exercises are prescribed to strengthen muscles and reduce pain. The patient's SE on how to do the exercises safely without hurting their back is low, as they have an expectation that all movement makes their back condition worse. This is a barrier to adherence, potentially leading to poorly controlled pain, impaired mobility and reduced quality of life. To increase SE, the physiotherapist needs to explain why the exercises are important (social persuasion), use step-by-step instructions to teach the patient the steps necessary to carry out each specific exercise (mastery) and get the patient to watch them demonstrate each exercise (vicarious learning). To assist in mastery, the patient will be asked to complete each exercise, while the physiotherapist observes, provides positive encouragement and comments (social persuasion). These factors should help reduce the patient's negative expectations about exercise making their back pain (physiological experience) worse. According to Bandura, use of these processes should help to improve the patient's SE about being able to complete the exercises at home, but to be successful, the patient needs to believe that the exercises will bring about a reduction in their

Using the scale below, circle the number that best describes how confident you are that you will be able to complete your exercises at home

Not confident at all	A little bit confident	Moderately confident	Fairly highly confident	Absolutely confident

0 1 2 3 4 5 6 7 8 9 10

Figure 7.4
Numerical rating scale for self-efficacy

Source: Author

back pain, this is known as the outcome expectancy. Many healthcare professionals recognise that low SE is a barrier to health behaviours, but do not formally assess it before and after providing instructions for home-based exercises (Picha et al., 2021). Assessment of SE may help to gauge how to tailor treatment to meet individual needs, as some patients may require further instructions to understand what they are being asked to do, or exercises that are simpler or just need encouragement. If a patient believes they can complete the exercises, they are more likely to do them at home; research shows that high SE is associated with better health outcomes (Martinez-Calderon et al., 2018), less emotional distress and disability (Martinez-Calderon et al., 2020).

A range of measures can be used to assess SE within health contexts, these can be disease specific, for example, the Pain Self-Efficacy Questionnaire (Nicholas, 2007) and the Self-Efficacy to Manage Chronic Disease (SEMCD) Scale (Ritter & Lorig, 2014). Questionnaires can also target specific health behaviours to assess intentions to quit smoking (the Smoking Self-Efficacy Questionnaire (SEQ); Etter et al., 2000) or to assess confidence in weight control and healthy eating (Healthy Eating and Weight Self-Efficacy (HEWSE) Scale; Wilson-Barlow et al., 2014). It is not always essential to use disease- or condition-specific measures, as simple numerical rating scales can also provide a quick measure of SE (see Figure 7.4).

Social cognitive models of health behaviour

Locus of Control

The Locus of Control Theory (Rotter, 1966) is based on social learning theory, it states that people hold beliefs about whether they have control over own successes and failures (outcomes). These beliefs, referred to as locus of control (LOC), are based on attributions that people make about what caused or who caused something to happen and are influenced by learning and past experience. Rotter identified two aspects of LOC, internal, in which people believe that they are responsible for their own successes and failures and external, which devolves responsibility for success and failures, to external factors that can be related to chance (fate) or other people (powerful others).

Health locus of control applied to diabetes

Locus of control (LOC) was adapted for use in health contexts (Wallston et al., 1978) and termed **Health Locus of Control** (HLOC). It tries to explain how people determine the cause of health and disease and how their beliefs influence their health behaviours. A person who has high internal HLOC believes that their health is mainly determined by their own lifestyle and health-related behaviours. Such people are more likely to engage in health enhancing behaviours that are reinforced by the health expectancy outcome and the value of the health behaviour. For example, 'I have diabetes, checking my blood glucose and reducing my intake of sugary foods, will help me to control my diabetes (expectancy). The results will be better glucose control (outcome) and this is important to me, as it will improve my overall health (value)'. In contrast, people with high external HLOC believe that their health outcomes are due to powerful others or chance. Hence, the individual believes that family members, friends, God and/or health professionals are responsible for helping to control their health. Such individuals may follow a health professional's advice but will not be proactive in searching for health information or making changes to lifestyle behaviours, unless they are suggested to them. Taking the example of diabetes, I may believe that 'my blood glucose will only improve if my doctor monitors it at regular intervals and my partner knows what foods I should eat or avoid (expectancy). My blood glucose will only get better if the doctor does their job and tells my partner about my dietary needs (outcome). The roles of my doctor and my partner are important because I want to stay healthy' (value; see Figure 7.5).

In chance-based external HLOC, the individual believes that it is just bad luck or fate that they have a disease, they have no control over their health and what will be, will be. These people may state that there is no point in stopping smoking, because getting a disease such as lung cancer is just bad luck. They may rationalise this by stating that there are lots of people who have smoked all their lives, lived until they were one hundred and did not develop lung cancer! In examining the relationship between HLOC, physical activity, alcohol consumption and smoking in patients with heart disease, Mercer et al. (2018) found people who scored highly on chance HLOC had a higher likelihood of smoking and sedentary behaviour, internal HLOC was associated with greater physical activity and based on advice from healthcare professionals, those high on powerful others HLOC were less likely to smoke.

While research generally indicates that internal HLOC is consistently linked to better physical health outcomes due to proactive health behaviours, factors such as the health condition being studied, the population, gender and self-efficacy may influence control beliefs. External HLOC (especially chance-based) often correlates with poorer health behaviours and outcomes, but it must be remembered beliefs about control may be influenced by situational factors, such as whether a disease is acute or chronic and also influenced by factors that are outside an individual's control. For example, an individual who has high internal HLOC believes that the lifestyle they lead (being a non-smoker, does not drink alcohol, eats a healthy diet and engages in regular physical activity) means they are at low risk of getting sick, but suddenly, they have a heart attack, this may change their HLOC beliefs. Despite having a healthy lifestyle, they had an unknown genetic predisposition to heart disease, which is outside their control. In this situation, the individual may think 'what is the point in looking after my health, it did not stop me from having a heart attack', their beliefs about controlling their own health may become more external and they may shift to being more dependent on health professionals (powerful others HLOC).

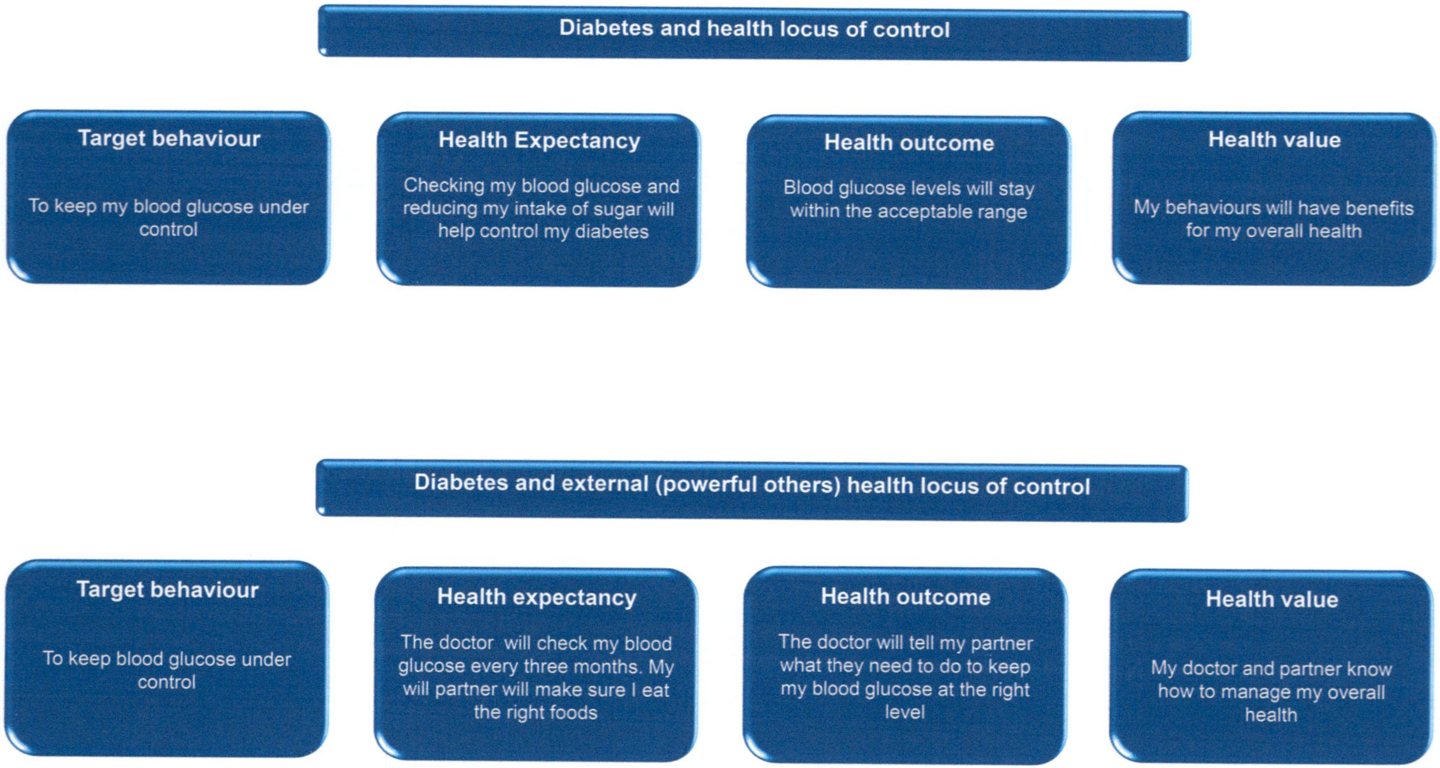
Diabetes and health locus of control
Target behaviour
To keep my blood glucose under control
Health Expectancy
Checking my blood glucose and reducing my intake of sugar will help control my diabetes
Health outcome
Blood glucose levels will stay within the acceptable range
Health value
My behaviours will have benefits for my overall health
Diabetes and external (powerful others) health locus of control
Target behaviour
To keep blood glucose under control
Health expectancy
The doctor will check my blood glucose every three months. My will partner will make sure I eat the right foods
Health outcome
The doctor will tell my partner what they need to do to keep my blood glucose at the right level
Health value
My doctor and partner know how to manage my overall health

Figure 7.5
Internal and external (powerful others) HLOC in diabetes

Source: Author based on Wallston et al. (1978)

The heath belief model applied to screening for breast cancer

The **Health Belief Model** (HBM; Rosenstock, 1974) was developed to understand why people did not take up the offer of screening tests to detect disease at an asymptomatic stage. The model consists of a personal appraisal of the perceived threat, individual health beliefs about personal susceptibility to getting a disease and how the individual views the severity of the consequences of the disease. Whether or not an individual engages in health screening can be influenced by modifying factors, these include demographic variables and **cues to action**, which may be internal, for example symptoms, or external, for example health invitations, media campaigns and diseases that friends have been diagnosed with. The likelihood of action (engaging in screening behaviour) is influenced by perceived benefits and perceived barriers, which can be thought of as a cost versus benefits analysis of engaging in the health behaviour.

To illustrate the model in action, we will use the example of screening for breast cancer (see Figure 7.6). When an individual receives an invitation to go for breast screening, their attendance may be influenced by perceived susceptibility, do they think they are at risk of breast cancer? Have any of their family members been diagnosed with breast or ovarian cancer? Do they have the *BRCA1* (*Breast Cancer Gene 1*) or *BRCA 2* (*Breast Cancer Gene 2*) genetic mutation that increases the likelihood of them developing breast cancer? The individual may consider the severity of breast cancer, in relation to it being a serious disease. If screening detects something suspicious, what might the consequences be, e.g. a lumpectomy, mastectomy, chemotherapy, radiotherapy or there may be more

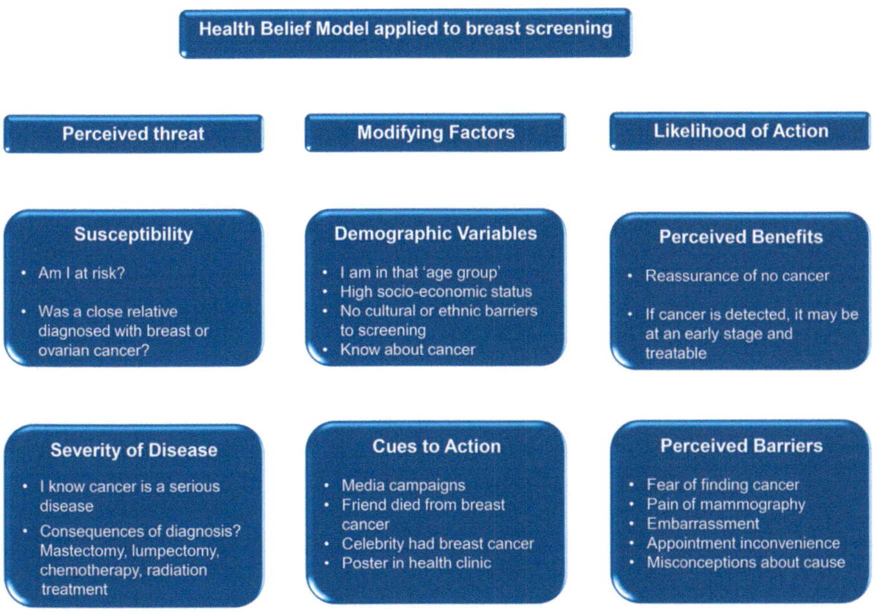

Figure 7.6
Health Belief Model applied to breast cancer screening

Source: Author based on Rosenstock (1974)

serious consequences if diagnosed with advanced disease. A diagnosis of breast cancer may mean time off work, it may have financial and social consequences, it may also cause concerns about being able to care for their family or the need to be cared for. Demographic variables may help in decisions to take up the offer of screening, this can be influenced by living in a deprived area, ethnicity, ability to read and speak English, as translators may not be available and documents may not be translated into the woman's language. Culture may be a barrier to screening (this can include the religious, ethnic, gender identity) and level of education may impact on health literacy (see Chapter 6), e.g. being unaware of the importance of breast screening and detection of cancer at an asymptomatic stage. Cues to action that can influence decisions to attend screening include, having a friend who was diagnosed early or who had a late diagnosis, seeing posters, leaflets, social media campaigns and high-profile role models talking about their diagnosis. The likelihood of action of going for screening can be influenced by the perceived benefits of when results come through, it will be reassuring to know that no cancer has been detected, or if detected, it may be at an early stage, with no spread and it will be curable. The perceived barriers to screening may include the inconvenience of the appointment time or place, weather, embarrassment of having to undress, discomfort of **mammography**, fear of finding something wrong and misconceptions about cancer being punishment from God for wrongdoing (Breast Cancer Now, 2023).

Later, the construct of self-efficacy (SE) was added to the HBM, (Rosenstock et al., 1988), as noted previously in this chapter SE is concerned with how well an individual thinks they will be able to complete a specific task or achieve a goal. Attendance for breast screening involves a range of interrelated behaviours that may be impacted on by SE, these include confidence that a person has navigating through the healthcare system, in making the appointment, finding a suitable time, arranging transport, parking and finding their way to the clinic area. During the appointment, SE comes into play in relation to the person overcoming any anxiety and/or embarrassment about having to undress, someone touching their breasts and discomfort involved in the screening test. Women who have high negative attitudes about cancer tend to have lower SE about taking part in breast screening (Kandemir et al., 2025).

The HBM has been used to study a range of preventative and risky health-related behaviours. After reviewing around 50 studies, Janz and Becker (1984) concluded that perceived barriers were the best predictor for non-engagement in health behaviours and perceived severity of a disease was an inconsistent predictor. Adoption of preventative health behaviours (e.g. screening for disease at an asymptomatic stage) was more likely to occur if the individual believed they were susceptible to the disease and that the perceived benefits outweighed the perceived barriers. In terms of engagement in risky health behaviours (e.g. smoking), reductions in the behaviour were more likely when the benefits (e.g. coughing less and it being easier to breathe) were perceived to be greater than the continued risk (susceptibility to chest infections and lung cancer).

Several criticisms have been levelled at the HBM, it is unclear how the variables within model interact with each other, if one aspect is more important than another and the variables within the model can be difficult to measure (Abraham & Sheeran, 2015). The HBM does not take emotional factors, such as a person being in denial about a health issue into account. In addition, health beliefs are not static, what a person thinks about a health behaviour at one time in their life may not hold true when the person is older. For example, children initially brush their teeth due to parental instruction, but as they move into their teenage years, they may become more concerned about their appearance, they want bright white teeth and brush their teeth to prevent bad breath. In adulthood, brushing of teeth may be due to fear of tooth decay and losing teeth. The model cannot account for the social determinants of health on behaviour, such as people wanting to brush their teeth, but due to a lack of money or environmental factors (e.g. war or displacement), this is not possible. Likewise, to ensure good oral health, many people will visit their dentist on a regular 6- or 12- monthly basis for screening to prevent dental decay at an asymptomatic stage, but within the UK, cost is a barrier to care for around 41% of adults and access to National Health Service (NHS) dentistry is problematic (Oral Health Foundation, 2024).

Stage model of health behaviour

The Transtheoretical Model applied to physical activity

The **Transtheoretical Model** ([TTM]; Prochaska & DiClemente, 1983) is a stage model of behaviour change that includes self-efficacy, decisional balance and processes of change. The TTM was originally used for smoking cessation, but it has been applied to a broad range of health-related contexts, including drug use, weight control, healthy eating, safer sex, condom use, sun protection, breast screening and physical activity (Prochaska et al., 1994). The desired health behaviours in each stage of the TTM are quite distinctive, as shown in Figure 7.7.

Five stages of the TTM

The TTM will be illustrated using the target behaviour of becoming more physically active. In the precontemplation stage, the individual has no plans to become physically active within the next six months. They may be unaware of the deleterious consequences of being sedentary or the health benefits of becoming physically active and be resistant to advice about taking up physical activity. In the contemplation stage, they may know about the benefits of becoming physically active but have doubts about how beneficial it would be. However, they intend to take action within the next six months and will consider the pros and cons associated with becoming physically active. During the preparation stage, the individual starts getting ready to take part in physical activity within the next 30 days. This may involve making decisions about the type of physical activity, looking for groups to join, buying clothing and footwear, purchasing gym membership and setting a date to start the activity. Within the action stage, the individual will have tried to commence physical activity, this can be on their own, with a group or by joining a gym and they may have set themselves goals and associated rewards. For example, to go out walking at least five times a week at a set time for the next month and celebrate reaching that goal by purchasing a new audiobook to listen to when out walking. In the action stage, engagement in physical activity may not yet be a regular occurrence, hence changes are considered as short term. Only when physical activity has been sustained for more than six months can an individual be said to have entered the maintenance stage (DiClemente & Hughes, 1990).

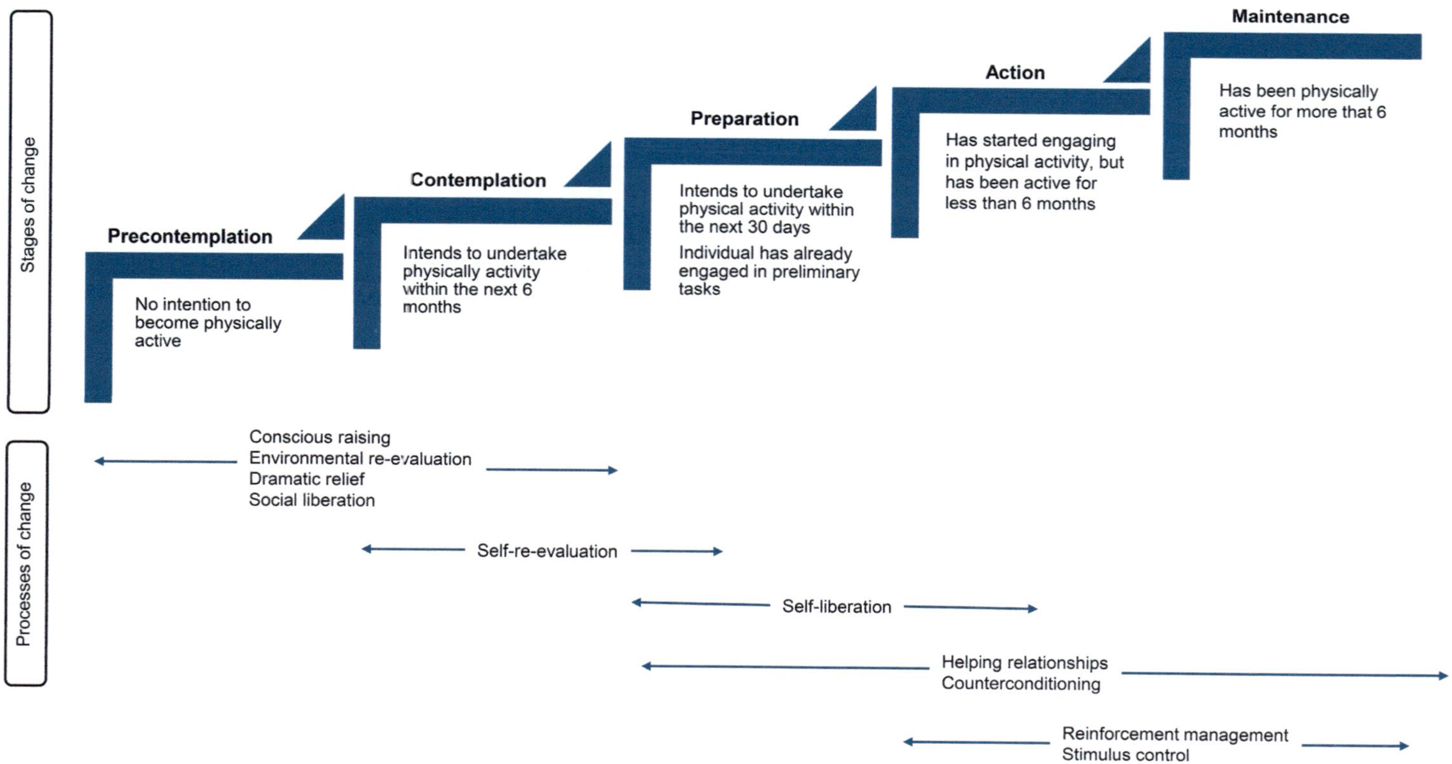

Figure 7.7
The Transtheoretical Model applied to physical activity

Source: Author based on Prochaska and DiClemente (1983)

At each stage of the TTM, people will need various types and amounts of information to help in moving through subsequent stages of the model. Reaching the target behaviour is a gradual process and completion of each stage is necessary to move on to the next. An individual in the precontemplation stage will have health informational needs about the negative health implications of sedentary behaviour and benefits of physical activity. This is a health promotional stage, role models and advice from healthcare professionals can be important prompts for change. This contrasts with the action stage, which is about helping people to continue with physical activity. This can include setting longer-term goals, such as increasing the activity time, effort or step count, which can be tracked on a smart device and celebrated.

Self-efficacy

Progression through the stages of the TTM is linked with self-efficacy (SE), decisional balance and processes of change. SE refers to how confident a person is that they will be able to achieve the target behaviour. SE can change over time, in relation to how much effort is required to maintain physical activity, getting advice from others on how to set goals and improve, the weather and according to the stage of the model the person is in. SE is a good indicator of behaviour change, as it indicates that an individual is confident that they can achieve a goal and people tend to exhibit higher levels of SE in the action and maintenance stages of the model. Low SE can be a barrier to physical activity, as despite knowing that physical activity is beneficial to health, the individual may not believe they can complete a set goal. Hence it is essential that goals are realistic and achievable, there is no point in setting the goal of running a marathon for an individual who has just started jogging! Goal setting will involve setting smaller goals that build up to bigger achievements.

Decisional balance

Decisional balance within the TTM refers to the 'pros' and cons', that is, weighing up positive and negative aspects of undertaking the health behaviour (see Table 7.2).

Table 7.2 The pros and cons of engaging in physical activity

Pros	Cons
Improve my sleep pattern	People will laugh at me
Help to relieve stress	I feel embarrassed
Weight reduction	Cost of joining a gym
Improved mood	Time constraints, I'm too busy
Make me feel good about myself	Weather too cold to go outside or too nice to go to the gym
Help me become fit	I do not want to get big muscles

Processes of change

Other factors that can influence an individual's thought processes about engaging in physical behaviour are known collectively as the processes of change (see Table 7.3). The importance of these five cognitive and five behavioural processes varies according to the stages of the model (Adams & White, 2003; see Figure 7.7). During the precontemplation and contemplation stages, cognitive processes are important to help the person move from having no intention to become physically active to considering it and forming intentions. Consciousness raising is concerned with awareness and education about the positive aspects of physical activity and the negative health consequences of sedentary behaviours. Environmental re-evaluation may involve thinking about how physical activity may impact on significant others, such as family members and the benefits of walking or taking public transport instead of driving. Dramatic relief is about emotional change, feelings of achievement that might be associated with physical activity and the potential to achieve a goal of being active for x minutes on x days of the week. Self re-evaluation is a characteristic of the move from the contemplation to preparation stage and indicates a change in values, to being more positive and developing a strengthening commitment about becoming physically active. Self-liberation is linked to the move from the preparation to into action stage, the realisation that being physically active is a normative behaviour, this includes recognition of other people out walking or going to the gym to improve their health.

Table 7.3 Processes of change within the TTM

Cognitive processes	Explanation
Consciousness raising	Searching for information on physical activity, how often, intensity, type of footwear, safety considerations and where to go.
Environmental re-evaluation	Thinking about the benefits to the environment of undertaking physical activity, which may include not adding to traffic congestion or parking problems. Encouraging others to join in to become more physically active.
Dramatic relief	Feeling of pride in achieving a new physical activity goal.
Social liberation	Realising that being physically active is the norm, seeing others going to the gym or walking before work or in the evening.
Self-re-evaluation	Feelings of positivity associated with being physically active.
Behavioural processes	**Explanation**
Self-liberation	Making a commitment to maintain the health choice of becoming more physically active.
Helping relationships	Seeking and using social support from others to help health behaviour change.
Counterconditioning	Substituting unhealthy behaviours for healthier ones.
Reinforcement management	Increasing rewards for engaging in physical activity, these may be intrinsic or extrinsic.
Stimulus control	Adding cues or reminders to engage in physical activity.

Behavioural processes feature more prominently in the action and maintenance stages. These include the formation of helping relationships in which social support from others may be sought, which can include taking physical activity with family members, peers or groups and/or receiving positive feedback from others about starting and continuing to be physically active. Counterconditioning is where healthier behaviours such as walking are substituted for sedentary activities. For example, getting out of bed earlier to go to the gym, walking or cycling to work instead of taking the car and being physically active after dinner instead of watching television. As the individual continues to engage in physical activity, stimulus control can be of use by adding cues or reminders to be more active, for example, putting a list of organised walks on the kitchen wall, searching for a list of Park Runs, using the stairs instead of a lift. The use of reinforcement management can act as an incentive and reward, this includes charting progress in a diary, phone app or chart, purchasing new headphones specifically to listen to podcasts or music when being physically active, buying new clothing when a specific goal has been reached and setting future goals.

The TTM does provide an explanation for the readiness processes and stages that individuals go through in changing their behaviour. Identifying the stage an individual is in permits the delivery of tailored information that considers the pros and cons of the target behaviour and the processes of change. This model also recognises that people may relapse into a previous stage, even if someone has started being physically active, for various reasons, they may move back into the preparation stage, this is seen as a normal occurrence, or they may move back into the contemplation stage. That said, the stage approach within the TTM has been criticised, as motivation to engage in a health behaviour is said to be continuous rather than based on discrete units and people can fall between stages (West, 2005). For example, a person who is in the preparation stage may decide to take action within the next 30 days, what happens if they do not take action for 31 days, are they still classified as being within this stage of the model or do they fall somewhere between the precontemplation and preparation stages? The model cannot account for this. To take up a health behaviour, the TTM suggests that people engage in a formal process of decision-making, this may work when people make New Year's resolutions, but for the rest of the year, most people do not set a date to prepare for a change in behaviour. Sometimes behaviour change can be spontaneous or in relation to a cue to action, such as seeing a poster about a walking group or an invite from a friend to start walking. Evidence to support the TTM in assisting behaviour change is weak, Sutton (2001) suggests that development of interventions based on the stage that an individual is in, does not have a higher rate of success than non-stage-based interventions. Additionally, Bridel (2005) reviewed 37 studies based on the TTM and found minimal evidence to show that use of interventions that specifically targeted the stage the person was at in the model resulted in behaviour change, a point echoed by Prestwich et al. (2014). Other criticisms of the model include the role of motivations and external factors. For example, the model also ignores social determinants of health such as income, if the target behaviour is to eat more fresh fruit, vegetables and lean cuts of meat, this can be hampered by food poverty, which is outside an individual's control. Despite these criticisms, the TTM remains a popular choice on which to base interventions, as it helps to tailor interventions according to an individual's needs. For example, health promotional advice in the early stages to motivational advice and goal setting in the later stages of the TTM.

Behaviour prediction model of health

Theory of Planned Behaviour applied to weight loss

The **Theory of Planned Behaviour** ([TPB]; Ajzen, 1991) has been used to explain and predict how individuals make decisions about specific health (target) behaviours (NICE, 2014). According to this model, the strongest predictor of a target behaviour is an individual's intention to engage in that behaviour (see Figure 7.8). Intentions are influenced by three factors, attitudes towards the target behaviour (considers advantages and disadvantages), subjective norms (what others think about the target behaviour and how much these opinions are valued) and perceived behavioural control (barriers and facilitators to engaging in the target behaviour). The model will be explained using the example target behaviour of weight loss.

An individual's attitude towards weight loss is based on their beliefs of what will happen if they engage in weight loss and how much they value the outcomes of losing weight. The individual believes that weight loss will help them become heathier, it will reduce their chances of developing type 2 diabetes (T2DM), give them more energy and weight loss means they can wear nicer clothes. Evaluation of outcomes relate to how much the individual values each potential outcome, feeling healthier and having more energy are very important to the individual and being able to wear nicer clothes will improve confidence. All the outcomes of the individual's beliefs are positive, leading towards the attitude that the behaviour (weight loss) will have lots of benefits. The second factor is subjective norms, these relate to the social pressure that the individual feels to lose weight. Their doctor wants them to lose weight for health reasons, not only will it reduce the risk of T2DM, but it will also reduce the risks of developing hypertension, cardiovascular disease and reduce wear and tear on joints. This is echoed by parents who worry about the individual's mental and physical wellbeing. The individual's peers are also trying to lose weight, so they have positive beliefs about this being a good health behaviour. An individual's motivation to comply with others' beliefs is concerned with how much they care about others' opinions. Valued opinions make it more likely that the individual will engage in weight loss. The final factor that influences intention is perceived behavioural control, this includes control beliefs and perceived power. Control beliefs reflect how much control the individual believes that they have over losing weight, as well as the impact of external factors. They know about healthy foods, how to cook from scratch, however, buying fresh fruit, vegetables and lean cuts of meat may affect perceived power to make the necessary changes, as there is limited availability of these foods where they live and what is available is quite expensive (referred to as a food desert). They are also worried about giving in to cravings for chocolate, biscuits and potato crisps. While they find that their knowledge of what and how to cook nutritious low-calorie meals is empowering and will help to control what they eat, there is an acknowledgement that healthy food availability, cost and cravings could be their main barriers to weight loss. Taken together, their positive attitude towards weight loss and the encouragement from others result in a moderately strong behavioural intention, but they are pragmatic about needing some help with control issues. In general, higher behaviour intentions are associated with a greater likelihood that individual will engage in weight loss-related activities.

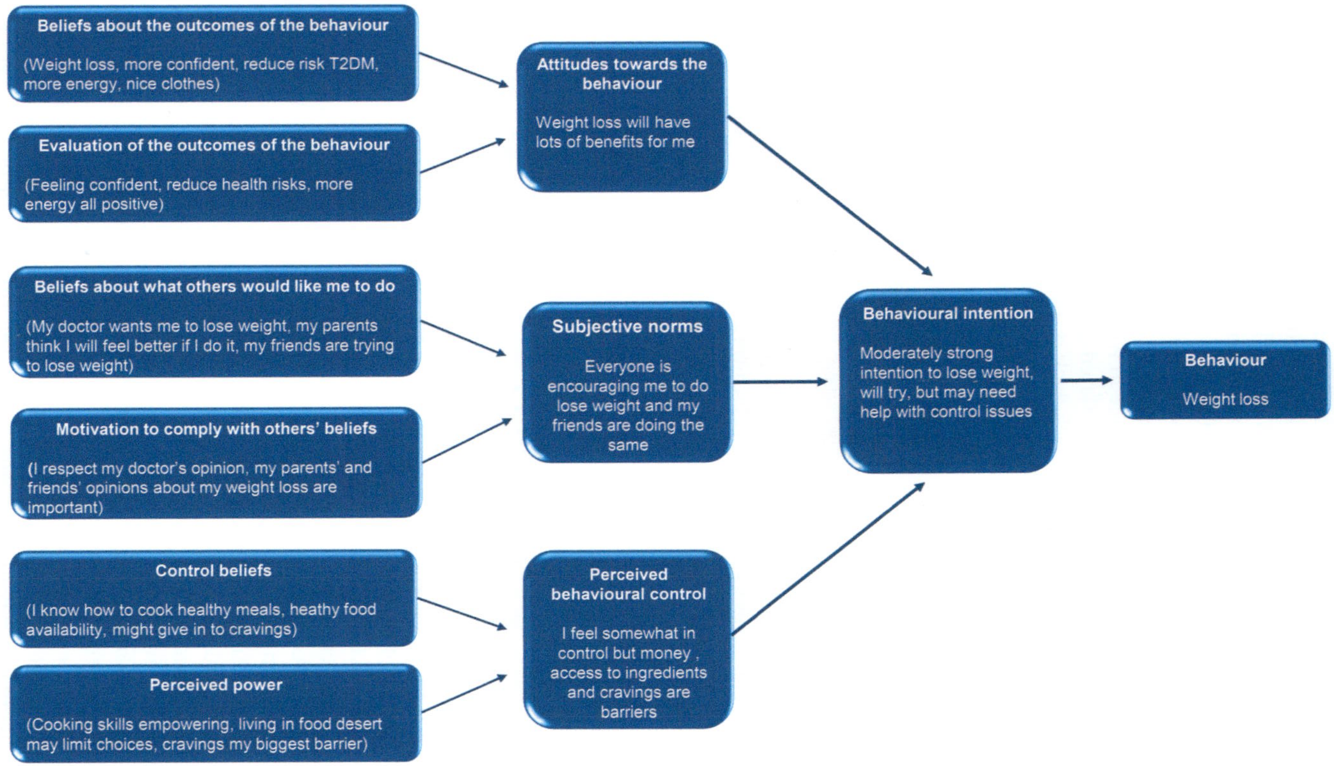

Figure 7.8
The Theory of Planned Behaviour applied to weight loss

Source: Author, based on Ajzen (1991)

The TPB constructs have be used to predict many health-related behaviours, for example food choices (McDermott et al., 2015), physical activity (Norman et al., 2010; Shafieinia et al., 2016) and smoking (Tapera et al., 2020; Zhao et al., 2022). In a systematic review of how the TBP had been applied to behaviour change interventions, Hardeman et al. (2002) highlighted that when used to develop interventions, it was unclear which parts of the TPB had been targeted and how they were used within the respective interventions. While the TPB can be used to predict intentions to engage in specific health behaviours, it cannot account for why most people do not follow through with the target behaviour, this is known as the **intention-behaviour gap** (Amireault et al., 2008; Conner & Norman, 2022). The individual may intend to engage in weight loss, but other factors may intervene to stop the intention being translated into action, for example, feeling too fatigued to cook, lack of time to cook, lack of ingredients and food poverty. Thus, a more holistic way of changing behaviour is required and one that looks beyond the individual, their family, peers and healthcare professionals.

BOX 7.4
CRITICAL THINKING

Many people make New Year's resolutions to become more physically active or stop eating sweets and start to eat a more healthy diet. Based on what you have learned so far about theories and models of health behaviour, why are so many people unable to keep to their resolutions?

Multisystem model of health behaviour

The behaviour change wheel applied to eating more fruits and vegetables

There are an array of models and theories used to predict and inform behaviour change and there is some overlap between models. They can focus on different aspects of behaviour, but many do not include emotional and habitual influences on behaviour. In addition, it is difficult to make comparisons between models and intervention effectiveness, leaving researchers and health professionals struggling to decide on which model is best when designing behaviour change interventions at an individual and population level. Michie et al. (2011) merged insights from 19 frameworks of behaviour change to develop the **Behaviour Change Wheel** (BCW) as a structured way to describe, design interventions and evaluate behaviour change interventions (see Figure 7.9). The BCW can help bridge the intention-behaviour gap, as it provides the structure to move people from intention (I want to change) to action (change in behaviour) by focusing on what actually influences behaviours.

The first step in using the BCW is to identify the target behaviour, this needs to be very specific, for example, an individual may have a goal to lose x amount of weight, but that needs to be broken down into how it will be achieved. For example, weight loss usually involves food choices and can also include becoming more physically active, thus, to enact behaviour change, interventions may focus on more than one behaviour. The example used here to explain the BCW will focus

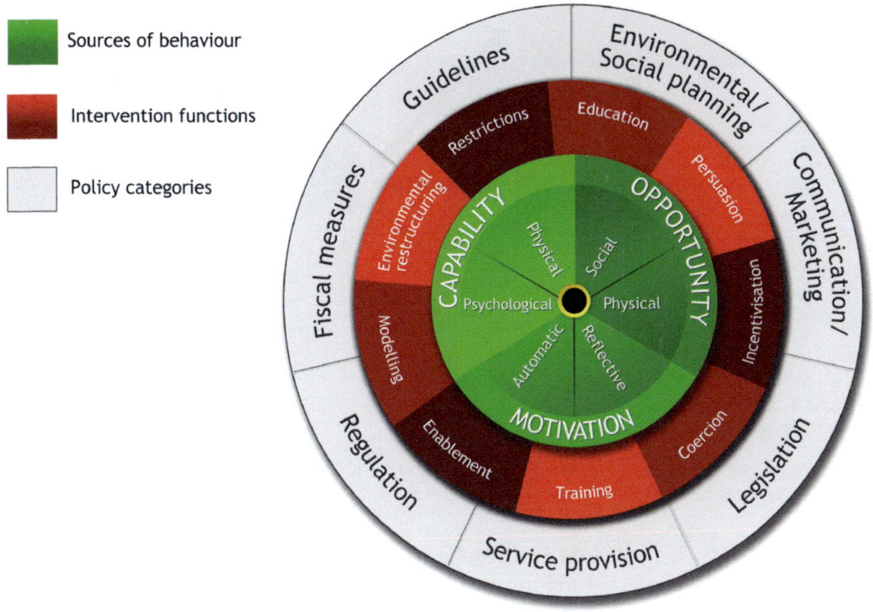

Figure 7.9
The Behaviour Change Wheel

Source: The Behaviour Change Wheel with permission from Michie et al. (2011) under Creative Commons CC BY

on weight loss through eating more fresh fruits and vegetables (FV). Various questions must be explored in relation to the behaviour. For example, the advice about what needs to change may include increasing portions of FV at mealtimes, replacing snacks such as biscuits and sweets with FV. There is need to identify where the behaviour happens. This may be dependent on the individual's work situation, ideally the dietary changes should happen at home, at work and if possible, when eating out, by selecting salads as a main course and fruit for dessert. This may not be achievable due to limited food choices or when eating meals that are prepared by friends and family. How often should the behaviour occur? This can cover all days of the week or Monday to Friday. Time factors must also be considered, as making dietary changes may involve more food preparation time and this needs to fit in with individual, family and work commitments. Who else will be involved? It is important to think about who does the shopping and cooks the meals and if this behaviour change will require additional work to prepare different meals for other family members. For some individuals, this weight loss intervention may seem too burdensome and a starting point may involve eating more FV for breakfast and at midday, when there is no need to cater for family meals, along with substituting morning and afternoon biscuits with FV. Once the target behaviour has been agreed on, it is time to move on to the COM-B part of the BCW.

COM-B

The COM-B model is located at the centre of the BCW and it is essential for behaviour change. It represents an individual's capability, opportunity and motivation (see Figure 7.10) to engage in the behaviour. For behaviour to change,

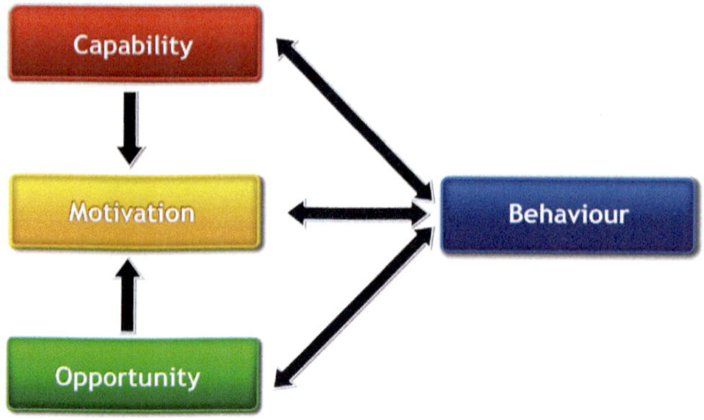

Figure 7.10
The COM-B

Source: The Capability, Opportunity, Motivation and Behaviour (COM-B) behaviour system, reproduced with permission from Michie et al. (2011) under Creative Commons CC BY

all three aspects of the COM-B must be in place, as they help to identify what aspect of the person's behaviour needs to change for them to succeed, with capability and opportunity having direct impacts on motivation. Capability is concerned with the individual's knowledge and skills to change their behaviour, which involves physical and psychological capability. Physical capability includes having the skills to prepare different FV, the best way to cook them to preserve nutrients and varying recipes to reduce boredom with meals. Psychological capability involves knowledge of what different types of FV are available, understanding why FV are nutritionally beneficial and preferable compared to high fat and sugary biscuits, cakes and chocolate and decision making about what to eat.

Opportunity includes social aspects, such as family members joining in and replacing their snacks with FV. When going out to eat, family and friends can help by selecting restaurants that have menu choices that support the individual's FV intake, while also permitting a range of dining options for others. Physical aspects of opportunity can include time requirements; due to FV being perishable, it may be necessary to shop more often to ensure food freshness and many products require storage in a cool environment, which may be problematic due to limited refrigeration space at home. Purchasing more FV will have additional cost implications, especially when trying to purchase a wider range of products, which may not be in season and knowing where to purchase foods.

The third aspect of the COM-B is motivation, which can be reflective, involving beliefs about own intentions, goals, capabilities, optimism and confidence in being able to eat FV instead of snacking on biscuits. It also includes beliefs about the consequences of eating more FV and reducing high fat and sugar snacks. Understanding that weight loss is not instant and changes are a long-term behaviour but acknowledging that occasional lapses may happen. Automatic motivation can include reinforcement for maintaining FV intake, emotions such as pride for sticking with the dietary plan, breaking habitual and impulsive eating, overcoming cravings for chocolate and enhanced enjoyment when experimenting with new recipes. The COM-B model is used to diagnose the behavioural changes (barriers and enablers) that need to happen to engage in the target behaviour of eating more FV. Once this has been completed, development of the intervention can commence.

Intervention development

The BCW (see Figure 7.9) contains nine intervention functions. Once the COM-B model has been used to identify the behaviours needed to help the individual eat more FV, the intervention functions can be used as a guide on how to bring about the dietary changes. An example of how this works is provided in Table 7.4. For example, if the individual is unaware of how to prepare FV, training will be

Table 7.4 Intervention functions associated with the COM-B diagnosis of required behaviour changes for eating more FV

	Intervention functions								
	Education	Persuasion	Incentivisation	Coercion	Training	Enablement	Modelling	Environmental restructuring	Restrictions
Capability									
Physical									
How to prepare FV	✓				✓				
Cooking without loss of nutrients	✓								
Recipes	✓								
Psychological									
Types of FV available	✓								
Best place to buy FV						✓			
Benefits of eating more FV	✓								
Opportunity									
Physical									
Storage and shelf life	✓							✓	
Eating out in places serving FV on menu						✓		✓	
Time to prepare and cook FV						✓			
Social									
Family eating more FV						✓		✓	
Friend dinner invitations with FV menu choice						✓			
Motivation									
Reflective									
Feelings of doubt about being able to eat FV		✓				✓			
Consequences of eating FV	✓	✓							
Feeling of wellbeing eating FV		✓	✓						
Relapsing back to old dietary habits		✓				✓			
Automatic									
Feeling proud of achievements		✓	✓						
Rewarding yourself for eating more FV			✓						

required; being uncertain of how to cook FV, while retaining as much nutritional benefits as possible can be achieved through education; having doubts about being able to eat more FV may be enhanced through persuasion. Eating out will require environmental restructuring that involves finding out in advance, which restaurants can cater for the individual's dietary needs. Weight loss can be motivated by incentivisation, by purchasing new clothes when a weight loss goal has been reached.

Behaviour change techniques

Once the intervention functions have been identified, it is necessary to decide on the best way of turning them into actions, this can be facilitated by using **behaviour change techniques** (BCTs), which are the precise and smallest details of any intervention. Michie et al. (2013) devised the Behaviour Change Techniques Taxonomy v1 (BCTTv1) as a standardised way of describing BCTs, this covers 93 BCTs that are organised into 16 categories (see Box 7.1). For example, one of the intervention functions for the behaviour of how to prepare FV was training, this can be operationalised by BCT number 6.1, 'demonstration of the behaviour' and 8.1 'behavioural practice/rehearsal'. For the intervention function of education, BCT 4.1 'instructions on how to perform the behaviour' could be employed. The use of the BCTTv1 to describe the active ingredients of an intervention enables other researchers and healthcare practitioners to take successful interventions and apply them in another setting or with another population (see Box 7.1).

BOX 7.1
BEHAVIOUR CHANGE TECHNIQUES TAXONOMY V1 (BCTT V1)

When conducting behaviour change research or designing and delivering interventions, it is important to describe the precise details of the interventions, so that everyone knows what the intervention content was and how it was delivered. You may come across research studies where it states that 'participants were supported to increase their physical activity', this gives an indication of what they were asked to do, but it would be impossible to replicate as no information has been provided on the nature of support. To replicate and implement interventions that change behaviour, it is necessary to have some common way of describing the content of interventions. Michie et al. (2013) devised the Behaviour Change Techniques Taxonomy V1 (BCTTv1) to do just this.

The BCTTv1 consists of 93 behaviour change techniques (BCTs) grouped into 16 categories that include 1. Goals and Planning; 2. Feedback and Monitoring; 3. Social Support; 4. Shaping Knowledge; 5. Natural Consequences; 6. Comparison of Behaviour; 7. Associations; 8. Repetition and Substitution; 9. Comparison of Outcomes; 10. Reward and Threat; 11. Regulation; 12. Antecedents; 13. Identity; 14. Scheduled Consequences; 15. Self-Belief; and 16. Covert learning. Each BCT is clearly numbered and labelled and the BCTTv1 taxonomy also provides examples of each BCT.

A introduction to BCTs is provided by provided by Professor Susan Michie in the BCT workshop 2021 Session 1: The Behaviour Change Technique Taxonomy (BCTTv1) Website: https://www.youtube.com/watch?v=TJXUkSPNihc. In order to become familiar with BCTs and to learn how to identify them within interventions, there is an accompanying website for BCTTv1 and free self-paced online training, which can be accessed via this link: https://www.bct-taxonomy.com/

BCW policy categories

The BCW can be used at an individual and population level and the outer circle contains seven policy categories (see Figure 7.9) that help to determine how the intervention functions can be facilitated. For example, at a community- or population level, service provision could be used to fund or support cookery classes to enable training, education may be delivered through mass media advertising about the health benefits of eating five portions of FV per day (5-a-day) through persuasion using role models (see Figure 7.11).

A plethora of studies have used the BCW to design various health-related interventions, for example, increasing physical activity in the general population (Ojo et al., 2019), in those with spinal cord injuries (Haley et al., 2023), chronic obstructive pulmonary disease (Xiang et al., 2023) and cancer care (Webb et al., 2016). It has also been used to develop a culturally tailored educational and support intervention for Black British adults with T2DM, in which researchers considered the importance of community, use of informal networks for seeking information and advice, along with challenges in attending appointments due to work, travel and caregiving responsibilities (Goff et al., 2021). The BCW provides a very structured approach to intervention development and it helps researchers and healthcare professionals to understand the behaviour in the context in which it occurs; it can be applied to any health behaviour and can address system-level barriers, which include government policy and organisational barriers to healthcare.

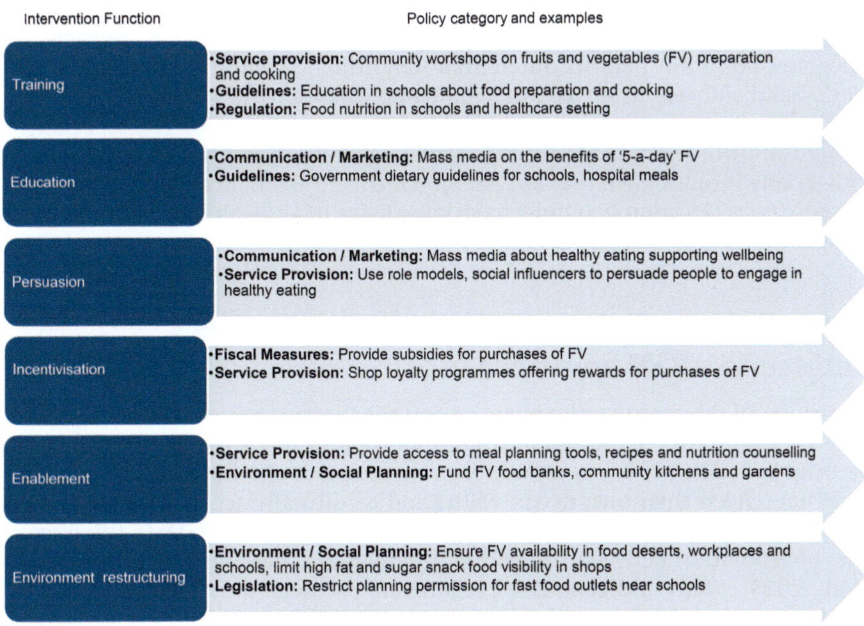

Figure 7.11

Intervention functions, policy categories and examples for eating more FV

Source: Author based on Michie et al. (2011)

Indigenous models of health

The theories and models of health reviewed so far within this chapter are Western centric, focused on individual behaviours and responsibility for behaviours. Such a view does not align with Indigenous understandings and knowledges about health, which are interconnected with their community, the spirit world and the land. This ethnocentrism has led to Indigenous knowledge being disregarded, devalued and viewed through a negative lens due to perceived deficiencies in scientific credibility (Kirkham et al., 2007). Moreover, systemic racism in healthcare has caused Indigenous mistrust of Western healthcare professionals and medical practices (Sylliboy et al., 2021).

Two-Eyed Seeing

To improve health equity, it is essential that health interventions are based on Indigenous cultural values and developed in partnership with Indigenous communities. While some acknowledgement of the coexistence of Indigenous health knowledge, beliefs, practice and contributions to health and wellbeing exists alongside Western viewpoints, there is a need to move from coexistence to integration. One way of linking these two viewpoints is through the use of the **Two-Eyed Seeing model** (TES). This was described by Indigenous Elder Albert Marshall, as representing one eye seeing Western knowledge and the other seeing Indigenous knowledge, these knowledges are then integrated to ensure that people receive the benefits from each (Bartlett et al., 2012). Researchers have echoed that synergies and differences between Indigenous and Western health knowledge may benefit from a multi-science approach that values, respects and integrates both, but permits differential weighting, depending on need (Ogawa, 1995; Sasakamoose et al., 2016). This helps to avoid the view of 'West being best' and may assist in reducing epistemic racism (Matthews, 2017), especially as recognising the legitimacy of Indigenous knowledge is central to the health of Indigenous Peoples (Seifert et al., 2025). For this to work, healthcare professionals who use a TES approach must have knowledge of and value both Western and Indigenous health knowledge.

Examples of collaborative healthcare that has embraced a TES approach

The causes of disease are more nuanced and the healthcare requirements of Indigenous communities are different to that in Western medicine. For healthcare to be truly beneficial, it is essential Indigenous populations have access to healthcare that reflects their own needs, values and is culturally acceptable. One way of facilitating this is through shared healthcare decision-making (SDM), this encourages collaboration between healthcare providers and patients (Dimopoulos-Bick et al., 2023). Many Indigenous-led healthcare partnerships have been based on SDM, prioritising traditional Indigenous knowledge from Elders, and Knowledge Keepers, with Western biomedical knowledge with treatments from each used as and when required (Allen et al., 2020). In Alaska, the Indigenous-led Nuka System of Care has been in operation for over 30 years, it was designed and is owned by Native Alaskans. It has been effective in reducing the number of visits for emergency care, led to reduced hospital stays, reduced staff turnover, improved vaccination rates and improved satisfaction with healthcare that is viewed as culturally safe (Gottlieb, 2013). In Ontario, Canada, the Anishinabe Peoples from Manitoulin Island have been provided with bicultural healthcare since 1998 at the Noojmowin Teg Health Centre. Western medical care has been coupled with traditional Indigenous health and wellbeing practices, including sensitivity to the importance of spirituality, offerings (gifts) associated with requests for traditional healing, along with specific healing ceremonies and teachings. The meaning of this was explored by Mantiowabi and Shawahnde (2011) who reported that these holistic aspects of traditional care addressed the four aspects of Indigenous well-being (mental, physical, emotional, spiritual), helping patients to regain balance and health associated with the inner spirit and connection with ancestors.

The Medicine Wheel

The Medicine Wheel is an Indigenous model and holistic approach to health and healing that was first used by Indigenous Peoples in the US (Robertson, 2021). It consists of four quadrants and may be used for teaching, health intervention development and research. The Medicine Wheel signifies values and principles related to living in harmony, connectedness in all aspects of life and the fundamental concepts within it are similar across Indigenous Peoples in the US. There is a recognition of the circular nature of life (infancy, youth adulthood and elder), but there are variations in the specific colour and content of each quadrant according to traditional teachings, stories and beliefs associated with different Indigenous nations. Each quadrant is signified with one of the four colours (yellow, red, black and white) and states of being, mental (mind), physical (body), emotional or spiritual wellbeing, with the latter referred to as the mind-body-spirit connection (Ford-Ellis, 2019). All elements of life and nature are interconnected within the Medicine Wheel, it can be used to represent the four compass points (East, South, West, North), seasons (Spring, Summer, Fall, Winter) and sacred medicines (tobacco, sage, sweetgrass, cedar).

Using the Medicine Wheel in an intervention for type 2 diabetes

The Medicine Wheel can be used to introduce nutrition-related interventions that illustrate the links between food, mental, emotional, spiritual and physical health. What an individual eats affects more than their physical body, as food is connected to the land, to ancestors and to the community. Traditional Indigenous foods (berries, beans, vegetables and wild game) are healing, meals are communal, hence they connect people and help emotional wellbeing. Often hunting and harvesting of food involve ceremonies and giving thanks to the land and the spirit world for producing food. Kattelmann et al. (2009) compared dietary adherence, education and glucose control within a sample of Indigenous People (Cheyenne River Sioux) who had T2DM. Participants were randomised into a control group who followed standard diabetes dietary education and the intervention group who, in addition, received six dietary lessons based on the Medicine Wheel Nutrition Model. This encouraged eating foods that were reflective of the macronutrient hunter-gatherer diet, typical of their Northern Plain Indian ancestors. Foods were categorised into four groups, based on the Medicine Wheel and included non-processed foods associated with hunter-gatherer ancestors. Participants were asked to consume daily diets that consisted of 25% protein, 45–50% carbohydrate and 25–30% of fat, respectively. At the end of six months, the intervention group showed significant reductions in weight and body mass index (BMI) compared to their baseline measures, but no significant difference was found for long-term blood glucose levels in either group. The intervention group did not manage to reach the 25% protein intake, with levels of around 14–18%, their carbohydrate intake remained similar to baseline and their fat consumption declined slightly. The authors of the study provided several suggestions for this, which included the duration of the trial (six months) being too short to result in effective dietary change, but interestingly they noted that the individual nature of the intervention may have been a barrier to dietary change. This was due to most intervention-group participants living in multigenerational families where food choices were based on the collective needs of the family, income and food availability. Even though the intervention included advice and input from tribal leaders, it highlighted that greater community and family involvement may have been required to make the required dietary changes more achievable for the intervention group. Indigenous health involves the extended family and community, rather being individually based, with an emphasis on collective responsibility for decision-making, underscoring the importance of family support and cognisance of culture in managing chronic health conditions such as T2DM (Epple et al., 2003).

He Pikinga Waiora

Within New Zealand, the **He Pikinga Waiora** (HPW) model, which means Enhancing Wellbeing, has been adopted as a guide to develop health interventions for the Māori (Oetzel et al., 2017). This approach includes four elements to ensure that Indigenous values are incorporated into health interventions. It requires a culture-centred approach, community engagement, systems thinking and the integration of Indigenous knowledge (see Figure 7.12).

The culture-centred approach involves listening to and acting on the views of the community, respecting Indigenous self-determination by challenging unfair power differentials and subjugation perpetuated by colonialism (Oetzel et al., 2017). This includes assurance that Western healthcare professionals and researchers are trained in cultural safety and that they reflect on their own beliefs and actions to ensure culturally safe practices. Such an approach situates Indigenous knowledge and views of health as being central to understanding health problems, which can then be used to co-design interventions to reduce health inequities (Dutta et al., 2013). Community engagement involves working in partnership with those who are affected by health issues, their families and healthcare professionals or support workers. This prioritises shared decision-making between the community and healthcare professionals, including leadership, as such an approach is more likely to result in the development of lasting health-related interventions (Cook, 2008). Systems thinking concentrates on the holistic view of health, it recognises that health problems are complex and stresses the necessity of considering multiple social determinants of health. These include the individual, their community and the healthcare system (services and healthcare policies), health literacy, food poverty and living in poor housing or in a rural location, all of which can directly and indirectly impact on heath. An essential aspect of systems thinking is valuing different world views by considering the perspectives of Indigenous Peoples and how different ways of working with healthcare systems can improve health outcomes and reduce health inequities (Frerichs et al., 2016). The use of Integrated Knowledge Translation ensures

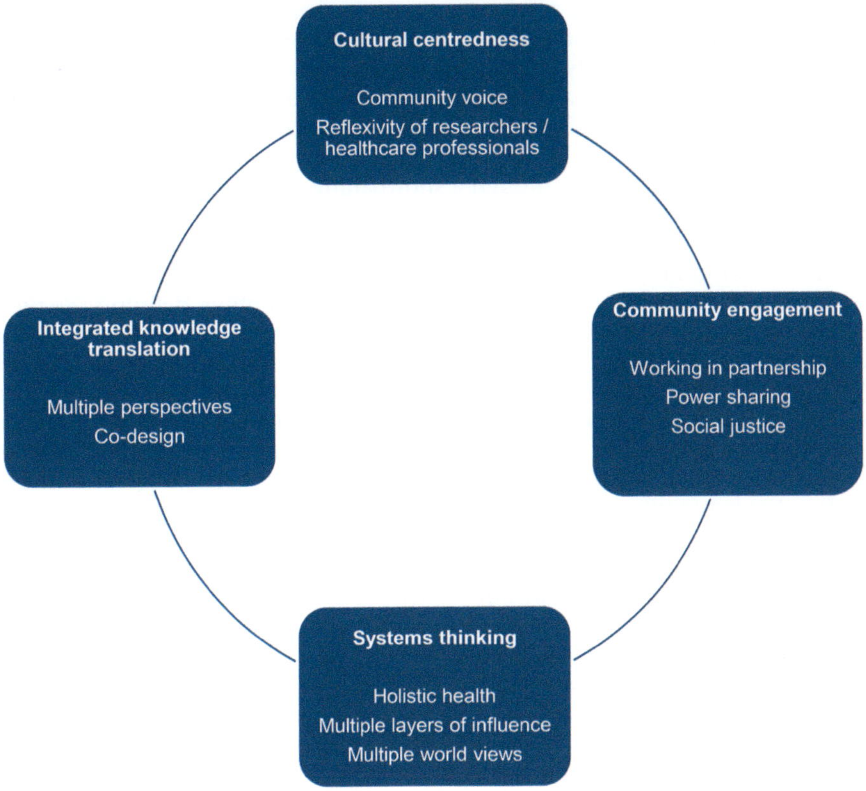

Figure 7.12
He Pikinga Waiora Model

Source: Author based on Oetzel et al. (2017)

that Indigenous knowledge and healthcare practices are respected and included in the co-design of healthcare interventions and services. This involves a range of views and contributions from those who will use the service, community leaders, healthcare professionals and policymakers. Taking this shared approach helps to identify barriers and facilitators to making interventions and services more effective and suited to the needs of Indigenous Peoples (Smylie et al., 2004).

Harding and Oetzel (2019) conducted a systematic review of how well the HPW was implemented within chronic disease interventions for Indigenous populations. They found that high use of community engagement and the culture-centred approach was associated with positive health outcomes at the individual and community levels for diabetes, cancer, weight loss and nutrition interventions. However, there was lower use of systems thinking and integrated knowledge translation, which may have implications for the sustainability of interventions, and it was not totally clear how strongly each element of HPW had to be within an intervention in order for it be successful and sustainable.

In using the HPW, Oetzel et al. (2020) employed a community-based participatory research approach in the co-design of an intervention for weight reduction in Māori men who were at risk of diabetes, cardiovascular disease and obesity. The 12-week lifestyle intervention included physical activity and nutrition, delivered to two groups, one facilitated by a Māori senior mentor and the other by a Māori peer community health worker. Stakeholders who were involved in the co-design of the intervention identify participant recruitment avenues. Group 1 was centred in a Christian church, although belonging to the church was not part of the inclusion criteria. The men's partners were also invited to the intervention, as it was thought that they could help promote attendance. Group 2 was recruited via a trainer at a local gym, through a snowballing sampling, with most participants not being active gym members at the time of recruitment. Co-design of the intervention involved a four-step process between researchers at a local university and a community-based Māori health provider. Step one was mainly about researchers and health providers getting to know each other, defining the project, identifying shared goals, along with provision of further information by the researchers and the Māori health provider. One stipulation at this stage from the Māori health provider was that the intervention needed to be sustainable. The second step involved decisions about the target population, along with discussions and drafting of the potential intervention. Step three included the views of other stakeholders, including those who would take part in the intervention and their extended families. Step four was intervention implementation. All those who started the intervention completed baseline and final weight measures, giving 100% retention, but not all men completed every week of the intervention. Both groups experienced significant reductions in weight and body mass index, improvements in health-related quality of life and a doubling of self-rated health. In evaluating the process of the intervention, the authors reported that it was consistent with the HPW framework, as it involved community engagement and culture-centredness, it integrated knowledge engagement with all stakeholders and included systems thinking. At the outset of the study, researchers were open about their inability to commit to longer-term resourcing, but did work with Māori healthcare providers who agreed to fund another run of the intervention, although continued feasibility was unclear.

BOX 7.5
CRITICAL THINKING

Why might the application of a Western model of health behaviour be inappropriate if applied to Indigenous populations?

Looking to the future

In developing interventions that take culture into account, Barrera et al. (2013) outlined four approaches. The first is researcher led, it assesses the risks to health that are pertinent for a specific group, this provides a basis on which to design, deliver and assess the outcomes of the intervention. In the second approach, researchers design the main aspects of a theory-based intervention and then invite the community to make suggestions for adding cultural aspects to the intervention. In the third approach, the community and their affiliated organisations use Indigenous models, knowledge and practices to create interventions that are evaluated by researchers. The final approach, which is the most commonly used, takes existing interventions and adjusts them to fit the culture that they are to be delivered in. This involves changes to intervention language, considering intervention delivery by staff who are from the same cultural background as participants and the inclusion of cultural traditions, without altering the core aspects of the intervention.

To adapt and change an existing intervention, it is necessary to gather information about the population and the target behaviour, this is used to create a draft version of the intervention, followed by pilot testing and making necessary changes based on the outcome of piloting (Barrera & Castro, 2006). Gathering information will help to determine whether cultural adaptation is required and identify what parts of the intervention need to be changed. For example, there may be different links between risk factors and health outcomes in a minority group compared to the majority population. Within the UK, breast cancer is often diagnosed at a more advanced stage in Black women of African and Caribbean descent, compared to their White counterparts. Marcu et al. (2022) conducted focus groups with Black women to explore if a booklet targeted at promoting early prevention of breast cancer (including information on symptoms and breast self-examination) was suitable for this population and what changes were necessary to make the booklet more culturally relevant. Data gathering about breast cancer showed that Black women tended not to discuss cancer, as they associated it with stigma and considered it to be a White person's disease. In the past, the latter may have been perpetuated in breast screening and self-examination messaging, as there was an absence of ethnic minority representation in public health information images. Women suggested changes to the booklet, which included making it more inclusive through the use of images and language that was more culturally relevant to women from ethnic minority groups. Furthermore, messaging was needed to highlight that some breast cancers are curable, which could be helped by focusing on Black women as survivors of breast cancer. A final point from this study was that dissemination of health information could be enhanced by using trusted Black communities to share the booklet and to raise cancer awareness.

Lessons learned

Within this chapter, we have reviewed a range of theories and models, including Indigenous frameworks, to inform intervention design. When working in partnership to design and implement interventions for minority groups, it is essential that cultural knowledge, community values and lived experiences are considered. This helps to develop more meaningful and sustainable health services and interventions that may reduce health inequities so commonly found in historically underserved populations. For services and interventions to work, they must include partnership working with the communities in which the intervention will be used. With good intent, researchers and healthcare professionals have made cultural adaptations to existing interventions designed for the 'dominant' group; however, research shows that these adaptations have limited effectiveness for Indigenous and some minority groups (Dixon et al., 2007; Okamoto et al., 2014). The use of participatory research practices (see Chapter 3) is now becoming more prevalent, recognising the important role and knowledge that communities and groups of people who use services (service users or experts by experience) can bring to partnership working (see Box 7.2). This will help to enable researchers, healthcare professionals and organisations to design and implement effective and culturally safe healthcare interventions and services for all groups within society.

BOX 7.2
PATIENT AND PUBLIC INVOLVEMENT (PPI) IN RESEARCH

The people who take part in health intervention research can provide researchers and healthcare professionals with important and valuable information about health conditions, treatments and the services received. Including patients, family members, carers and public views on research helps to capture diverse perspectives, which can make research relevant to a wider range of population groups. Including patient and public involvement (PPI) can help to ensure that research is focused on what matters to users of services and research participants. Most grant awarding bodies now stipulate that research funding applications must have PPI built into their research in a meaningful way.

PPI can happen at all stages of the research process, including identification of priority areas to study. This can commence at the planning stages, in helping to identify funders of research, in the development of research proposals and co-design of interventions, decisions about the intervention components, in gaining ethical approval, writing of participant information sheets, consent forms and study documentation, data collection, analysis, evaluation and dissemination of results.

For PPI to be successful, participants may need training to help them get up to speed with the way research or an intervention design works. This can also be beneficial for researchers, as they will have to learn how to talk to non-researchers and use terminology that is understood by everyone. Training can also make PPI participants feel that they are part of the research team and that their contributions are valued and listened to.

If you would like to know more about PPI in UK health research, follow the link to find out about the National Institute for Health and Care Research (NIHR): https://www.peopleinresearch.org/public-involvement/

Chapter summary

Discuss how classical conditioning, operant conditioning and social learning theory may influence health behaviours

Classical conditioning can be used to explain how in a healthcare setting neutral stimuli can become associated with reflexive behaviours such as fear or the vomit reflex, behaviour therapy can be used as a way of desensitising people to stimuli that elicit a reflexive behaviour. The frequency and timing of reinforcement in operant condition can be used to shape health behaviours. Social learning theory helps to explain how vicarious learning may be important in health enhancing and risky behaviours.

Outline the main components of the social cognitive models of health

Internal and external (powerful other and chance) locus of control help to explain people's beliefs in the causes of disease and how beliefs influence their health behaviours. The Health Belief Model was developed to understand why people did not engage in screening behaviours. It is based on perceived threat (susceptibility, severity of disease), modifying factors (demographic factors and cues to action), likelihood of action (perceived benefits and perceived barriers) and self-efficacy.

Examine the stages and associated processes of change in the Transtheoretical Model?

This model has five stages, precontemplation, contemplation, preparation, action and maintenance, associated with five cognitive and five behavioural processes of change. Cognitive processes of change are associated with education and health promotion in the first two stages of the model. The latter stages of the model are characterised by use of behavioural processes of change.

Discuss factors that influence behaviour intention in the Theory of Planned Behaviour?

Behaviour intention is the strongest predictor of engaging in a health behaviour, it is influenced by attitudes towards the behaviour (beliefs about the outcome of the behaviour and evaluations of the outcome of the behaviour); subjective norms (beliefs about what others would like me to do and motivation to comply with others' beliefs) and perceived behavioural control (control beliefs and perceived power).

Outline the COM-B model and how it is related to intervention functions and policy categories in the Behaviour Change Wheel

Behaviour is influenced by capability, opportunity and motivation, which are linked with the intervention functions of education, persuasion, incentivisation, coercion, training, enablement, environmental restructuring and restrictions. Identification of intervention functions enables the identification of behaviour change techniques to turn functions into actions. Intervention functions can be facilitated through implementation of policy categories.

Explain the Two-Eyed Seeing model and discuss why it is important to Indigenous health?

This model involves the integration of Western healthcare approach with that of Indigenous healing practices. It values, respects and integrates both, but permits differential weighting to benefit the needs of this population.

Outline why the Medicine Wheel is of use when designing an intervention for Indigenous communities

It emphasises holistic healing incorporating mental, emotional, spiritual and physical healing and the interconnection with nature that are intertwined with the four seasons and the cycle of life.

Discuss how the He Pikinga Waiora model has been used as a guide to develop health interventions in New Zealand

This model ensures that Indigenous values and knowledge of cultural centeredness, community engagement, systems thinking and integrated knowledge translation are incorporated into intervention development.

Keywords

Health enhancing behaviours: Behaviours that are beneficial to health e.g. healthy eating, physical activity, vaccinations and preventative screening.
Health compromising behaviours: Behaviours that are detrimental to health e.g. smoking, binge drinking and risky sexual behaviours.
Classical conditioning: A type of associative learning based on reflexive behaviours.
Operant conditioning: A type of learning based on voluntary behaviours that can be shaped by schedules of reinforcement.
Social Learning Theory: Observational learning that includes modelling the behaviour of others.
Vicarious learning: Learning from the experience of others.
Self-efficacy: A person's belief in their own ability to accomplish a task or behaviour.
Health Locus of Control: The beliefs that people have over the control of their own health and health behaviours.
Health Belief Model: A social cognition model that tries to understand why people engage in health behaviours, based on perceived threat, modifying factors and likelihood of action.
Cues to action: Internal (symptoms) or external factors (the media or healthcare invitations) that influence health behaviours.
Mammography: X-rays that are used to examine the breasts for cancer.
Transtheoretical model: A five-stage model used to explain behaviour that includes processes of change, self-efficacy and decisional balance.
Theory of Planned Behaviour: A model used to predict behavioural intention, based on attitudes towards the behaviour, subjective norms and perceived behavioural control.
Intention-behaviour gap: The inability to convert intentions into actions.
Behaviour Change Wheel: A structured way to describe, design and evaluate interventions that moves people from intention to action by focusing on factors that influence behaviour.
Behaviour change techniques: The smallest precisely defined active ingredients used in interventions.
Two-Eyed Seeing: A model that incorporates Western and Indigenous knowledges, values and beliefs, so that Indigenous Peoples can benefit from both.
The Medicine Wheel: Represents a holistic Indigenous approach to health and healing that values harmony and connectedness in all aspects of life.
He Pikinga Waiora: An Indigenous model that has been used to guide the development of health interventions in New Zealand.

Key readings

Harding, T., & Oetzel, J. (2019). Implementation effectiveness of health interventions for indigenous communities: A systematic review. *Implementation Science, 14*(1), 76. https://doi.org/10.1186/s13012-019-0920-4

Marcu, A., Marke, L., Armes, J., Whitaker, K. L., & Ream, E. (2022). Adapting a breast cancer early presentation intervention for Black women: A focus group study with women of Black African and Black Caribbean descent in the United Kingdom. *European Journal of Cancer Care, 31*(6), e13652. https://doi.org/10.1111/ecc.13652

Michie, S., van Stralen, M. M. & West, R. (2011). The behaviour change wheel: A new method for characterising and designing behaviour change interventions. *Implementation Science, 6*, 42. https://doi.org/10.1186/1748-5908-6-42

These reflective questions are designed to encourage you to think about the material presented in this chapter

1 Have you ever planned to change something (like diet or exercise) but did not follow through? What do you think stopped you and how could you use a psychological theory or model to explain this?

2 Why might health locus of control be an important concept to consider when trying to help an individual to change their health behaviours?

3 How do Indigenous models like the Medicine Wheel or Two-Eyed Seeing give us a different way to think about health?

4 Why is it important to include patients' and the public views when conducting health research or designing interventions?

References

Abraham, C., & Sheeran, P. (2015). The health belief model. In M. Conner & P. Norman (Eds.), *Predicting and changing health behaviour: Research and practice with social cognition models* (3rd ed., pp. 30–69). Open University Press.

Adams, J., & White, M. (2003). Are activity promotion interventions based on the transtheoretical model effective? A critical review. *British Journal of Sports Medicine, 37*(2), 106–114. https://doi.org/10.1136/bjsm.37.2.106

Ajzen, I. (1991). The theory of planned behavior. *Organizational Behavior and Human Decision Processes, 50*(2), 179–211. https://doi.org/10.1016/0749-5978(91)90020-T

Allen, L., Hatala, A., Ijaz, S., Courchene, E. D., & Bushie, E. B. (2020). Indigenous-led health care partnerships in Canada. *Canadian Medical Association Journal, 192*(9), E208–E216. https://doi.org/10.1503/cmaj.190728

Amireault, S., Godin, G., Vohl, M. C., & Pérusse, L. (2008). Moderators of the intention-behaviour and perceived behavioural control-behaviour relationships for leisure-time physical activity. *The International Journal of Behavioral Nutrition and Physical Activity, 5*, 7. https://doi.org/10.1186/1479-5868-5-7

Bandura, A. (1977a). *Social learning theory*. Prentice-Hall.

Bandura, A. (1977b). Self-efficacy: Toward a unifying theory of behavioral change. *Psychological Review, 84*(2), 191–215. https://doi.org/10.1037/0033-295X.84.2.191

Bandura, A., Ross, D., & Ross, S. A. (1961). Transmission of aggression through imitation of aggressive models. *The Journal of Abnormal and Social Psychology, 63*(3), 575–582. https://doi.org/10.1037/h0045925

Barrera, M. Jr., & Castro, F. G. (2006). A heuristic framework for the cultural adaptation of Interventions. *Clinical Psychology: Science and Practice, 13*(4), 311–316. https://doi.org/10.1111/j.1468-2850.2006.00043.x

Barrera, M. Jr, Castro, F. G., Strycker, L. A., & Toobert, D. J. (2013). Cultural adaptations of behavioral health interventions: A progress report. *Journal of Consulting and Clinical Psychology, 81*(2), 196–205. https://doi.org/10.1037/a0027085

Bartlett, C., Marshall, M., & Marshall, A. (2012). Two-Eyed Seeing and other lessons learned within a co-learning journey of bringing together indigenous and mainstream knowledges and ways of knowing. *Journal of Environmental Studies and Sciences, 2*, 331–340. https://doi.org/10.1007/s13412-012-0086-8

Bertoni, A., Rapelli, G., Parise, M., Pagani, A. F., & Donato, S. (2023). "Cardiotoxic" and "cardioprotective" partner support for patient activation and distress: Are two better than one? *Family Relations, 72*(3), 1335–1350. https://doi.org/10.1111/fare.12694

Breast Cancer Now (2023). *Barriers to breast cancer screening*. Retrieved July 4, 2025, from https://breastcancernow.org/about-us/campaign-news/barriers-breast-cancer-screening

Conner, M., & Norman, P. (Eds.). (2015). *Predicting and changing health behaviour: Research and practice with social cognition models* (3rd eds.). Open University Press.

Conner, M., & Norman, P. (2022). Understanding the intention-behavior gap: The role of intention strength. *Frontiers in Psychology, 13*, 923464. https://doi.org/10.3389/fpsyg.2022.923464

Cook, W. K. (2008). Integrating research and action: A systematic review of community-based participatory research to address health disparities in environment and occupational health in the USA. *Journal of Epidemiology and Community Health, 62*(8), 668–676. https://doi.org/10.1136/jech.2007.067645

Coxon, J., Hosey, M. T., & Newton, J. T. (2017). What reward does a child prefer for behaving well at the dentist? *British Dental Journal Open, 3*, 17018. https://doi.org/10.1038/bdjopen.2017.18

DiClemente, C. C., & Hughes, S. O. (1990). Stages of change profiles in outpatient alcoholism treatment. *Journal of Substance Abuse, 2*(2), 217–235. https://doi.org/10.1016/s0899-3289(05)80057-4

Dimopoulos-Bick, T., Follent, D., Kostovski, C., Middleton, V., Paulson, C., Sutherland, S., Cawley, M., Files, M., Follent, S., Osten, R., & Trevena, L. (2023). Finding Your Way - A shared decision making resource developed by and for Aboriginal people in Australia: Perceived acceptability, usability, and feasibility. *Patient Education and Counseling, 115*, 107920. https://doi.org/10.1016/j.pec.2023.107920

Dixon, A. L., Yabiku, S. T., Okamoto, S. K., Tann, S. S., Marsiglia, F. F., Kulis, S., & Burke, A. M. (2007). The efficacy of a multicultural prevention intervention among urban American Indian youth in the Southwest U.S. *The Journal of Primary Prevention, 28*(6), 547–568. https://doi.org/10.1007/s10935-007-0114-8

Dutta, M., Anaele, A., & Jones, C. (2013). Voiced of hunger: Addressing health disparities through the culture-centered approach. *Journal of Communication, 63*(1), 159–180. https://doi.org/10.1111/jcom.12009

Epple, C., Wright, A. L., Joish, V. N., & Bauer, M. (2003). The role of active family nutritional support in Navajos' type 2 diabetes metabolic control. *Diabetes Care, 26*(10), 2829–2834. https://doi.org/10.2337/diacare.26.10.2829

Etter, J. F., Bergman, M. M., Humair, J. P., & Perneger, T. V. (2000). Development and validation of a scale measuring self-efficacy of current and former smokers. *Addiction, 95*(6), 901–913. https://doi.org/10.1046/j.1360-0443.2000.9569017.x

Figueroa-Moseley, C., Jean-Pierre, P., Roscoe, J. A., Ryan, J. L., Kohli, S., Palesh, O. G., Ryan, E. P., Carroll, J., & Morrow, G. R. (2007). Behavioral interventions in treating anticipatory nausea and vomiting. *Journal of the National Comprehensive Cancer Network, 5*(1), 44–50. https://doi.org/10.6004/jnccn.2007.0006

Ford-Ellis, A. G. (2019). How is the Medicine Wheel considered in therapeutic practice. *Journal of Concurrent Disorders, 1*(3), 78–93. https://doi.org/10.54127/ALJJ4787

Frerichs, L., Lich, K. H., Dave, G., & Corbie-Smith, G. (2016). Integrating systems science and community-based participatory research to achieve health equity. *American Journal of Public Health, 106*(2), 215–222. https://doi.org/10.2105/AJPH.2015.302944

Glanz, K., & Rimer, B. K. (2005). Theory at a glance: A guide for health promotion practice (2nd ed.). National Cancer Institute, MIH, Public Health Services. U.S. Government Printing Office. Retrieved September 9, 2025, from https://cancer-control.cancer.gov/sites/default/files/2020-06/theory.pdf

Goff, L. M., Moore, A. P., Harding, S., & Rivas, C. (2021). Development of healthy eating and active lifestyles for diabetes, a culturally tailored diabetes self-management education and support programme for Black-British adults: A participatory research approach. *Diabetic Medicine, 38*(11), e14594. https://doi.org/10.1111/dme.14594

Gottlieb, K. (2013). The Nuka System of Care: Improving health through ownership and relationships. *International Journal of Circumpolar Health, 72*, 21118. https://doi.org/10.3402/ijch.v72i0.21118

Hailey, B. J., & White, J. G. (1983). Systematic desensitization for anticipatory nausea associated with chemotherapy. *Psychosomatics, 24*(3), 287–291. https://doi.org/10.1016/s0033-3182(83)73231-7

Haley, J. A., Rhind, D. J. A., & Maidment, D. W. (2023). Applying the behaviour change wheel to assess the theoretical underpinning of a novel smartphone application to increase physical activity in adults with spinal cord injuries. *mHealth, 9*, 10. https://doi.org/10.21037/mhealth-22-52

Hardeman, W., Johnston, M., Johnston, D. W., Bonetti, D., Wareham, N. J., & Kinmonth, A. L. (2002). Application of the Theory of Planned Behaviour in behaviour change interventions: A systematic review. *Psychology & Health, 17*(2), 123–158. https://doi.org/10.1080/08870440290013644a

Harding, T., & Oetzel, J. (2019). Implementation effectiveness of health interventions for indigenous communities: A systematic review. *Implementation Science, 14*(1), 76. https://doi.org/10.1186/s13012-019-0920-4

Hatzenbuehler, M. L., Corbin, W. R., & Fromme, K. (2008). Trajectories and determinants of alcohol use among LGB young adults and their heterosexual peers: Results from a prospective study. *Developmental Psychology, 44*(1), 81–90. https://doi.org/10.1037/0012-1649.44.1.81

Hickok, J. T., Roscoe, J. A., & Morrow, G. R. (2001). The role of patients' expectations in the development of anticipatory nausea related to chemotherapy for cancer. *Journal of Pain and Symptom Management, 22*(4), 843–850. https://doi.org/10.1016/s0885-3924(01)00317-7

Itkowitz, N. I., Kerns, R. D., & Otis, J. D. (2003). Support and coronary heart disease: The importance of significant other responses. *Journal of Behavioral Medicine, 26*(1), 19–30. https://doi.org/10.1023/a:1021790921471

Janz, N. K., & Becker, M. H. (1984). The Health Belief Model: A decade later. *Health Education Quarterly, 11*(1), 1–47. https://doi.org/10.1177/109019818401100101

Kandemir, D., Yüksel, S., Kanbay, Y., Temiz, Z., Altun Uğras, G., & Akyolcu, N. (2025). The mediating role of mammography self-efficacy in the effect of cancer attitudes on fear of breast cancer in women. *Seminars in Oncology Nursing, 41*(3), 151896. https://doi.org/10.1016/j.soncn.2025.151896

Kasl, S. V., & Cobb, S. (1966). Health behavior, illness behavior, and sick role behavior: I. Health and illness behavior. *Archives of Environmental Health, 12*(2), 246–266. https://doi.org/10.1080/00039896.1966.10664365

Kattelmann, K. K., Conti, K., & Ren, C. (2009). The Medicine Wheel nutrition intervention: A diabetes education study with the Cheyenne River Sioux Tribe. *Journal of the American Dietetic Association, 109*(9), 1532–1539. https://doi.org/10.1016/j.jada.2009.06.362

Kirkham, S. R., Baumbusch, J. L., Schultz, A. S. H., & Anderson, J. M. (2007). Knowledge development and evidence based practice: Insights and opportunities from a postcolonial feminist perspective for transformative nursing practice. *Advances in Nursing Science, 30*(1), 26–40. https://doi.org/10.1097/00012272-200701000-00004

Mantiowabi, D., & Shawahnde, M. (2011). The meaning of Anishinabe healing and wellbeing on Manitoulin Island. *Pimatisiwin: A Journal of Aboriginal & Indigenous Community Health, 9*(2), 441–458. https://journalindigenouswellbeing.co.nz/media/2018/12/10_Manitowabi.pdf

Marcu, A., Marke, L., Armes, J., Whitaker, K. L., & Ream, E. (2022). Adapting a breast cancer early presentation intervention for Black women: A focus group study with women of Black African and Black Caribbean descent in the United Kingdom. *European Journal of Cancer Care, 31*(6), e13652. https://doi.org/10.1111/ecc.13652

Martinez-Calderon, J., Zamora-Campos, C., Navarro-Ledesma, S., & Luque-Suarez, A. (2018). The role of self-efficacy on the prognosis of chronic musculoskeletal pain: A systematic review. *The Journal of Pain, 19*(1), 10–34. https://doi.org/10.1016/j.jpain.2017.08.008

Martinez-Calderon, J., Flores-Cortes, M., Morales-Asencio, J. M., Fernandez-Sanchez, M., & Luque-Suarez, A. (2020). Which interventions enhance pain self-efficacy in people with chronic musculoskeletal pain? A systematic review with meta-analysis of randomized controlled trials, including over 12 000 participants. *The Journal of Orthopaedic and Sports Physical Therapy, 50*(8), 418–430. https://doi.org/10.2519/jospt.2020.9319

Matthews, R. (2017). The cultural erosion of Indigenous people in health care. *Canadian Medical Association Journal, 189*(2), E78–E79. https://doi.org/10.1503/cmaj.160167

McDermott, M. S., Oliver, M., Svenson, A., Simnadis, T., Beck, E. J., Coltman, T., Iverson, D., Caputi, P., & Sharma, R. (2015). The Theory of Planned Behaviour and discrete food choices: A systematic review and meta-analysis. *The international Journal of Behavioral Nutrition and Physical Activity, 12*, 162. https://doi.org/10.1186/s12966-015-0324-z

Mercer, D. A., Ditto, B., Lavoie, K. L., Campbell, T., Arsenault, A., & Bacon, S. L. (2018). Health locus of control is associated with physical activity and other health behaviors in cardiac patients. *Journal of Cardiopulmonary Rehabilitation and Prevention, 38*(6), 394–399. https://doi.org/10.1097/HCR.0000000000000350

Michie, S., Richardson, M., Johnston, M., Abraham, C., Francis, J., Hardeman, W., Eccles, M. P., Cane, J., & Wood, C. E. (2013). The Behavior Change Technique Taxonomy (v1) of 93 hierarchically clustered techniques: Building an international consensus for the reporting of behavior change interventions. *Annals of Behavioral Medicine, 46*(1), 81–95. https://doi.org/10.1007/s12160-013-9486-6

Michie, S., van Stralen, M. M., & West, R. (2011). The behaviour change wheel: A new method for characterising and designing behaviour change interventions. *Implementation Science, 6*, 42 https://doi.org/10.1186/1748-5908-6-42

National Institute for Health and Care Excellence. (2014). *Behaviour change: Individual approaches* (Public health guideline; PH49). https://www.nice.org.uk/Guidance/PH49

Nicholas, M. K. (2007). The pain self-efficacy questionnaire: Taking pain into account. *European Journal of Pain, 11*(2), 153–163. https://doi.org/10.1016/j.ejpain.2005.12.008

Nilsen, P. (2015). Making sense of implementation theories, models and frameworks. *Implementation Science, 10*, 53. https://doi.org/10.1186/s13012-015-0242-0

Norman, P., Conner, M., & Bell, R. (2010). The Theory of Planned Behaviour and exercise: Evidence for the moderating role of past behaviour. *British Journal of Health Psychology, 5*(3), 249–261. https://doi.org/10.1348/135910700168892

Oetzel, J., Scott, N., Hudson, M., Masters-Awatere, B., Rarere, M., Foote, J., Beaton, A., & Ehau, T. (2017). Implementation framework for chronic disease intervention effectiveness in Māori and other indigenous communities. *Globalization and Health, 13*(1), 69. https://doi.org/10.1186/s12992-017-0295-8

Oetzel, J., Rarere, M., Wihapi, R., Manuel, C., & Tapsell, J. (2020). A case study of using the He Pikinga Waiora Implementation Framework: Challenges and successes in implementing a twelve-week lifestyle intervention to reduce weight in Māori men at risk of diabetes, cardiovascular disease and obesity. *International Journal of Equity in Health, 19*, 103. https://doi.org/10.1186/s12939-020-01222-3

Ogawa, M. (1995). Science education in a multiscience perspective. *Science Education, 79*(5), 583–593. https://doi.org/10.1002/sce.3730790507

Ojo, S. O., Bailey, D. P., Brierley, M. L., Hewson, D. J., & Chater, A. M. (2019). Breaking barriers: Using the Behavior Change Wheel to develop a tailored intervention to overcome workplace inhibitors to breaking up sitting time. *BMC Public Health, 19*, 1126. http://doi.org/10.1186/s12889-019-7468-8

Okamoto, S. K., Kulis, S., Marsiglia, F. F., Holleran Steiker, L. K., Dustman, P., Steiker, L. K. H., & Dustman, P. (2014). A continuum of approaches toward developing culturally focused prevention interventions, from adaptation to grounding. *The Journal of Primary Prevention, 35*(2), 103–112. https://doi.org/10.1007/s10935-013-0334-z

Oral Health Foundation (2024). UK could face dental health crisis as costs soar, says Oral Health Foundation. Retrieved July 7, 2025, from https://www.dentalhealth.org/news/uk-could-face-dental-health-crisis-as-costs-soar-says-oral-health-foundation

Pavlov, I. P. (1927). *Conditioned reflexes: An investigation of the physiological activity of the cerebral cortex*. Oxford University Press.

Picha, K. J., Valier, A. S., Heebner, N. R., Abt, J. P., Usher, E. L., Capilouto, G., & Uhl, T. L. (2021). Physical therapists' assessment of patient self-efficacy for home exercise programs. *International Journal of Sports Physical Therapy, 16*(1), 184–194. https://doi.org/10.26603/001c.18957

Prestwich, A., Sniehotta, F. F., Whittington, C., Dombrowski, S. U., Rogers, L., & Michie, S. (2014). Does theory influence the effectiveness of health behavior interventions? Meta-analysis. *Health Psychology, 33*(5), 465–474. https://doi.org/10.1037/a0032853

Prochaska, J. O., & DiClemente, C. C. (1983). Stages and processes of self-change of smoking: Toward an integrative model of change. *Journal of Consulting and Clinical Psychology, 51*(3), 390–395. https://doi.org/10.1037/0022-006X.51.3.390

Prochaska, J. O., Velicer, W. F., Rossi, J. S., Goldstein, M. G., Marcus, B. H., Rakowski, W., Fiore, C., Harlow, L. L., Redding, C. A., & Rosenbloom, D. (1994). Stages of change and decisional balance for 12 problem behaviors. *Health Psychology, 13*(1), 39–46. https://doi.org/10.1037//0278-6133.13.1.39

Ritter, P. L., & Lorig, K. (2014). The English and Spanish Self-Efficacy to Manage Chronic Disease Scale measures were validated using multiple studies. *Journal of Clinical Epidemiology, 67*(11), 1265–1273. https://doi.org/10.1016/j.jclinepi.2014.06.009

Robertson, L. H. (2021). The Medicine Wheel revisited: Reflections on indigenization in counseling and education. *SAGE Open, 11*(2). https://doi.org/10.1177/21582440211015202

Rosenstock, I. M. (1974). Historical origins of the Health Belief Model. *Health Education Monographs, 2*(4), 328–335. https://doi.org/10.1177/109019817400200403

Rosenstock, I. M., Stretcher, V. J., & Becker, M. H. (1988). Social learning theory and the Health Belief Model. *Health Education Quarterly, 15*(2), 175–183. https://doi.org/10.1177/109019818801500203

Rotter, J. B. (1966). Generalized expectancies for internal versus external control of reinforcement. *Psychological Monographs: General and Applied, 80*(1), 1–28. https://doi.org/10.1037/h0092976

Sasakamoose, J., Scerbe, A., Wenaus, I., & Scandrett, A. (2016). First Nation and Métis youth perspectives of health: An Indigenous qualitative inquiry. *Qualitative Inquiry, 22*(8), 636–650. https://doi.org/10.1177/1077800416629695

Seifert, G., Boujnah, H., Ghods, R., Wieland, S., Aginam, O., Chuthaputti, A., Ghelman, R., Goh, C. S., Matsabisa, M. G., Tu'itahi, S., Kim, S., Kuruvilla, S., & Patwardhan, B. (2025). Promoting planetary health and well-being for all: Harnessing indigenous knowledges for health with traditional, complementary and integrative health systems. *Frontiers in Medicine, 12*, 1543687. https://doi.org/10.3389/fmed.2025.1543687

Shafieinia, M., Hidarnia, A., Kazemnejad, A., & Rajabi, R. (2016). Effects of a theory based intervention on physical activity among female employees: A quasi-experimental study. *Asian Journal of Sports Medicine, 7*(2), e31534. https://doi.org/10.5812/asjsm.31534

Skinner, B. F. (1953). *Science and human behavior*. Macmillian.

Skivington, K., Matthews, L., Simpson, S. A., Craig, P., Baird, J., Blazeby, J. M., Boyd, K. A., Craig, N., French, D. P., McIntosh, E., Petticrew, M., Rycroft-Malone, J., White, M., & Moore, L. (2021). A new framework for developing and evaluating complex interventions: Update of Medical Research Council guidance. *British Medical Journal, 374*, n2061. https://doi.org/10.1136/bmj.n2061

Smylie, J., Martin, C. M., Kaplan-Myrth, N., Steele, L., Tait, C., & Hogg, W. (2004). Knowledge translation and indigenous knowledge. *International Journal of Circumpolar Health, 63*(2), 139–143. https://doi.org/10.3402/ijch.v63i0.17877

Stockhorst, U., Steingrueber, H.-J., Enck, P., & Klosterhalfen, S. (2006). Pavlovian conditioning of nausea and vomiting. *Autonomic Neuroscience, 129*(1–2), 50–57. https://doi.org/10.1016/j.autneu.2006.07.012

Sutton, S. (2001). Back to the drawing board? A review of applications of the transtheoretical model to substance use. *Addiction, 96*(1), 175–186. https://doi.org/10.1046/j.1360-0443.2001.96117513.x

Sylliboy, J. R., Latimer, M., Marshall, E. A., & MacLeod, E. (2021). Communities take the lead: Exploring Indigenous health research practices through Two-Eyed Seeing & kinship. *International Journal of Circumpolar Health, 80*(1), 1929755. https://doi.org/10.1080/22423982.2021.1929755

Tapera, R., Mbongwe, B., Mhaka-Mutepfa, M., Lord, A., Phaladze, N. A., & Zetola, N. M. (2020). The Theory of Planned Behavior as a behavior change model for tobacco control strategies among adolescents in Botswana. *PloS One, 15*(6), e0233462. https://doi.org/10.1371/journal.pone.0233462

Wallston, K. A., Wallston, B. S., & DeVellis, R. (1978). Development of the Multidimensional Health Locus of Control (MHLC) Scales. *Health Education Monographs, 6*(2), 160–170. https://doi.org/10.1177/109019817800600107

Webb, J., Foster, J., & Poulter, E. (2016). Increasing the frequency of physical activity very brief advice for cancer patients. Development of an intervention using the behaviour change wheel. *Public Health, 133*, 45–56. https://doi.org/10.1016/j.puhe.2015.12.009

West, R. (2005). Time for change: Putting the Transtheoretical Model (Stages of Change) Model to rest. *Addiction, 100*(8), 1036–1039. https://doi.org/10.1111/j.1360-0443.2005.01139.x

Wilson-Barlow, L., Hollins, T. R., & Clopton, J. R. (2014). Construction and validation of the healthy eating and weight self-efficacy (HEWSE) scale. *Eating Behaviors, 15*(3), 490–492. https://doi.org/10.1016/j.eatbeh.2014.06.004

World Health Organization. (2003). *Indigenous peoples and participatory health research.* World Health Organization. https://www.mcgill.ca/cine/files/cine/partreresearch_english.pdf

Xiang, X., Han, M., Luo, X., Yu, Y., Lu, X., Cai, S., & Huang, L. (2023). Development of a behavior change intervention to improve physical activity in patients with COPD using the Behavior Change Wheel: A non-randomized trial. *Scientific Reports, 13*(1), 22929. https://doi.org/10.1038/s41598-023-50099-z

Zhao, X., Dichtl, F. F., & Foran, H. M. (2022). Predicting smoking behavior: Intention and future self-continuity among Austrians. *Psychology, Health & Medicine, 27*(5), 1042–1051. https://doi.org/10.1080/13548506.2020.1842898

8 Stress and coping

Chapter contents

- What is stress?
- Stress as a stimulus.
- Stress as a physiological response.
- Transactional model of stress.
- Coping with stress.
- Stress and disease.
- Stress and health compromising behaviours.
- Disease as a source of stress.
- Stress, personality and disease.
- Colonisation, intersectionality and stress.
- Measuring stress.

Chapter objectives

After reading this chapter, you should be able to answer the following questions:

- Outline the ways in which stress has been defined.
- Explain what is meant by primary and secondary appraisal of stress.
- What types of social support can help mediate the effects of stress?
- Examine the role of stress in disease.
- Discuss the link between stress and personality.
- Explain how colonisation and intersectionality contribute to stress.

What is stress?

Stress is a word that most people are familiar with however, it is difficult to define and can mean different things to different people. Stress can be described as a stimulus, which is something that is external to the individual, such as an event, a situation or a demand that triggers a stress response. We experience physiological and psychological responses to stress. The ways in which various physiological systems respond to stress are universal and automatic, but the extent of the response and how long it persists varies according to how the stressor is interpreted. Interpretation is a dynamic process and emphasises the interaction between the person, their environment and their perceived ability to cope. Sources of stress can include relationships, life events, such as examinations and examination results, starting university, financial issues including poverty, relationship problems, health conditions and everyday interactions with others. Environmental stressors may include noise, the impact of the weather, catastrophic flooding, earthquakes, wildfires,

DOI: 10.4324/9781003423157-8

climate change, wars and living in deprived neighbourhoods. Stress can be caused by the experience of **discrimination** and/or **stigma** associated with belonging to a marginalised group, due to ethnicity, disability, gender identity, sexual orientation, religious beliefs, the impacts of colonisation and social injustice. This chapter examines some of the sources of stress and models that explain the physiological and psychological impacts of stress and explores how people cope with stress.

What one person defines as stressful may be an enjoyable experience for others. Think about going on to a stage to give a talk, many people would find this incredibly stressful, yet for others it can be an enjoyable experience, which they get great satisfaction from! A rollercoaster ride at the funfair may be an exhilarating and enjoyable experience for one person, while others who have a fear of heights would find it quite stressful. Going on holiday is something that most people look forward to, but the stress of booking transport, hotels, flights, etc., tasks that need to be completed before leaving home, getting to the airport and through security can be quite stressful, yet the end result of being on holiday is great. These examples show that stress does not always involve something that is negative; Selye (1956) referred to 'eustress' as being a positive enjoyable type of stress and 'distress' as being the negative form of stress that could have detrimental health consequences.

Stress as a stimulus

When people talk about stress, they sometimes mention that they are feeling under 'pressure' or a situation is causing them 'strain'. To help us think about the impact of external sources of stress, an analogy can be made with a principle in physics called Hooke's Law of Elasticity. Imagine you have an elastic band, which you keep stretching, it will be able to withstand a certain amount of stretching and return to normal (the elastic limit), but after a while some of the fibres will start to break (yielding), especially if it is overstretched, when this happens the elastic band will not be capable of returning to normal and it may rupture. Any repeated overstretching will result in more fibres breaking and eventually the elastic band will snap (breakdown). So how can we apply this to human stress? People have to deal with various types of issues (e.g. work, financial, relationship and health) that may cause stress, they manage to deal with stressors and carry on as normal. However, there is a limit to the amount or degree of stress that most people can deal with at a time, going beyond this can be detrimental to physical and mental health. Some people can return to normal once the stressor has been removed, but just in the same way an elastic band can become damaged. When stress is repeatedly applied beyond the elastic limit, individuals who experience chronic stress may be unable to return to their normal unstressed state, culminating in mental and physical health issues. While the analogy of Hooke's Law of elasticity is useful in understanding the potential impact of external stressful events, it cannot account for individual psychological, emotional, social, cultural, historical and physiological factors that may affect how people respond to and cope with stress. In addition, it presupposes that greater force or demand is associated with increased stress, but that is not always the case, as an undemanding boring job may be just as stressful as a working in a highly demanding and pressured job environment.

Stress as a physiological response

Cannon (1932) provided one of the earliest explanations of stress, referring to it as the 'fight or flight' response. When faced with a threat (stressor), the individual tries to deal with it (fight) or escape (flight), which is viewed as an adaptive response, necessary to keep an individual safe. You may remember from Chapter 4 that a whole array of physiological processes are involved with the recognition of a stressor and the body's response to it. When confronted with a source of stress, the amygdala sends a signal to the posterior hypothalamus, which in turn triggers the sympathetic nervous system, which alerts the adrenal medulla, resulting in secretion of adrenaline and noradrenaline. In addition, the anterior hypothalamus releases corticotrophin-releasing factor (CRF), activating the pituitary gland, which secretes adrenocorticotropic hormone (ACTH), resulting in the adrenal cortex secreting glucocorticoids and mineralocorticoids. What Cannon was describing was activation of the sympathetic-adrenal-medullary (SAM) response and the hypothalamic-pituitary-adrenal (HPA) response, as described in Chapter 4. Cannon believed that once the person dealt with the stressor, the body's internal natural state gradually returned to the normal pre-stressed state, called **homeostasis**.

General Adaptation Syndrome

Selye (1956) was interested in how animals coped with anything that affected their homeostasis, including stressors, such as heat, cold, infections, physical activity and toxins, but thought that Cannon's explanation of the 'fight or flight' response was too simplistic. By studying the effects of various stressors on animals, Selye developed a three-stage model of stress, called the **General Adaptation Syndrome** (GAS). Selye found that regardless of the type of stress that rats were exposed to, they exhibited a similar physiological pattern, marked by increases in the size of the adrenal cortex (involved in HPA activation), stomach ulceration and shrinkage of the thymus gland (see Chapter 4). From these experiments, Selye proposed that stress had similar negative physiological responses in humans, regardless of whether the stressful experience was good (eustress) or bad (distress). This led Selye to conclude that prolonged exposure to anything that caused stress would disrupt the body's biological systems and over time lead to disease and or death.

Selye's three stage General Adaptation Syndrome

Stage 1 Alarm

This is the initial stage the body goes through when exposed to any stressor. Being confronted by a large aggressive dog or hearing a very loud noise are quite different experiences, but according to Selye they result in the same initial shock response. The body is surprised and momentarily stunned by the event; this is rapidly followed by the countershock phase. During this part of the alarm stage, the physiological effects of stress commence automatically via the SAM response to get the individual ready for fight or flight, followed slightly later by HPA response. Physiological responses to stress will cause sweaty palms, a sick (nausea) or a nervous sensation in the stomach (due to slowing down of the gastrointestinal tract to allow more blood to be diverted to the muscles), shaking or trembling of muscles, awareness of increased heart rate and breathing. When the stressful event has ended, the parasympathetic nervous system will try and calm everything down to bring the body back to its naturally resting state (homeostasis). The HPA response will also return to normal, but due to stress hormones taking time to dissipate, the effects of the stressful experience may be felt for a period after the stressful event has ended (see Chapter 4).

Stage 2 Resistance

Chronic stress occurs when an individual is subjected to prolonged stress or a perceived threat. During chronic stress, the initial physiological stress response is attenuated by the parasympathetic nervous system, but the body will not fully return to the normal homeostatic resting state. Due to sustained HPA activity, cortisol will fluctuate, but remain higher than normal, although an individual will adapt to being in a heightened state of readiness, to deal with the stressor. As we will see later in this chapter, increased levels of cortisol can have negative health consequences.

Stage 3 Exhaustion

Individuals differ in how long they can tolerate the chronicity of stressful situations and events. The prolonged physiological and psychological impact of stress hormones can contribute to decreased immune functioning, gastrointestinal problems, aches and pains, fatigue, mental health problems, exacerbate pre-existing diseases and pain, contribute to hypertension, cardiovascular disease and even death.

Cannon's views on stress and Selye's GAS model have been influential in explaining the physiological effects of stress and influences on disease, but it must be remembered that Selye's work was based on experiments with animals and generalised to humans. Implicit within Selye's theory is the idea that everyone will have the same level of physiological response to a stressor, but factors such as genetics and adverse childhood experiences can impact stress responsiveness, which may predispose people to stress-related diseases (Nelson et al., 2020). In addition, a stressor can be viewed as a challenge that can be overcome or a threat that is overwhelming (Lazarus & Folkman, 1984).

Allostatic load

McEwen and Stellar (1993) and Schulkin et al. (1994) extended the physiological explanations of chronic stress and introduced the term **allostatic load** to describe the effects of long-term and repeated effects of stress on the body, especially from the HPA. It has been suggested that prolonged HPA activation has more deleterious effects on health than the SAM response, as the former leads to alterations in daily cortisol production. Cortisol is usually highest in the morning around 30 minutes after waking up, it then reduces, showing a slight increase after lunch and then declines throughout the rest of the day. Cortisol is helpful during a stress response, it increases blood glucose helping the body to meet the physiological energy demands to deal with the stressor, in addition it promotes blood flow and increases blood pressure by narrowing the blood vessels. When an individual experiences sustained stress, persistent HPA activity means that cortisol levels do not readily return to the normal 24-hour cycle (cortisol dysregulation), which can be detrimental to health. Heightened cortisol contributes to sleep problems and weight gain, especially fat accumulation around the abdomen, it is linked to higher risks of developing coronary heart disease, stroke, hypertension, type 2 diabetes (T2DM) and mental health problems (Friedli, 2009; Girod & Brotman, 2004). Cortisol also suppresses inflammation, which inhibits healing, leading to negative impacts on immune functioning, and increasing the individual's vulnerability to infection. According to McEwen and Stellar (1993), chronic and repeated exposure to stress hormones means that the body becomes less efficient at turning physiological responses on and off and in returning to a normal resting state of homeostasis, which leads to a type of 'wear and tear' on the body called allostatic load.

Transactional model of stress

Lazarus and Folkman (1984) believed that stress could not be considered solely in terms of physiological responses to external stimuli (events or situations), as people's perceptions of the same stressful event varied. What may be considered as threatening for one person may be viewed by someone else as a welcome challenge. These researchers explained that it is not the event or situation that is fundamentally stressful, rather it is the person's perception of the stressor and their perceived ability to cope with it that determine whether something is deemed as being stressful. A central aspect of the transaction model of stress is cognitive appraisal, which can be influenced by a range of factors, including past experience, mood, health status, work-life balance, finances and how motivated a person feels at a particular time. This model helps to explain individual variations in assessing the threat of a stressor and ability to cope with it.

Cognitive appraisal

When faced with a potentially stressful event, an individual will engage in primary and secondary appraisal to consider how meaningful and demanding the stressor is for them. **Primary appraisal** is all about assessing how harmful the external stressor is and deciding whether further action is needed, while **secondary appraisal** involves assessment of the internal resources (coping strategies) to help deal with the stressor. There are four potential outcomes to primary appraisal (see Figure 8.1). 1. The event is irrelevant and there is no cause for concern, hence no action is necessary. For example, your friend has told you that they had a recent health checkup, which revealed a diagnosis of hypertension and high cholesterol, putting them at risk of a stroke or heart attack. You are a bit alarmed as both are serious and potentially life threatening and both of your parents had hypertension; however, you get your cholesterol and blood pressure checked regularly and know they were within normal limits, hence the potential threat is appraised as irrelevant, not stressful and no action be required. 2. An event may be considered as benign and positive, for example, a lecturer is providing verbal feedback on an assignment to a student group and your work is singled out as being of a very high standard. This may cause

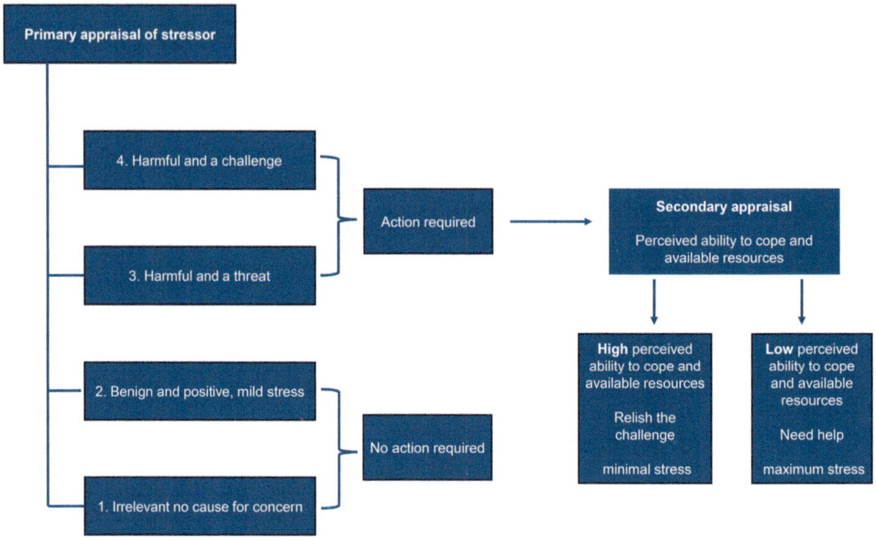

Figure 8.1
Primary and secondary appraisal of a threat

Source: Author, based on Lazarus and Folkman (1984)

you some mild stress in terms of feeling embarrassed, but it is a positive outcome, no action is necessary, it causes no further stress and can be ignored. 3. You are struggling with statistics, your primary appraisal is that this is a threat, which is harmful, as you are at risk of failing your statistics examination and this will prevent you from proceeding to the next year of your course. Action is required, you engage in secondary appraisal and decide to spend more time reading about statistical concepts, but after several hours, you are still confused, stressed and reappraise the situation. There is a need to change your coping strategy from reading to getting advice and practical help from peers or lecturing staff. Reappraisal happens several times and coping strategies may change. 4. You have been appointed as the project leader on a group task. Even though this is stressful and will require secondary appraisal, you may relish the challenge and consider it as an opportunity for personal growth. For Lazarus and Folkman (1984), the individual's cognitive appraisal of the event and their perceived ability to cope are important and they are influenced by the resources that the individual can use.

Resources to help deal with stress can include personal factors, such as previous experience, self-efficacy, self-esteem, problem-solving and knowledge. There may be a need to seek help from others, because an individual's own coping strategies are not sufficient to deal with the event. This includes help from friends and family, professional help and sourcing of information. The transactional model of stress was developed for and by Western populations, as such, it may overlook cultural differences in how stress is experienced and managed within diverse cultural contexts. This is especially true within Indigenous populations, where there is greater reliance on community support, family networks and cultural specific practices. However, the transactional model has stimulated research and helps to explain individual differences in stress appraisal.

Coping with stress

Coping styles in response to stress

Coping is a process, which is concerned with how an individual views and deals with specific events or situations and their perceptions about the event or situation being a challenge or potentially overwhelming to their available resources (Lazarus & Folkman, 1984). Coping is an active process that involves appraisal, reappraisal, evaluation and re-evaluation of own ways of coping. There are two basic **coping styles** for dealing with stress, called **approach** and **avoidant**, both can be adaptive or maladaptive (Roth & Cohen, 1986), but that depends on the nature of the event that is causing stress. When a person uses an approach coping style, they tackle the stressor directly through actions, such as purposeful planning. For example, a student is overwhelmed and struggling to write up a practical experiment. In this situation, the problem can be tackled by using purposeful planning to break the write-up into smaller manageable steps through setting achievable goals, completing each one before moving onto the next part of the assignment. The method section is a good place to start, as it can be subsectioned into design, participants, materials and procedure. Purposeful planning also involves time management to identify specific time periods to complete each part of the write-up. The opposite is **avoidant coping**, which includes trying not to think about the assignment or the consequences of nonsubmission in the hope that it will go away. Avoidance may include engaging in other activities, such as not going to class to avoid being asked why the assignment is late. Shuster et al. (2023) examined perceived stress and coping styles in university students during the COVID-19 pandemic and found that higher perceived stress was associated with greater use of avoidant coping and those who had lower perceived stress tended to make use of approach coping.

Coping strategies in response to stress

Styles of coping and **coping strategies** are related concepts, the former provides an indication of how people generally respond to stressful events, whereas coping strategies are techniques used to manage specific stressors. Coping strategies may vary according to the nature of the stressor and are divided into problem-focused and emotion-focused coping (Lazarus & Folkman, 1984).

Problem-focused coping strategies involve dealing with the actual stressor, trying to reduce or remove it. The student who is struggling with an assignment may seek informational help from friends, lecturing staff or search the internet for a solution. This contrasts with **emotion-focused coping** where the emphasis is on trying to change the emotional response to the stressor. Using the same example, rather than seeking informational support from others, the student may engage in procrastination or watch a movie to try block out thoughts about the assignment. Individuals tend to make use of both problem- and emotion-focused coping, which can depend on the cause or type of stress they are dealing with. In a health situation, an individual who finds a lump underneath their arm may be worried (stressed) that it is a symptom of cancer. Rather than employing a problem-focused strategy of seeking medical advice and getting a diagnosis, they try to reduce their stress by engaging in the emotion-focused strategy of hopeful thinking, willing the lump to go away. In this situation, emotion-focused coping would not be appropriate and any delay in seeking help could be detrimental to health. When something constructive (e.g. medical tests and treatment) can be done about the stressor (finding a lump), a problem-focused strategy is useful. However, the dichotomy between problem- and emotion-focused strategies is not always as simple as in this example. Folkman and Lazarus (1988) examined 67 types of cognitive and behavioural strategies that people used to cope with stress and refined them into eight ways of coping that could be assessed by the Ways of Coping Questionnaire (WCQ). This questionnaire is designed to measure problem- and emotion-based ways of coping and has been applied across a range of stressful life events, including cancer diagnoses (see Box 8.1 for some examples of the types of coping strategies that may be used by a person with a newly diagnosed cancer). It is important to note that how people cope with stress is not static, they may use several ways of coping according to the situation or event and this can change over time (Stone & Neale, 1984).

BOX 8.1

AN EXAMPLE OF PROBLEM- AND EMOTION-FOCUSED COPING STRATEGIES OF SOMEONE NEWLY DIAGNOSED WITH CANCER

Problem-focused coping strategies

1 Planful problem-solving – reading about the type and stages of cancer and available treatments, making action plans to manage travelling to medical appointments and how to cope with the side effects of treatment.
2 Seeking social support – informational support from others, such as family members or friends. Talking to others who are living with and beyond cancer to share experiences and get practical advice.
3 Confrontative coping – advocating for a specific type of treatment or asking for a second opinion.

Emotion-focused coping strategies

1 Self-control – hiding true feelings by not wanting family members to know how worried they are about their cancer diagnosis.
2 Distancing – trying not to think about cancer, downplaying how serious the diagnosis is or avoiding the topic of cancer completely.
3 Positive re-appraisal – feeling fortunate that their cancer was diagnosed before it had spread. The diagnosis may have been a 'wake-up' call providing opportunities to make healthier lifestyle choices, re-establish or improve relationships with family and friends.
4 Accepting responsibility – acceptance (rightly or wrongly) that 'it is my own fault I got cancer due to my lifestyle choices'; hence, the individual may feel a sense of guilt.
5 Escape/avoidance – engaging in wishful thinking that the cancer will go away or using drugs or alcohol to try and 'forget' about the cancer.

The way in which one individual copes with stress may not work for another person, as coping is not only influenced by individual coping strategies, external resources also have a role to play. These include time, finances, educational level, socioeconomic status, social support and the absence of other life stressors (Taylor & Stanton, 2007); what may work in one situation may not work in another. For example, when feeling stressed about an impending examination, using a coping strategy of deep breathing and practising relaxation may help reduce feelings of stress, but on its own relaxation would not be sufficient to help an individual cope with financial problems, they may need to seek help from others in the form of advice and social support.

BOX 8.1
CRITICAL THINKING

Think about a recent mildly stressful situation. What coping strategies did you use, were they problem- or emotion focused? Are there situations where one type of coping strategy is better than another?

Social support

One aspect of coping with stress that has received quite a lot of interest is **social support**; this can provide an individual with the feeling of being cared for in a personal relationship or through being a part of a group or community. An individual may have several people who can provide social support, but it is the satisfaction that the individual feels with the support which is important (De Maria et al., 2020; Fernández-Peña et al., 2020). House (1981) proposed four types of social support, which included emotional, instrumental, informational and appraisal, with companionship added by Cohen and Wills (1985). Emotional support includes empathy, trust, concern and love, which is characteristic of close relationships that offer reassurance and a sense of belonging. This type of support may be of use when an individual is coping with personal problems including disease and death of a loved one. Instrumental support is usually offered when a person needs some type of direct practical help to deal with a problem. It can include offering to get the shopping for someone who is too ill to go out and providing transport to get to a medical appointment. Informational support involves giving advice, sourcing advice or providing suggestions to help an individual solve a problem, make a decision or to cope with a stressful situation. Informational support is often used in healthcare interactions when healthcare professionals offer explanations about diagnosis, treatment or the likely course of a disease. Appraisal support can help an individual evaluate their situation by providing feedback on their capabilities or strengths, which can help to boost self-esteem. For example, a healthcare professional may praise a patient for the way in which they are managing various aspects of their disease and this can have a positive impact on self-efficacy ('I can do this'). Companionship support, which helps create a sense of belonging, may involve a friend or a member of a group spending time with an individual to help reduce feelings of loneliness and create social cohesion. This type of support is often a feature of walking for health groups, whereby people with various diseases come together to support each other while they engage in physical activity.

Social support can be beneficial to health, Berkman and Syme (1979) explored the relationship between social support and mortality rates in men and women, aged 30–69 years. Participants were asked to complete questionnaires on sources of social support (e.g. from spouse, close friends and relatives, members of the church community, formal and informal groups). Data were collected on general physical health, socioeconomic status (derived from educational level and income) and health practices (smoking status, alcohol consumption, obesity and physical activity and use of medical services). Follow-up data were collected over a nine-year period, along with information on mortality. After statistically controlling for physical health, socioeconomic status and health practices at baseline, people who had fewer social and community supports were more than twice as likely to die compared to those with more social supports.

Social support can be of help to people who are living with chronic disease. Graven and Grant (2014) found that support from family members was a key factor in helping people with heart problems to sustain health-enhancing behaviours. However, a recent systematic review of 54 randomised controlled trials investigating social support interventions for people with heart disease found no indication that interventions enhance health-related quality of life, decreased hospital admissions or mortality rates (Purcell et al., 2023). Oversolicitous family social support in chronic disease can have negative consequences for the uptake of health rehabilitative behaviours. After a heart attack, when an individual has been discharged from hospital, it is quite normal for the patient and family members to be fearful of another heart attack or death. This can result in well-meant social support that is overprotective and controlling. Family members may discourage physical activity or independence in tasks, which can limit a patient's autonomy, making them feel helpless, dependent and less likely to engage in self-care (Boutin-Foster, 2005).

Knowing about the types of social support identified by House (1981) and Cohen and Wills (1985) can help healthcare professionals support patients at specific times in their disease trajectory. For example, when a patient is recently diagnosed with type 2 diabetes (T2DM), offering informational support is essential, but people can feel a bit overwhelmed by their diagnosis and may not retain verbal information, hence there is a need to supplement this with written information. As people become more comfortable with managing their diet and avoiding peaks in blood glucose, the use of appraisal support during review appointments can be an effective way of helping the patient to realise that they can self-manage their diabetes. Engaging in physical activity is an important self-management strategy in T2DM but people may struggle to go out walking on their own, due to safety concerns, the weather or due to lack of motivation. Signposting patients to local walking for health groups may provide companionship support to encourage regular walking. In summary, social support can be health enhancing, but to avoid overloading the patient, it is paramount that the type of social support offered by healthcare professionals is tailored and matched to the patient's specific needs.

ACTIVITY 8.1

Take some time to consider a few recent stressful events or situations that you have experienced. What types of things did you do to cope with the stressor? Did this involve dealing directly with the stressor (problem-focused coping) or doing something to distract yourself from the stressor (emotion-focused coping). Also consider the different social support strategies that you used.

Stress and disease

Psychoneuroimmunology

Research into the effects of stress on the immune system was pioneered accidently by two researchers, Ader and Cohen (1975, 1981). They were conducting classical conditioning experiments (see Chapter 7) on rats using taste aversion. Ader and Cohen gave laboratory rats a sweet saccharine solution, which the rats had not tasted before, the rats engaged in a natural response by drinking the solution. The rats were then injected with a chemotherapy drug called cyclophosphamide, which caused immune suppression and made the rats feel unwell. After a single pairing of the saccharine solution and the drug, the rats made an association between the taste of saccharine and feeling unwell, just giving the rats the saccharin solution on its own led to the rats feeling unwell and had negative impacts on their immune systems. This provided evidence that learning could influence immune functioning and illustrated the potential role that psychological factors had on the immune responses. Ader and Cohen's work was the starting point for further studies into links between psychological processes, the nervous and immune systems, referred to as **psychoneuroimmunology** (PNI).

The impact of stress and PNI has involved viral challenge trials. Research has focused on cytokines to explain the link between psychological stress and development of respiratory illnesses. There are different types of cytokines, if you remember from Chapter 4, these are chemical messengers involved in the body's immune response. When faced with pathogens, such as viruses, bacteria and fungi or tissue damage through injury, cytokines helped create an inflammatory response to assist the body in fighting off pathogens and assist with healing tissue damage. When challenged with a respiratory virus (e.g. the cold or flu), the immune system becomes activated and cytokines are released, they in turn signal to other cells within the immune system to try and kill the virus. The release of cytokines contributes to bodily aches and muscle pains, fever and fatigue, these are symptoms that the body is mounting an immune response.

Kiecolt-Glaser et al. (1987) were interested in the impacts of stress on wound healing. Two groups of volunteers, those with high stress levels, caring for a relative with Alzheimer's disease and a low stress group with no caring responsibilities, were asked to complete baseline questionnaires to measure their perceived stress. Experimental wounds were created on the forearms of all volunteers, using a 3.5-mm punch biopsy (a special device used to cut out a small circle of skin). Photographs were taken each day until the wounds were completely healed. On average, it took 24% longer for wounds to heal in the group with high stress levels, compared to the low stress group. When blood samples were assessed, the high stress group had a lower percentage of total lymphocytes and T-helper cells, indicating lower immune functioning, making them more susceptible to bacteria and viruses.

Correlational evidence suggests that examination stress can have detrimental impacts on immune functioning, with students reporting increased acute infections during this time (Kiecolt-Glaser et al., 1987). Marucha et al. (1998) investigated the effects of examination stress on the healing time for experimentally created wounds in students. Punch biopsies (3.5 mm) were taken from the hard palate (roof of mouth) during the summer holiday time and later in the year, three days before an important academic examination. Results showed that wounds made closer to exam time took 40% longer to heal compared to those made in the summer, providing evidence that short-term stress could have a negative impact on wound healing. Other research has confirmed that students who experience elevated levels of anxiety, stress and loneliness or who spend time thinking about past stressful events have greater reductions in immunological functioning compared to low anxiety, low stressed students during examination time (Marshall et al., 1998).

Cohen et al. (1999) exposed healthy volunteers to the flu virus and monitored the relationship between psychological stress and cytokine production. They found that volunteers who had high levels of psychological stress prior to being infected with the flu had higher levels of cytokines and symptoms. These researchers reported that two important sources of stress were associated with higher cytokine production, which were problematic interpersonal relationships between friends and family and extremes of employment, that is, being unemployed or being overworked. In a later study, Cohen et al. (2005) measured if there were any associations between participants perceived stress, mood, recent stressful life events and development of respiratory symptoms in healthy volunteers who had been experimentally exposed to the common cold virus. They found that people who had higher levels of stress appeared to have an increased risk of developing the common cold and the longer the duration of stress, the more susceptible people were to infective types of disease. However, it must be remembered that susceptibility to infectious respiratory disease during periods of long-term stress can also be influenced by other behaviours, such as lack of restful sleep, sedentary behaviours, dietary changes and smoking (Cohen, 2005).

In a systematic review, the negative impacts of stress on delayed and poor wound healing were confirmed in 17 out of 21 studies (Walburn et al., 2009). This evidence suggests there is a link between experience of distress (bad stress) and reduced immune functioning, but the relationship is not straightforward. In Chapter 4, we learned that the immune system was quite complex and consists of a range of different cells, hence measuring just one specific type of cell may not be representative of total immune functioning. Added to this is the temporal (time) relationship between the stressful experience and taking a blood or saliva sample and the reliability of various biochemical markers to quantify the extent of the stress response. Iqbal et al. (2021) have questioned whether it is possible to use biochemical markers as a way of quantifying the extent of the stress response, highlighting that the relationship between stress and immune functioning is quite complex. In addition, factors other than stress may have negative effects on immune functioning. For example, when people feel stressed, they tend to eat unhealthy snacks such as high fat and sugary foods, rather than consuming a balanced diet (Zellner et al., 2006). In addition, they may consume more drinks that contain caffeine, smoke more (Minichiello et al., 2016) and consume higher amounts of alcohol (Lovall et al, 2019) and/or drugs, all of which have detrimental impacts on health. While research shows that the interaction between stress and immune functioning may contribute to disease, as noted in Chapter 6, disease can also be modified by health literacy, adherence, lifestyle behaviours (see Chapter 9) and inequities in healthcare (see Chapter 5). We know there is a direct relationship between stress and activation of the SAM and HPA axes, but not everyone who experiences long-term stress goes on to develop disease. Hence, there are physiological and psychological differences in how people respond to and recover from stressful encounters.

Stress and heart disease

Some individuals have greater **physiological reactivity** to stress, while others show a longer period of stress recovery. Large increases in heart rate and blood pressure, because of acute stress, are known as **cardiovascular reactivity** (Orbist, 1981). People who exhibit such responses are at greater risk of developing hypertension (al'Absi & Wittmers, 2003). Chronic stress is also associated with systemic inflammation that affects the normal functioning of blood vessels, which can result in the build-up of atherosclerosis, increase the risk of blood clots and cardiovascular disease (Dar et al., 2019).

The INTERHEART study was conducted in 52 countries across Africa, Asia, Australia, Europe, the Middle East and North and South America. Researchers compared psychosocial stress over the past 12 months in 11,119 patients who had experienced a first heart attack (cases) and a similar number of people who were matched for age and sex without heart disease (controls). After considering socioeconomic status, sex, ethnicity, education, income, smoking and geographical location, results showed that those who had heart attacks, had higher work, home, financial stress and major life events over the previous 12 months than controls. Furthermore, those with high levels of psychosocial stress were at double the risk of a heart attack (Rosengren et al., 2004).

Evidence links catastrophic natural disasters, such as earthquakes, to an increased risk of heart-related deaths in people who already have some degree of atherosclerosis. Leor et al. (1996) examined causes of death in coroner reports for the week preceding an earthquake in Los Angeles, on the day of the earthquake and six days after the earthquake. They found that the mean number of daily deaths in the weak preceding the earthquake was 4.6, compared to 24 on the day of the earthquake and 2.7 in the subsequent week. These researchers concluded that acute psychological stress was a major factor for the high death rates in people with existing heart disease. While the risks to cardiovascular health are higher from smoking, obesity and hypertension, psychosocial stress has the potential to lead to disease progression in those who have pre-existing cardiovascular disease (Kivimäki & Steptoe, 2018). This has been acknowledged by The European Society of Cardiology Guidelines (Visseren et al., 2021) who recommend that screening patients for multiple sources of stress should be considered as part of psychosocial assessment.

Stress and headaches

Stress is also implicated in non-life-threatening conditions, such as headaches. Around 70% of people who have repeated debilitating migraines state that daily stressors or repeated hassles are precipitating factors for triggering attacks (Maleki et al., 2012). In addition, it is thought that increased activity of the sympathetic nervous system can lead to greater muscular tension in the neck and shoulders, which probably contributes to tension headaches (Buse & Lipton, (2015). HPA activation linked to chronic stress makes people more sensitive to pain, causes vascular changes and neuroinflammation (Beech et al., 2023), which sets up a cyclical process of stress that can cause headaches and repeated headaches are also a source of stress.

Stress and health compromising behaviours

Chronic stress can also contribute indirectly to disease by impacting unhealthy behaviours, such as diet, increased alcohol consumption, sedentary behaviour and smoking.

Diet

Overeating and eating foods high in fat and sugars have been linked to becoming overweight or obese, the development of T2DM, hypertension and to some cancers (Epner et al., 2022). Zellner et al. (2006) compared the effects of experimentally induced high stress (trying to work out the correct answers to unsolvable puzzles) and low stress (solvable puzzles) on healthy (grapes and nuts) and unhealthy (M&M chocolate sweets and potato chips) food choices. They found that women with high stress scores tended to eat snacks higher in fat and sugar (M&Ms) compared to the low stress group. These researchers repeated the same study with men and found that the low-stressed group ate more of the unhealthy snacks, suggesting that stress and snacking differ by gender (Zellner et al., 2007). Caution is required in the interpretation of these two studies as the sources of stress were experimental and in the artificial setting of a laboratory, it is unclear if the findings can be applied to real-life stress. However, a meta-analysis of 54 studies showed links between stress and eating more unhealthy foods and reductions in healthy food consumption (Hill et al., 2022). O'Connor et al. (2008) investigated the impact of daily hassle stress on eating by asking participants to keep diaries of the snacks consumed between meals, along with fruit and vegetable intake. They found a positive relationship between increased hassles and snacking on high fat and sugary foods, along with a decreased intake of fruits, vegetables and main meals. More specifically, daily hassles that were associated with relationships, work problems or affected self-esteem were linked with a higher likelihood of unhealthy snacking. Physical stress associated with illness, led to less snacking, which suggested that people tend to snack more when they are experiencing emotion- related stress.

Ethnic minority groups experience multiple stressors that have been linked to discrimination stigma, **microaggressions** and low socioeconomic status (Hatch & Dohrenwend, 2007), which can result in maladaptive coping in the form of unhealthy eating. It has been suggested that the higher burden of obesity among non-Hispanic Black women in the US is associated with experiences of higher levels of chronic stress (e.g. persistent discrimination and childhood socioeconomic disadvantages) compared to other ethnic minority groups (Pickett et al., 2020). A more recent systematic review of 30 studies found that stress was linked to overeating or eating unhealthy foods in African American and Hispanic/Latino groups, but to date no studies have examined stress-induced eating in Indigenous Americans or other Indigenous groups (Kazmierski et al., 2021). People who are overweight or obese also face weight-based stigma in healthcare settings. Advice provided is usually to 'exercise more and eat less', with the focus on weight and body mass index as indicators of success or failure. However, healthcare professionals need to be aware that unsuccessful weight loss may increase an individual's stress due to feelings of shame and self-reproach (Tomiyama et al., 2018).

The experience of minority stress, such as fear of rejection in lesbian and bisexual women, has been associated with social isolation and emotion-focused coping, contributing to binge eating (Mason & Lewis, 2015). Minority stress in gay, bisexual and queer men has been linked to a greater likelihood of disordered eating (binge eating, food restriction, bulimic behaviours) and excessive exercise with the goal of weight loss, compared to heterosexual men (Parker & Harriger, 2020). Often, men from sexual minority groups feel pressured into being muscular, lean and athletic, which can lead to a type of within-group stress that can contribute to disordered eating (Soulliard et al., 2025).

Smoking

Smoking is one of the main causes of death and disease across the world (WHO, 2025), it is linked with cancer, cardiovascular and lung diseases. In a study spanning 41 countries across Africa, the Americas, Asia and Europe, Stubbs et al. (2017) found evidence of higher perceived stress being associated with heavier smoking (more than 30 cigarettes per day). An Action on Smoking and Health report (ASH, 2019) in England (UK) found that smoking tends to be more common in people who have low incomes, those who live in the north of the country, looked after children and in those who belong to LGBT (lesbian, gay and bisexual with the addition of transgender) groups. Many of these groups are subjected to chronic stressors associated with belonging to disadvantaged or marginalised groups and turn to smoking to cope with stress or smoke due to intergenerational transmission of smoking. The higher prevalence of smoking in LGBT groups, compared to their heterosexual and cisgender counterparts, is thought to be due to stress related to stigma, discrimination and microaggressions (Lick et al., 2013).

People from Indigenous communities across the world have higher rates of smoking compared to non-Indigenous populations (Minichiello et al., 2016). In Australia, the higher prevalence of smoking within Indigenous groups is thought to be linked with the intergeneration impacts of colonisation, systemic discrimination, the dispossession of land and continued marginalisation (Nguyen & Doan, 2025). According to Markwick et al. (2014), the intersection of poverty, low educational attainment and high rates of unemployment also contribute to stress and is associated with higher rates of smoking. Helping Indigenous Peoples to quit smoking is not as simple as implementing a standard stop-smoking intervention designed for the non-Indigenous population, as action is required to address the stressors associated with social injustice and social determinants of health (Dilley et al., 2013).

Smoking is more prevalent in gender and sexual minority individuals compared with cisgender and heterosexual people; transgender women have some of the highest rates of smoking (Vogel et al., 2019). Transgender women are more inclined to use smoking as a maladaptive coping strategy for gender identity-related discrimination, stigma, microaggressions, violence (Shires & Jaffee, 2016) and concealment of identity (Menino et al., 2018). A more recent study by Culbreth et al. (2023) found that smoking prevalence among transgender women in the US was almost three times higher than that of the cisgender population. Surprisingly, this study found no relationship between smoking and stress associated with gender identity discriminations or internalised stigma of being transgender, rather, smoking was linked with homelessness, sex working and intimate partner violence. However, these factors are not addressed in smoking cessation interventions.

BOX 8.2
CRITICAL THINKING

Think back over the past year about any time that you felt stressed, did you notice any changes in your physical health, such as feeling run down or more prone to getting colds. Were there any other factors that could have influenced how susceptible you were to illness (diet, sleep, social support)? How likely are you to over- or underestimate the link between stress and illness, how reliable is this type of retrospective self-report for studying the effects of stress on acute illnesses?

Disease as a source of stress

Disease can be described as acute or chronic. Living with a chronic disease over a period of years or decades may be an ongoing source of stress, as disease can involve physical limitations, emotional challenges, chronic pain, financial and housing concerns. All these factors may impact an individual's lifestyle, family and personal relationships, leisure and work roles. Lack of control over health may be a major source of stress for individuals and family members, as the rate of disease progression, possible remission of symptoms and extent of lifestyle limitations imposed by chronic diseases, such as cancer, arthritis, dementia, multiple sclerosis and motor neuron disease, may be hard to predict (Helgeson & Zajdel, 2017). In addition, individuals may also have to cope with the side effects of medication, surgery and other treatments, all of which can have negative consequences for quality of life (Helgeson & Zajdel, 2017). When adjusting to a chronic disease diagnosis, the individual may have to deal with a myriad of challenges to their identity. This can include, going from a person who was the main wage earner to being financially dependent on the state or other family members. Stress can be caused by disease adaptions, for example, from being very physically active to being disabled due to pain or other symptoms and from being independent to becoming dependent on others for everyday basic care. Such transitions can be a cause of stress due to negative impacts on relationships, possible changes in living arrangements and adaptations to the home environment. Such adjustments may be an ongoing feature of progressive chronic diseases.

Stress, personality and disease

Type A behaviour pattern

Friedman and Rosenman (1959) believed there was an association between personality, how people react to stress and heart disease. **The Type A behaviour pattern** (TABP) is characterised by competitive, ambitious, perfectionists, who are time driven, hostile and have aggressive tendencies. The opposite to the TABP is the **Type B behaviour pattern** (TBBP), which is characterised as having low levels of competitiveness, urgency and hostility and a tendency to have an 'easy going' attitude to life. The longitudinal Western Collaborative Group study followed 3,200 males over an 8.5-year period and found that men with a TABP were 2.5 times more prone to developing coronary artery disease (CAD) than men with the TBBP (Rosenman et al., 1975). The Framingham Heart study (Haynes et al., 1980) suggested that the TABP was more prevalent in men who worked in managerial, professional or administrative jobs and women who worked outside of the home. However, subsequent research (Matthews & Haynes, 1986) refuted a link between overall TABP and CAD and singled out hostility as the best predictor of CAD (Siegman & Smith, 1994). Hostility refers to a cynical attitude, which involves antagonism, being cynical about the intentions of others, which can lead to aggression. It was thought that people who exhibited hostility and aggression associated with the TABP had greater physiological stress reactions, which had longer-lasting impacts on blood pressure leading to cardiac damage (Brydon et al., 2010). Subsequent research into the anger aspect of the TABP found that anger that is outwardly expressed by shouting, walking off or slamming doors is less harmful than internalised anger. The internalisation of anger characterised by brooding over problems and suppressing feelings of anger is more toxic to health and has been associated with CAD. This is due to activation of stress pathways, which results in increased blood pressure, cortisol levels and the development of atherosclerotic plaques (Player et al., 2007). However, as we will see in Chapter 9, there are many other factors that contribute to the development of heart disease.

Hardiness

Hardiness (Kobasa, 1979) is a personality trait characterised by three beliefs, control (ability to control or exert some influence over experience of life events/situations, rather than being passive observers), commitment (having a sense of purpose and staying engaged, rather than withdrawal) and challenge (seeing stress as an opportunity for growth and learning, rather than a threat). While a person who is hardy may view stressful events as a threat, they will be more likely to appraise them as benign or as a challenge that can be overcome by the use of an approach coping style that involves problem- rather than emotion-focused coping strategies (Kobasa, 1979; Maddi, 2002). Hardiness has been used to explain why some people can cope well with stress and remain healthy, with Brooks (2003) reporting that hardiness was associated with better adherence and health outcomes across a range of diseases including multiple sclerosis, rheumatoid arthritis, HIV/AIDS, lung disease and diabetes.

Dispositional optimism

People who are optimistic have a general view that when faced with a stressful situation or event, the outcomes will tend to be good rather than bad (Scheier & Carver, 1992). Research indicates that **dispositional optimism** is associated with having a lower risk of heart attacks, strokes and lower distress (Rozanski et al., 2019). Optimism has also been linked with slower progression of disease in the human immunodeficiency virus (HIV), due to lower avoidant coping (Ironson et al., 2005). A systematic review of studies that examined the relationship between optimism, acute and chronic post-surgical pain in patients with cancer found those who scored highly on optimism reported lower pain (Forte et al., 2022). While the exact reasons behind the links between optimism and better health outcomes are not totally understood, there is evidence to suggest that people who are optimistic tend to consume less alcohol, are less likely to smoke and when faced with stress, they tend to adopt problem-focused coping strategies (Taylor & Stanton, 2007).

While there is evidence to link the TAPB, hardiness, optimism and stress with coping, factors such as socioeconomic status, educational level, access to healthcare and social injustice all have a role to play in coping behaviours. In addition, theories and measurements of personality are based on Western populations, which may limit generalisability to Indigenous and non-Western communities, especially when stress, coping and health are conceptualised as collective rather than individualistic matters.

Colonisation, intersectionality and stress

Colonisation

Across the world, Indigenous Peoples have experienced higher mental, physical health problems and lower life expectancy compared to their non-Indigenous counterparts (Anderson et al., 2016). They have been forced to move away from their ancestral lands, their ways of living and knowledge have been undermined, contributing to multiple stressors that include discrimination, loss of identity, poverty, unemployment, inadequate housing and healthcare (Berger & Sarnyai, 2015; Marmot, 2011). The separation of Indigenous People from their ancestral lands has also led to a disconnect with traditional spiritual, cultural and healing practices. The intergeneration trauma of colonisation lives on, as many children were forcibly taken away from their parents to be educated in residential or boarding schools, forbidden to use their own languages and had to adopt Western cultures and religions. In Australia, the enduring nature of these stressors is thought to be linked with higher rates of cardiovascular disease (CVD), metabolic syndrome and greater alcohol abuse in the Indigenous population (Brunner, 2007). Intergeneration trauma and stress have been linked with a greater likelihood of becoming obese and smoking in adulthood (Najman et al., 2006). Many people from Indigenous communities face a lifetime of stress that is based on direct discrimination and negative stereotypic attitudes from others (Lewis et al., 2021). The effects of chronic stress may help explain the disproportionately poorer health outcomes and higher mortality of Indigenous compared to non-Indigenous populations (Ketheesan et al., 2020). This may be explained through the link between chronic stress and increased allostatic load, which may have many long-term health consequences for Indigenous populations (Sarnyai et al., 2016).

Intersectionality and stress

Meyer's (2003) minority stress theory proposed that people from gender and sexual minority groups experience discrimination, external stigma from others', self-stigma through internalising others' views and a fear of rejection that can lead to identity concealment. Examination of health can overlook intersectionality relating to LGBTQI+ discrimination and health needs (Day et al., 2023). The intersection of multiple social statuses, for example, disability, ethnicity, sexual orientation, gender identity, social class, age, etc., can contribute to multiple stressful experiences. Over 20 years on from Meyer's theory, LGBTQI+ groups still experience stigma and discrimination (Adamczyk & Liao, 2019) that are linked to the development of physical (Flentje et al., 2020; Hoy-Ellis, 2023) and mental health problems (Sattler et al., 2017). We know that individuals respond to stress in different ways, but there are also intersectional variations in stress appraisal and reactions to stress.

In some countries, LGBTQI+ populations face added stress due to cultural norms and religious beliefs. For example, Sekoni et al. (2022) referred to LGBTQI+ individuals in Nigeria being as being a 'hidden healthcare population'. In order to conform to societal norms and avoid negative attitudes, stigma and discrimination, LGBTQI+ individuals have to conceal their sexual orientation and/or gender identities from family members and healthcare professionals These individuals talked about experiencing stress due to healthcare providers not being trained to deal with their identities, along with fears of being rejected or confidentiality not being respected, especially in healthcare settings. This is not a new finding, as negative reactions to LBGTQI+ populations have included parental rejection and bullying by peers, contributing to internalisation of negative societal perceptions, social isolation and **identity concealment** (Testa et al., 2015). This is of concern, as negative experiences may result in people not seeking medical help due to anticipatory stigma or fears surrounding the illegality of same-sex relationships in some countries (Samad et al., 2025).

In a review of research studies conducted with Asian Americans who also identified as belonging to LGBTQI+ groups, Ching et al. (2018) reported that many people experienced intersectional stress due to their ethnicity, sexual and gender minority statuses. Stress took the form of overt **structural oppression**, as evidenced by LGBTQI+ Asian Americans having lower incomes, living in poverty, fewer being employed in managerial positions and living in segregated neighbourhoods compared with their White American counterparts (Lee & Kye, 2016). Due to laws against same-sex marriage, which were in place until 2015, LGBTQI+ individuals faced additional constraints, as their personal relationships have been shaped and stigmatised by cisgenderism and heterosexualism. Stigma emanated from cultural norms, as Asian American LGBTQI+ relationships were viewed as damaging to the family and ethnic reputation, leading to discouragement of openly identifying as LGBTQI+ (Choudhury et al., 2009). In addition, the internalised stress associated with fear of disappointing parents and bringing shame on the family resulted in conflicted thinking about 'coming out' or staying silenced about their LGBTQ+ identity (Sarno et al., 2015). The structural and cultural discrimination, stigma, microaggressions and internalisation of these experiences led to negative self-perceptions, isolation and limited social support, which negatively impacted physical health (Molina et al., 2014; Wei et al., 2012). Intersectional stress has also been linked to maladaptive coping, resulting in risky sexual behaviours, increased alcohol consumption, smoking and recreational drug use.

Microaggressions as a source of stress

Minority ethnic communities, Indigenous populations, people with disabilities and LGBTQI+ individuals not only experience discrimination, but they are also often on the receiving end of subtle day-to-day discriminatory events, referred to as microaggressions (Mercer et al., 2011), which can be displayed by unintended actions or words (Sue, 2010). Research into the impact of stress on minority communities has mainly used standardised measures of self-reported stress in assessing the extent of situational stressors in a person's life (Cohen et al., 1983). These have included the impact of various life events on stress levels (Holmes & Rahe, 1967); the frequency and intensity of daily hassles (Delongis et al., 1982); job stress (Karasek, 1985) and burnout (Maslach & Jackson, 1981). However, these scales do not include the specific nature of the stress experienced by minority groups. Based on past experiences of rejection, LGBTQI+, Indigenous and non-White populations have heightened vigilance related to expectations of rejection, from having to conceal their true identities and the stress from self-contempt related to **internalised stigma** (Meyer, 2003). Some questionnaires do claim to measure minority stress, but they tend to focus on singular aspects such as discriminatory events (Huebner & Davis, 2007) or stigma (Balsam & Mohr, 2007), overlooking subtle everyday sources of stress and humiliation. While microaggressions may be quite subtle and can be intentional, they usually consist of daily unintentional forms of prejudice that can be verbal and nonverbal. Microaggressions have been explored in sexual and gender minorities (Nadal et al., 2016), Indigenous groups (Walls et al., 2015) and people with disabilities. Individuals can experience several types of microaggressions related to each of their singular identities, for example, a lesbian woman who is Black, of a low socioeconomic status and has a disability, may experience microaggressions that are targeted at their sexual orientation, ethnicity, social status and disability. Intentional microaggressions may include the use of derogatory language and making racist or sexist jokes, but they can also involve unintentional microinsults that impact a person's identity, even though an individual is trying to be complementary. For example, saying, 'you speak English very well for someone who is from China', implying that they do not expect them to be fluent, or telling someone from an Indigenous population 'coming from your background, you have done so well to get a university degree', may be taken to imply that they are not expected to be well educated due to being Indigenous.

Such microaggressions can build up over time and contribute to minority stress, which is associated with poorer physical and mental health within Indigenous communities in the US (Walls et al., 2015) and digestive problems, anxiety and re-traumatisation of racial experiences in Black Americans (Hall & Fields, 2015). Minority stress has negative implications for mental health and alcohol abuse in people from LGBTQI+ communities, with more marked impacts on transgender individuals (Marchi et al., 2024) and has been shown to have negative impacts on self-belief in own academic ability for Black students with disabilities (Lett et al., 2020). Additionally, the minority stress of microaggressions can contribute to health compromising behaviours that include increased smoking, alcohol intake, use of recreational drugs, poor diet and low levels of physical activity.

BOX 8.3
CRITICAL THINKING

From what you have learned in this chapter, how might stress be experienced not just by personal circumstances, but also by the combination of social identities, such as ethnicity, gender identity and sexual orientation?

Measuring stress

At the current time, there is no agreed gold standard way of measuring stress, but there are a range of ways to measure stress objectively and subjectively. Objective measures include heart rate, blood pressure and biochemical markers, which are perceived to be more reliable than subjective measures. Questionnaires are a quick and inexpensive way to measure subjective stress, with a range of standardised scales that include general and specific aspects of stress. For example, in relation to work, parenting, school, student life, daily hassles, life events and specific diseases. When using questionnaires, it is important to ensure that they are standardised, reliable, valid, culturally appropriate and when possible, the scales used, should avoid response bias and social desirability.

Questionnaires

Social Readjustment Rating Scale

In the Holmes and Rahe (1967) Social Readjustment Rating Scale (SRRS), people are asked to select major life events experienced over the past year; these range from major stressful events to minor ones. For example, marriage, death of a family member, taking out a large financial loan, examinations, going on holiday, etc. Each life event is associated with a numerical life change unit that is said to indicate the extent of stress caused by the event. The life units are summed to give a total score, which is used to determine the likelihood of the individual becoming ill or having an accident due to the impact of their stressful experiences. This scale has been criticised as the numerical value given to each of the life events seems to be arbitrary. It does not differentiate between positive and negative life events, with both viewed as causing the same degree of stress. For example, two people who have retired, score the same life change units, but their experiences of the stress of retirement may have been quite different. One individual may have viewed retirement with dread, as they felt they no longer had a purpose in their life, their days lacked structure and retirement was associated with decreased income. For someone else, retirement was a welcomed life stage due to the end of stressful work activities and viewed as a new exciting chapter in their life, looking forward to engagement in new activities and travel.

Hassles and Uplifts Scale

While the SRRS deals with big life events, Kanner et al. (1981) created a way to measure the accumulated minor stressors that people experience each day, called the Hassles and Uplifts scale. The individual is asked to rate the degree to which each item on the scale is a hassle (causes annoyance or stress) or an uplift (minor positive events). This includes interacting with children, peers, co-workers and subjective aspects of the individual's health. Zautra (2003) and Almeida (2005) reported that hassles are more predictive of poor health than uplifts and may involve activation of the HPA axis. Furthermore, daily hassles may increase greater symptom reporting in chronic conditions, such as irritable bowel syndrome (Dancey et al., 1998), rheumatoid arthritis (Fifield et al., 2004), and have negative impacts on blood glucose control in people with type 1 diabetes (Riazi et al., 2004).

The Perceived Stress Scale

The Perceived Stress Scale (PSS; Cohen et al., 1983) has been used to assess individuals' perceptions of how stressful their life has been over the past month. This is based on the transactional model of stress; therefore, it is concerned with the person's subjective appraisal of stressful situations or events and their ability to cope. Kiecolt-Glaser et al. (1995) used the PSS to assess levels of carer stress on wound healing and found that those who scored highly on the PSS had longer healing times. The PSS has been used in a range of studies that link stress and health outcomes. In a longitudinal study of 10,232 women aged 70–75 years, over a 3-year period, higher perceived stress was a significant predictor of coronary heart disease symptoms (Strodl et al. (2003).

The decision on which stress questionnaire to use will very much depend on the research question. If a health psychologist is interested in the impact of work stress and self-reported physical health, rather than use the PSS, it would be more valid to use a specific scale, such as the Work Stress Questionnaire (Holmgren et al., 2009). This measures stress associated with work conflicts, individual time demands and commitments, the impact of work on leisure time and responsibility at work. It must be remembered that questionnaire-based measurements of stress are usually based on life events or used to assess recent stressful situations or hassles, they do not give an indication of cumulative stress or predict the longer-term health outcomes of stress. However, the results of a stress questionnaire may provide some indication of the way in which an individual typically deals with a stressor in terms of their emotional responses. In a longitudinal study, Piazza et al. (2013) assessed the extent of emotional stress (affective reactivity) to everyday stressors and physical health status and did the same 10 years later. They found that participants who reported emotional reactions to daily stressors were more likely to develop chronic health problems, suggesting that how people respond to stress may have important consequences for health. However, the researchers cautioned that due to the self-report nature of stress responses and health outcomes, there was a potential for results to be contaminated by negative response bias, i.e. people who are more emotionally reactive may be more likely to report more health problems, but that does not necessarily mean that they have more health issues.

Physiological measures of stress

There is no single physiological or biological measure of stress or allostatic load. Physiological measures of stress can include metabolic markers that provide an insight into the utilisation of blood glucose over several months (HbA1c), inflammatory and/or immune markers. Due to the physiological response of the body to stress being universal, biomarkers of stress can be measured in blood, sweat and urine, but intensity and duration of the stress response varies across people. It must be remembered that many factors can intersect to influence physiological responses to stress, including socioeconomic status, culture, early life experiences, coping skills, gender, past and current stress and health behaviours, meaning that results are often correlation in nature and not cause and effect.

Cortisol has been used in numerous studies as a biomarker of stress. Levels of cortisol are at their highest around 30–40 minutes after experiencing a stressful event or situation, they then slowly return to normal once the stressor has gone. Cortisol levels can be measured in saliva, which has the advantage of convenience, it is a non-invasive method and salivary cortisol correlates well with blood levels of cortisol. The collection of salivary cortisol works well in laboratory settings where the storage temperature of samples can be regulated, but the unstable nature of salivary cortisol can be problematic when conducting research outside of a controlled environment. Cortisol can also be collected from the shaft of a person's hair (closest to the scalp) and this non-invasive method permits assessment of the longer-term effects of stress. Cortisol may also be collected via urine sampling, but requires total urine output over a 24-hour period. This can pose some problems for people in relation to collecting samples at work and urine needs to be stored in a refrigerator until it is transferred to the laboratory for analysis. Pregnancy and some medications can interfere with this type of cortisol measurement. Cortisol can be collected in blood samples, but this is resource intensive and requires a trained person to take the sample, with collection taking place in a clean environment. Blood cortisol collection is invasive, involving insertion of a needle into a vein, which can be unpleasant and cause increases in cortisol due to the stress of the procedure. In addition, there are specific requirements for storage of blood and refrigeration is required. Of all the methods outlined here, the most commonly used is salivary cortisol (Iqbal et al., 2023).

When experiencing acute stress, sympathetic nervous system activation usually results in the production of sweat. Galvanic skin response (GSR) makes use of small electrodes that are attached to the fingertips to measure the electrical conductance of the skin caused by increased sweating. GSR is often used in conjunction with other non-invasive ways of measuring stress, such as heart rate, blood pressure and respiration, all of which can be influenced by stress. With the increase in the use of mobile sensors, some physiological indicators of stress, such as heart rate, respiration and blood pressure, can be monitored by wearable devices, such as smart watches and rings.

Chapter summary

Outline the ways in which stress has been defined

Stress has been defined as an external stimulus or event that makes a demand on the person, which can result in a stress response. This response can be physiological in nature, activating the sympathetic-adrenal-medullary and the hypothalamic-medullary-adrenal pathways. Stress is also considered as a transaction between the person and their environment, with perceived ability to cope being a determinant of whether the event is deemed to be stressful.

Explain what is meant by primary and secondary appraisal of stress

Primary appraisal involves consideration of the relevance of the threat, which can be irrelevant and benign, leading to no action being required. The other two primary appraisals are harmful, with one being considered as a challenge and the other as a threat, both will involve secondary appraisal. Challenge usually means the individual has a high perceived ability to cope, which will result in minimal stress. If the threat is deemed harmful, it suggests that the individual has low perceived ability to cope, which may lead to maximum stress.

What types of social support can help mediate the effects of stress?

There are various types of social support that include emotional (feeling cared for), instrumental (direct practical help), informational (provision of explanations), appraisal (help with evaluation of the situation) and companionship (the provision of company or friendship). Social support can be beneficial to health, but the type of support must match the individual's needs.

Examine the role of stress in disease

Research indicates that stress can have determinantal impacts on immune functioning, with evidence from experimentally-induced wounds taking longer to heal in people who have higher levels of stress. Studies have suggested a link between high levels of stress and susceptibility to viruses, but people who are stressed may also engage in behaviours that can have detrimental effects on health, such as smoking and eating unhealthy diets. Stress is also indirectly associated with the development of chronic diseases and disease can be a source of stress.

Explain how colonisation and intersectionality contribute to stress

Colonisation has caused both direct and intergeneration stress, contributing to poorer health and high rates of chronic disease among Indigenous Peoples. The effects of stress have also been linked with obesity and higher rates of smoking. Other minority groups face ongoing intersectional stress, stigma, discrimination and microaggressions, which have been linked to unhealthy coping behaviours, such as increased alcohol consumption, smoking and risky sexual practices. Over time, chronic stress can have determinantal impacts on health.

Keywords

Discrimination: The unfair or unequal treatment of individuals or groups based on ethnicity, gender, gender identity, sexual orientation, religion, socioeconomic status, disability and being from an Indigenous group.

Stigma: A negative attitude or belief that someone holds about others who are perceived to be different.

Stress: A stimulus or event that is external to the person that triggers a stress response. Stress can also be a physiology response of the body to a stressful event or situation. Stress can be a results of the relationship between the stressor and the person's perceived ability to cope with it.

Homeostasis: The body's stable internal (resting) environment.

General Adaptation System: A three-stage model (alarm, resistance and exhaustion) to explain how the body responds physiologically to stress.

Allostatic load: The cumulation of the wear and tear on the body because of exposure to chronic stress.

Primary appraisal: The initial stage in the cognitive evaluation of a stressor, that is used to judge whether the stressor is irrelevant, benign and positive, a threat and harmful or a threat and a challenge.

Secondary appraisal: After primary appraisal, secondary appraisal involves the assessment of perceived ability to cope and available resources.

Coping styles: How people generally respond to stressful events.

Approach coping: Directly dealing with the stressful event.

Avoidant coping: Trying to ignore the stressful event by engaging in other activities.

Problem focused coping: Taking direct action by focusing on the stressor.

Emotion-focused coping: Trying to change the emotional response to stress, rather than dealing with the problem directly.

Social support: Help received from others to buffer stress that can be emotional, instrumental, informational, appraisal and companionship.

Psychoneuroimmunology: How psychological factors, the immune system and nervous system are interrelated and exert impacts on immune status.

Physiological reactivity: The extent to which an individual's physiological systems respond to stress.

Cardiovascular reactivity: Changes to heart rate and blood pressure because of stress.

Microaggressions: Subtle day-to-day discriminatory events that can be intentional or unintentional.

Type A behaviour pattern: Associated with individuals who are competitive, ambitious, perfectionists and time driven.
Type B behaviour pattern: Associated with individuals who have low levels of competitiveness, relaxed and easy going.
Hardiness: People who are resilient to stress due to commitment, control and challenge.
Dispositional optimism: People who have a general expectation that good things will happen in the future, if they focus on positive outcomes.
Identity concealment: Intentionally hiding some aspect of identity, often to avoid discrimination or stigma.
Structural oppression: Laws, systems and organisations in society unfairly disadvantage minoritised groups.
Internalised stigma: The individual believes and feels ashamed and accepts the negative beliefs that others express about some aspect of their identity.

Key Readings

Hall, J. M., & Fields, B. (2015). "It's killing us!" Narratives of Black adults about microaggression experiences and related health stress. *Global Qualitative Nursing Research, 2*, 2333393615591569. https://doi.org/10.1177/2333393615591569
Jacob, G., Faber, S. C., Faber, N., Bartlett, A., Ouimet, A. J., & Williams, M. T. (2023). A systematic review of Black people coping with racism: Approaches, analysis, and empowerment. *Perspectives on Psychological, 18*(2), 392–415. https://doi.org/10.1177/17456916221100509
O'Connor, D. B., Thayer, J. F., & Vedhara, K. (2021). Stress and health: A review of psychobiological processes. *Annual Review of Psychology, 72*, 663–688. https://doi.org/10.1146/annurev-psych-062520-122331

Reflective Questions

1 How does the way that you think about stress affect how you deal with it?
2 What types of stressors do people from different cultural, ethnic, sexual or gender minority groups experience?
3 How might long-term exposure to microaggressions or chronic stressors impact unhealthy coping behaviours and physical health over time?

References

Action on Smoking and Health (ASH) (2019). ASH annual report. Retrieved August 8, 2025, from https://ash.org/wp-content/uploads/2020/06/ASH-Annual-Report-2019.pdf
Adamczyk, A., & Liao, Y. C. (2019). Examining public opinion about LGBTQ-related issues in the United States and across multiple nations. *Annual Review of Sociology, 45*(1), 401–423. https://doi.org/10.1146/annurev-soc-073018-022332
Ader, R., & Cohen, N. (1975). Behaviorally conditioned immunosuppression. *Psychosomatic Medicine, 37*(4), 333–340. https://doi.org/10.1097/00006842-197507000-00007
Ader, R., & Cohen, N. (1981). Psychoneuroimmunology: Conditioning and stress. *Annual Review of Psychology, 32*(1), 527–558. https://doi.org/10.1146/annurev.ps.44.020193.000413
al'Absi, M., & Wittmers, L. E. Jr (2003). Enhanced adrenocortical responses to stress in hypertension-prone men and women. *Annals of Behavioral Medicine, 25*(1), 25–33. https://doi.org/10.1207/S15324796ABM2501_04

Almeida, D. M. (2005). Resilience and vulnerability to daily stressors assessed via diary methods. *Current Directions in Psychological Science, 14*(2), 64–68. https://doi.org/10.1111/j.0963-7214.2005.00336.x

Anderson, I., Robson, B., Connolly, M., Al-Yaman, F., Bjertness, E., King, A., Tynan, M., Madden, R., Bang, A., Coimbra, C. E. Jr, Pesantes, M. A., Amigo, H., Andronov, S., Armien, B., Obando, D. A., Axelsson, P., Bhatti, Z. S., Bhutta, Z. A., Bjerregaard, P., Bjertness, M. B., & Yap, L. (2016). Indigenous and tribal peoples' health (The Lancet-Lowitja Institute Global Collaboration): A population study. *Lancet, 388*(10040), 131–157. https://doi.org/10.1016/S0140-6736(16)00345-7

Balsam, K. F., & Mohr, J. J. (2007). Adaptation to sexual orientation stigma: A comparison of bisexual and lesbian/gay adults. *Journal of Counseling Psychology, 54*(3), 306–319. https://doi.org/10.1037/0022-0167.54.3.306

Beech, E. L., Riddell, N., Murphy, M. J., & Crewther, S. G. (2023). Sex and stress hormone dysregulation as clinical manifestations of hypothalamic function in migraine disorder: A meta-analysis. *The European Journal of Neuroscience, 58*(4), 3150–3171. https://doi.org/10.1111/ejn.16087

Berger, M., & Sarnyai, Z. (2015). More than skin deep: Stress neurobiology and mental health consequences of racial discrimination. *Stress, 18*(1), 1–10. https://doi.org/10.3109/10253890.2014.989204

Berkman, L. F., & Syme, S. L. (1979). Social networks, host resistance, and mortality: A nine-year follow-up study of Alameda County residents. *American Journal of Epidemiology, 109*(2), 186–204. https://doi.org/10.1093/oxfordjournals.aje.a112674

Boutin-Foster, C. (2005). In spite of good intentions: Patients' perspectives on problematic social support interactions. *Health and Quality of Life Outcomes, 3*, 52. https://doi.org/10.1186/1477-7525-3-52

Brooks, M. V. (2003). Health-related hardiness and chronic illness: A synthesis of current research. *Nursing forum, 38*(3), 11–20. https://doi.org/10.1111/j.0029-6473.2003.00011.x

Brunner, E. (2007). Biology and health inequality. *PLoS Biology, 5*, e267. http://doi.org/10.1371/journal.pbio.0050267

Brydon, L., Strike, P. C., Bhattacharyya, M. R., Whitehead, D. L., McEwan, J., Zachary, I., & Steptoe, A. (2010). Hostility and physiological responses to laboratory stress in acute coronary syndrome patients. *Journal of Psychosomatic Research, 68*(2), 109–116. https://doi.org/10.1016/j.jpsychores.2009.06.007

Buse, D. C., & Lipton, R. B. (2015). Primary headache: What's stress got to do with it? *Cephalalgia, 35*(10), 844–849. https://doi.org/10.1177/0333102414567382

Cannon, W. B. (1932). *The wisdom of the body*. Norton.

Ching, T. H. W., Lee, S. Y., Chen, J., So, R. P., & Williams, M. T. (2018). A model of intersectional stress and trauma in Asian American sexual and gender minorities. *Psychology of Violence, 8*(6), 657–668. https://doi.org/10.1037/vio0000204

Choudhury, P. P., Badhan, N. S., Chand, J., Chhugani, S., Choksey, R., Husainy, S., Lui, C., & Wat, E. C. (2009). Community alienation and its impact on help-seeking behavior among LGBTIQ South Asians in Southern California. *Journal of Gay & Lesbian Social Services, 21*(2–3), 247–266. https://doi.org/10.1080/10538720902772196

Cohen, S. (2005). The Pittsburgh common cold studies: Psychosocial predictors of susceptibility to respiratory infectious illness. *International Journal of Behavioral Medicine, 12*(3), 123–131. https://doi.org/10.1207/s15327558ijbm1203_1

Cohen, S., Doyle, W. J., & Skoner, D. P. (1999). Psychological stress, cytokine production, and severity of upper respiratory illness. *Psychosomatic Medicine, 61*(2), 175–180. https://doi.org/10.1097/00006842-199903000-00009

Cohen, S., Kamarck, T., & Mermelstein, R. (1983). A global measure of perceived stress. *Journal of Health and Social Behavior, 24*(4), 385–396. https://doi.org/10.2307/2136404

Cohen, S., & Wills, T. A. (1985). Stress, social support, and the buffering hypothesis. *Psychological Bulletin, 98*(2), 310–357. https://doi.org/10.1037/0033-2909.98.2.310

Culbreth, R. E., Salazar, L. F., Spears, C. A., Crosby, R., Hayat, M. J., & Aycock, D. M. (2023). Stressors associated with tobacco use among trans women. *Transgender Health, 8*(3), 282–292. https://doi.org/10.1089/trgh.2020.0168

Dancey, C. P., Taghavi, M., & Fox, R. J. (1998). The relationship between daily stress and symptoms of irritable bowel: A time-series approach. *Journal of Psychosomatic Research, 44*(5), 537–545. https://doi.org/10.1016/s0022-3999(97)00255-9

Dar, T., Radfar, A., Abohashem, S., Pitman, R. K., Tawakol, A., & Osborne, M. T. (2019). Psychosocial stress and cardiovascular disease. *Current Treatment Options in Cardiovascular Medicine, 21*(5), 23. https://doi.org/10.1007/s11936-019-0724-5

Day, M., Carlson, B., Bonson, D., & Farrelly, T. (2023). *Aboriginal and Torres Strait Islander LGBTQIASB+ people and mental health and wellbeing*. Australian Institute of Health and Welfare. Retrieved August 6, 2025, from https://www.aihw.gov.au/reports/indigenous-mental-health-suicide-prevention/aboriginal-torres-strait-islander-lgbtqiasb-people/summary

DeLongis, A., Coyne, J. C., Dakof, G., Folkman, S., & Lazarus, R. S. (1982). Relationship of daily hassles, uplifts, and major life events to health status. *Health Psychology, 1*(2), 119–136. https://doi.org/10.1037/0278-6133.1.2.119

De Maria, M., Tagliabue, S., Ausili, D., Vellone, E., & Matarese, M. (2020). Perceived social support and health-related quality of life in older adults who have multiple chronic conditions and their caregivers: A dyadic analysis. *Social Science & Medicine, 262*, 113193. https://doi.org/10.1016/j.socscimed.2020.113193

Dilley, J. A., Peterson, E., Bobo, M., Pickle, K. E., & Rohde, K. (2013). Tobacco use prevalence–disentangling associations between Alaska Native race, low socio-economic status and rural disparities. *International Journal of Circumpolar Health, 72*, 10.3402/ijch.v72i0.21582. https://doi.org/10.3402/ijch.v72i0.21582

Epner, M., Yang, P., Wagner, R. W., & Cohen, L. (2022). Understanding the link between sugar and cancer: An examination of the preclinical and clinical evidence. *Cancers, 14*(24), 6042. https://doi.org/10.3390/cancers14246042

Fernández-Peña, R., Molina, J. L., & Valero, O. (2020). Satisfaction with social support received from social relationships in cases of chronic pain: The influence of personal network characteristics in terms of structure, composition and functional content. *International Journal of Environmental Research and Public Health, 17*(8), 2706. https://doi.org/10.3390/ijerph17082706

Fifield, J., McQuillan, J., Armeli, S., Tennen, H., Reisine, S., & Affleck, G. (2004). Chronic strain, daily work stress and pain among workers with rheumatoid arthritis: Does job stress make a bad day worse? *Work & Stress, 18*(4), 275–291. https://doi.org/10.1080/02678370412331324996

Flentje, A., Heck, N. C., Brennan, J. M., & Meyer, I. H. (2020). The relationship between minority stress and biological outcomes: A systematic review. *Journal of Behavioral Medicine, 43*(5), 673–694. https://doi.org/10.1007/s10865-019-00120-6

Forte, A. J., Guliyeva, G., McLeod, H., Dabrh, A. M. A., Salinas, M., Avila, F. R., & Perlman, A. (2022). The impact of optimism on cancer-related and postsurgical cancer pain: A systematic review. *Journal of Pain and Symptom Management, 63*(2), e203–e211. https://doi.org/10.1016/j.jpainsymman.2021.09.008

Folkman, S., & Lazarus, R. S. (1988). *Ways of coping questionnaire*. Consulting Psychologists Press.

Friedli, L. (2009). *Mental health, resilience and inequalities*. WHO Regional Office for Europe. Retrieved August 8, 2025, from https://iris.who.int/handle/10665/107925

Friedman, M., & Rosenman, R. H. (1959). Association of specific overt behavior pattern with blood and cardiovascular findings; blood cholesterol level, blood clotting time, incidence of arcus senilis, and clinical coronary artery disease. *Journal of the American Medical Association, 169*(12), 1286–1296. https://doi.org/10.1001/jama.1959.03000290012005

Girod, J. P., & Brotman, D. J. (2004). Does altered glucocorticoid homeostasis increase cardiovascular risk? *Cardiovascular Research, 64*(2), 217–226. https://doi.org/10.1016/j.cardiores.2004.07.006

Graven, L. J., & Grant, J. S. (2014). Social support and self-care behaviors in individuals with heart failure: An integrative review. *International Journal of Nursing Studies, 51*(2), 320–333. https://doi.org/10.1016/j.ijnurstu.2013.06.013

Hall, J. M., & Fields, B. (2015). "It's killing us!" Narratives of Black adults about microaggression experiences and related health stress. *Global Qualitative Nursing Research, 2*, 2333393615591569. https://doi.org/10.1177/2333393615591569

Hatch, S. L., & Dohrenwend, B. P. (2007). Distribution of traumatic and other stressful life events by race/ethnicity, gender, SES and age: A review of the research. *American Journal of Community Psychology, 40*(3–4), 313–332. https://doi.org/10.1007/s10464-007-9134-z

Haynes, S. G., Feinleib, M., & Kannel, W. B. (1980). The relationship of psychosocial factors to coronary heart disease in the Framingham Study. III. Eight-year incidence of coronary heart disease. *American Journal of Epidemiology, 111*(1), 37–58. https://doi.org/10.1093/oxfordjournals.aje.a112873

Helgeson, V. S., & Zajdel, M. (2017). Adjusting to chronic health conditions. *Annual Review of Psychology, 68*, 545–71. https://doi.org/10.1146/annurev-psych-010416-044014

Hill, D., Conner, M., Clancy, F., Moss, R., Wilding, S., Bristow, M., & O'Connor, D. B. (2022). Stress and eating behaviours in healthy adults: A systematic review and meta-analysis. *Health Psychology Review, 16*(2), 280–304. https://doi.org/10.1080/17437199.2021.1923406

Holmes, T. H., & Rahe, R. H. (1967). The social readjustment rating scale. *Journal of Psychosomatic Research, 11*(2), 213–218. https://doi.org/10.1016/0022-3999(67)90010-4

Holmgren, K., Hensing, G., & Dahlin-Ivanoff, S. (2009). Development of a questionnaire assessing work-related stress in women - identifying individuals who risk being put on sick leave. *Disability and Rehabilitation, 31*(4), 284–292. https://doi.org/10.1080/09638280801931287

House, J. S. (1981). *Work stress and social support*. Addison-Wesley.

Hoy-Ellis, C. P. (2023). Minority stress and mental health: A review of the literature. *Journal of Homosexuality, 70*, 806–830. https://doi.org/10.1080/00918369.2021.2004794

Huebner, D. M., & Davis, M. C. (2007). Perceived antigay discrimination and physical health outcomes. *Health Psychology, 26*(5), 627–634. https://doi.org/10.1037/0278-6133.26.5.627

Iqbal, T., Elahi, A., Redon, P., Vazquez, P., Wijns, W., & Shahzad, A. (2021). A review of biophysiological and biochemical indicators of stress for connected and preventive healthcare. *Diagnostics, 11*(3), 556. https://doi.org/10.3390/diagnostics11030556

Iqbal, T., Elahi, A., Wijns, W., & Shahzad, A. (2023). Cortisol detection methods for stress monitoring in connected health. *Health Sciences Review, 6*, 100079. https://doi.org/10.1016/j.hsr.2023.100079

Ironson, G., Balbin, E., Stuetzle, R., Fletcher, M. A., O'Cleirigh, C., Laurenceau, J. P., Schneiderman, N., & Solomon, G. (2005). Dispositional optimism and the mechanisms by which it predicts slower disease progression in HIV: Proactive behavior, avoidant coping, and depression. *International Journal of Behavioral Medicine, 12*(2), 86–97. https://doi.org/10.1207/s15327558ijbm1202_6

Kanner, A. D., Coyne, J. C., Schaefer, C., & Lazarus, R. S. (1981). Comparison of two modes of stress measurement: Daily hassles and uplifts versus major life events. *Journal of Behavioral Medicine, 4*(1), 1–39. https://doi.org/10.1007/BF00844845

Karasek, R. A. (1979). Job demands, job decision latitude, and mental strain: Implications for job redesign. *Administrative Science Quarterly, 24*, 285–306.

Kazmierski, K. F. M., Gillespie, M. L., Kuo, S., Zurita, T., Felix, D., & Rao, U. (2021). Stress-induced eating among racial/ethnic groups in the United States: A systematic review. *Journal of Racial and Ethnic Health Disparities, 8*(4), 912–926. https://doi.org/10.1007/s40615-020-00849-w

Ketheesan, S., Rinaudo, M., Berger, M., Wenitong, M., Juster, R. P., McEwen, B. S., & Sarnyai, Z. (2020). Stress, allostatic load and mental health in Indigenous Australians. *Stress, 23*(5), 509–518. https://doi.org/10.1080/10253890.2020.1732346

Kiecolt-Glaser, J. K., Glaser, R., Shuttleworth, E. C., Dyer, C. S., Ogrocki, P., & Speicher, C. E. (1987). Chronic stress and immunity in family caregivers of Alzheimer's disease victims. *Psychosomatic Medicine, 49*(5), 523–535. https://doi.org/10.1097/00006842-198709000-00008

Kiecolt-Glaser, J. K., Marucha, P. T., Malarkey, W. B., Mercado, A. M., & Glaser, R. (1995). Slowing of wound healing by psychological stress. *Lancet, 346*(8984), 1194–1196. https://doi.org/10.1016/s0140-6736(95)92899-5

Kivimäki, M., & Steptoe, A. (2018). Effects of stress on the development and progression of cardiovascular disease. *Nature Reviews. Cardiology, 15*(4), 215–229. https://doi.org/10.1038/nrcardio.2017.189

Kobasa, S. C. (1979). Stressful life events, personality, and health: An inquiry into hardiness. *Journal of Personality and Social Psychology, 37*(1), 1–11. https://doi.org/10.1037/0022-3514.37.1.1

Lazarus, R. S., & Folkman, S. (1984). *Stress, appraisal and coping*. Springer.

Lee, J. C., & Kye, S. (2016). Racialized assimilation of Asian Americans. *Annual Review of Sociology, 42*, 253–273. https://doi.org/10.1146/annurev-soc-081715-074310

Leor, J., Poole, W. K., & Kloner, R. A. (1996). Sudden cardiac death triggered by an earthquake. *The New England Journal of Medicine, 334*(7), 413–419. https://doi.org/10.1056/NEJM199602153340701

Lett, K., Tamaian, A., & Klest, B. (2020). Impact of ableist microaggressions on university students with self-identified disabilities. *Disability & Society, 35*(9), 1441–1456. https://doi.org/10.1080/09687599.2019.1680344

Lewis, M. E., Volpert-Esmond, H. I., Deen, J. F., Modde, E., & Warne, D. (2021). Stress and cardiometabolic disease risk for Indigenous populations throughout the lifespan. *International Journal of Environmental Research and Public Health, 18*(4), 1821. https://doi.org/10.3390/ijerph18041821

Lick, D. J., Durso, L. E., & Johnson, K. L. (2013). Minority stress and physical health among sexual minorities. *Perspectives on Psychological Science, 8*(5), 521–548. https://doi.org/10.1177/1745691613497965

Maddi, S. R. (2002). The story of hardiness: Twenty years of theorizing, research, and practice. *Consulting Psychology Journal, 54*(3), 173–185. https://doi.org/10.1037/1061-4087.54.3.173

Maleki, N., Becerra, L., & Borsook, D. (2012). Migraine: Maladaptive brain responses to stress. *Headache, 52*(2), 102–106. https://doi.org/10.1111/j.1526-4610.2012.02241.x

Marchi, M., Travascio, A., Uberti, D., De Micheli, E., Quartaroli, F., Laquatra, G., Grenzi, P., Pingani, L., Ferrari, S., Fiorillo, A., Converti, M., Pinna, F., Amaddeo, F., Ventriglio, A., Mirandola, M., & Galeazzi, G. M. (2024). Microaggression toward LGBTIQ people and implications for mental health: A systematic review. *The International Journal of Social Psychiatry, 70*(1), 23–35. https://doi.org/10.1177/00207640231194478

Markwick, A., Ansari, Z., Sullivan, M., Parsons, L., & McNeil, J. (2014). Inequalities in the social determinants of health of Aboriginal and Torres Strait Islander People: A cross-sectional population-based study in the Australian state of Victoria. *International Journal for Equity in Health, 13*(1), 91. https://doi.org/10.1186/s12939-014-0091-5

Marmot, M. (2011). Social determinants and the health of Indigenous Australians. *Medical Journal of Australia, 194*, 512–513. https://doi.org/10.5694/j.1326-5377.2011.tb03086.x

Marshall, G. D., Jr, Agarwal, S. K., Lloyd, C., Cohen, L., Henninger, E. M., & Morris, G. J. (1998). Cytokine dysregulation associated with exam stress in healthy medical students. *Brain, Behavior, and Immunity, 12*(4), 297–307. https://doi.org/10.1006/brbi.1998.0537

Marucha, P. T., Kiecolt-Glaser, J. K., & Favagehi, M. (1998). Mucosal wound healing is impaired by examination stress. *Psychosomatic Medicine, 60*(3), 362–365. https://doi.org/10.1097/00006842-199805000-00025

Maslach, C., & Jackson, S. E. (1981). The management of experienced burnout. *Journal of Organizational Behavior, 2*(2), 99–113. https://doi.org/10.1002/job.4030020205

Matthews, K. A., & Haynes, S. G. (1986). Type A behavior pattern and coronary disease risk. Update and critical evaluation. *American Journal of Epidemiology, 123*(6), 923–960. https://doi.org/10.1093/oxfordjournals.aje.a114347

Mason, T. B., & Lewis, R. J. (2015). Minority stress and binge eating among lesbian and bisexual women. *Journal of Homosexuality, 62*(7), 971–992. https://doi.org/10.1080/00918369.2015.1008285

Meyer, I. H. (2003). Prejudice, social stress, and mental health in lesbian, gay, and bisexual populations: Conceptual issues and research evidence. *Psychological Bulletin, 129*(5), 674–697. https://doi.org/10.1037/0033-2909.129.5.674

McEwen, B. S., & Stellar, E. (1993). Stress and the individual; mechanisms leading to disease. *Archives of Internal Medicine, 153*, 2093–2101. https://doi.org/10.1001/archinte.1993.00410180039004

Menino, D. D., Katz-Wise, S. L., Vetters, R., & Reisner, S. L. (2018). Associations between the length of time from transgender identity recognition to hormone initiation and smoking among transgender youth and young adults. *Transgender Health, 3*(1), 82–87. https://doi.org/10.1089/trgh.2018.0002

Mercer, S. H., Zeigler-Hil, V., Wallace, M., & Hayes, D. M. (2011). Development and initial validation of the inventory of microaggressions against Black individuals. *Journal of Counselling Psychology, 58*(4), 457–469. https://doi.org/10.1037/a0024937

Meyer, I. H. (2003). Prejudice, social stress, and mental health in lesbian, gay, and bisexual populations: Conceptual issues and research evidence. *Psychological Bulletin, 129*(5), 674–697. https://doi.org/10.1037/2329-0382.1.S.3

Minichiello, A., Lefkowitz, A. R., Firestone, M., Smylie, J. K., & Schwartz, R. (2016). Effective strategies to reduce commercial tobacco use in Indigenous communities globally: A systematic review. *BMC Public Health, 16*, 21. https://doi.org/10.1186/s12889-015-2645-x

Molina, Y., Lehavot, K., Beadnell, B., & Simoni, J. (2014). Racial disparities in health behaviors and conditions among lesbian and bisexual women: The role of internalized stigma. *LGBT Health, 1*(2), 131–139. https://doi.org/10.1089/lgbt.2013.0007

Nadal, K. L., Whitman, C. N., Davis, L. S., Erazo, T., & Davidoff, K. C. (2016). Microaggressions toward lesbian, gay, bisexual, transgender, queer, and genderqueer people: A review of the literature. *Journal of Sex Research, 53*(4–5), 488–508. https://doi.org/10.1080/00224499.2016.1142495

Najman, J. M., Toloo, G., & Siskind, V. (2006). Socioeconomic disadvantage and changes in health risk behaviours in Australia: 1989–90 to 2001. *Bulletin of the World Health Organization, 84*, 976–984. http://doi:10.2471/BLT.05.028928

Nelson, C. A., Scott, R. D., Bhutta, Z. A., Harris, N. B., Danese, A., & Samara, M. (2020). Adversity in childhood is linked to mental and physical health throughout life. *British Medical Journal, 371*, m3048. https://doi.org/10.1136/bmj.m3048

Nguyen, H., & Doan, T. (2025). What explains the smoking prevalence disparity between Indigenous and non-Indigenous Australians? *International Journal of Social Welfare, 34*, e70030. https://doi.org/10.1111/ijsw.70030

Orbist, P. A. (1981). *Cardiovascular psychophysiology: A perspective*. Plenum Press.

O'Connor, D. B., Jones, F., Conner, M., McMillan, B., & Ferguson, E. (2008). Effects of daily hassles and eating style on eating behavior. *Health Psychology, 27*(1), S20–S31. https://doi.org/10.1037/0278-6133.27.1.S20

Parker, L. L., & Harriger, J. A. (2020). Eating disorders and disordered eating behaviors in the LGBT population: A review of the literature. *Journal of Eating Disorders, 8*, 51. https://doi.org/10.1186/s40337-020-00327-y

Piazza, J. R., Charles, S. T., Sliwinski, M. J., Mogle, J., & Almeida, D. M. (2013). Affective reactivity to daily stressors and long-term risk of reporting a chronic physical health condition. *Annals of Behavioral Medicine, 45*(1), 110–120. https://doi.org/10.1007/s12160-012-9423-0

Pickett, S., Burchenal, C. A., Haber, L., Batten, K., & Phillips, E. (2020). Understanding and effectively addressing disparities in obesity: A systematic review of the psychological determinants of emotional eating behaviours among Black women. *Obesity Reviews 21*(6), e13010. https://doi.org/10.1111/obr.13010

Player, M. S., King, D. E., Mainous, A. G. 3rd, & Geesey, M. E. (2007). Psychosocial factors and progression from prehypertension to hypertension or coronary heart disease. *Annals of Family Medicine, 5*(5), 403–411. https://doi.org/10.1370/afm.738

Purcell, C., Dibben, G., Hilton Boon, M., Matthews, L., Palmer, V. J., Thomson, M., Smillie, S., Simpson, S. A., & Taylor, R. S. (2023). Social network interventions to support cardiac rehabilitation and secondary prevention in the management of people with heart disease. *The Cochrane Database of Systematic Reviews, 6*(6), CD013820. https://doi.org/10.1002/14651858.CD013820.pub2

Riazi, A., Pickup, J., & Bradley, C. (2004). Daily stress and glycaemic control in Type 1 diabetes: Individual differences in magnitude, direction, and timing of stress-reactivity. *Diabetes Research and Clinical Practice, 66*(3), 237–244. https://doi.org/10.1016/j.diabres.2004.04.001

Rosengren, A., Hawken, S., Ounpuu, S., Sliwa, K., Zubaid, M., Almahmeed, W. A., Blackett, K. N., Sitthi-Amorn, C., Sato, H., Yusuf, S.; INTERHEART investigators (2004). Association of psychosocial risk factors with risk of acute myocardial infarction in 11119 cases and 13648 controls from 52 countries (the INTERHEART study): Case-control study. *Lancet, 364*(9438), 953–962. https://doi.org/10.1016/S0140-6736(04)17019-0

Rosenman, R. H., Brand, R. J., Jenkins, D., Friedman, M., Straus, R., & Wurm, M. (1975). Coronary heart disease in the Western Collaborative Group Study: Final follow-up experience of 8½ years. *Journal of the American Medical Association, 233*(8), 872–877. https://doi.org/10.1001/jama.1975.03260080034016

Roth, S., & Cohen, L. J. (1986). Approach, avoidance, and coping with stress. *American Psychologist, 41*(7), 813–819. https://doi.org/10.1037/0003-066X.41.7.813

Rozanski, A., Bavishi, C., Kubzansky, L. D., & Cohen, R. (2019). Association of optimism with cardiovascular events and all-cause mortality: A systematic review and meta-analysis. *JAMA Network Open, 2*(9), e1912200. https://doi.org/10.1001/jamanetworkopen.2019.12200

Samad, S., Irving, S., Prankumar, S. K., Wong, H., Norr, M. N., & Saliba, B. (2025). Analysing the health of queer Muslims through the 4M framework: A scoping literature review. *Sexuality & Culture, 29*, 1971–1995. https://doi.org/10.1007/s12119-025-10342-3

Sarno, E. L., Mohr, J. J., Jackson, S. D., & Fassinger, R. E. (2015). When identities collide: Conflicts in allegiances among LGB people of color. *Cultural Diversity & Ethnic Minority Psychology, 21*(4), 550–559. https://doi.org/10.1037/cdp0000026

Sarnyai, Z., Berger, M., & Jawan, I. (2016). Allostatic load mediates the impact of stress and trauma on physical and mental health in Indigenous Australians. *Australasian Psychiatry, 24*(1), 72–75. https://doi.org/10.1177/1039856215620025

Sattler, F. A., Zeyen, J., & Christiansen, H. (2017). Does sexual identity stress mediate the association between sexual identity and mental health? *Psychology of Sexual Orientation and Gender Diversity, 4*(3), 296–303. https://doi.org/10.1037/sgd0000232

Scheier, M. F., & Carver, C. S. (1992). Effects of optimism on psychological and physical well-being: Theoretical overview and empirical update. *Cognitive Therapy and Research, 16*(2), 201–228. https://doi.org/10.1007/BF01173489

Schulkin, J., McEwen, B. S., & Gold, P. W. (1994). Allostasis, amygdala, and anticipatory angst. *Neuroscience and Biobehavioral Reviews, 18*(3), 385–396. https://doi.org/10.1016/0149-7634(94)90051-5

Sekoni, A. O., Jolly, K., & Gale, N. K. (2022). Hidden healthcare population; using intersectionality to theorise the experiences of LGBTQ+ people in Nigeria, Africa. *Global Public Health, 17*(1), 134–149. https://doi.org/10.1080/17441692.2020.1849351

Selye, H. (1956). *The stress of life*. McGraw-Hill.

Siegman, A. W., & Smith, T. W. (Eds.). (1994). *Anger, hostility, and the heart*. Lawrence Erlbaum Associates, Inc.

Shires, D. A., & Jaffee, K. D. (2016). Structural discrimination is associated with smoking status among a national sample of transgender individuals. *Nicotine & Tobacco Research, 18*(6), 1502–1508. https://doi.org/10.1093/ntr/ntv221

Shuster, C. L., Tate, M. C., Schulz, C. T., Reyes, C. T., Drohan, M. M., Astorini, A. G., Stamates, A. L., Yang, M., & Robbins, M. L. (2023). Perceived stress and coping among university students amidst COVID-19 pandemic. *COVID, 3*(10), 1544–1553. https://doi.org/10.3390/covid3100105

Soulliard, Z. A., Manning Iii, R. B., & Elbe, C. I. (2025). Intraminority stress, body image, and community connectedness: Associations with disordered eating among sexual minority men. *Journal of Eating Disorders, 13*(1), 99. https://doi.org/10.1186/s40337-025-01298-8

Stone, A. A., & Neale, J. M. (1984). New measure of daily coping: Development and preliminary results. *Journal of Personality and Social Psychology, 46*(4), 892–906. https://doi.org/10.1037/0022-3514.46.4.892

Strodl, E., Kenardy, J., & Aroney, C. (2003). Perceived stress as a predictor of the self-reported new diagnosis of symptomatic CHD in older women. *International Journal of Behavioral Medicine, 10*(3), 205–220. https://doi.org/10.1207/s15327558ijbm1003_02

Stubbs, B., Veronese, N., Vancampfort, D., Prina, A. M., Lin, P. Y., Tseng, P. T., Evangelou, E., Solmi, M., Kohler, C., Carvalho, A. F., & Koyanagi, A. (2017). Perceived stress and smoking across 41 countries: A global perspective across Europe, Africa, Asia and the Americas. *Scientific Reports, 7*(1), 7597. https://doi.org/10.1038/s41598-017-07579-w

Sue, D. (2010). Microaggressions, marginality, and oppression: An introduction. In D. Sue (Ed). *Microaggressions and marginality: Manifestations, dynamics, and impact* (pp. 3–22), John Wiley & Sons Inc.

Taylor, S. E., & Stanton, A. L. (2007). Coping resources, coping processes, and mental health. *Annual Review of Clinical Psychology, 3*, 377–401. https://doi.org/10.1146/annurev.clinpsy.3.022806.091520

Testa, R. J., Habarth, J., Peta, J., Balsam, K., & Bockting, W. (2015). Development of the gender minority stress and resilience measure. *Psychology of Sexual Orientation and Gender Diversity, 2*(1), 65–77. https://doi.org/10.1037/sgd0000081

Tomiyama, A. J., Carr, D., Granberg, E. M., Major, B., Robinson, E., Sutin, A. R., & Brewis, A. (2018). How and why weight stigma drives the obesity 'epidemic' and harms health. *BMC Medicine, 16*(1), 123. https://doi.org/10.1186/s12916-018-1116-5

Visseren, F. L. J., Mach, F., Smulders, Y. M., Carballo, D., Koskinas, K. C., Bäck, M., Benetos, A., Biffi, A., Boavida, J. M., Capodanno, D., Cosyns, B., Crawford, C., Davos, C. H., Desormais, I., Di Angelantonio, E., Franco, O. H., Halvorsen, S., Hobbs, F. D. R., Hollander, M., & Jankowska, E. A. ... ESC Scientific Document Group (2021). 2021 ESC Guidelines on cardiovascular disease prevention in clinical practice. *European Heart Journal, 42*(34), 3227–3337. https://doi.org/10.1093/eurheartj/ehab484

Vogel, E. A., Humfleet, G. L., Meacham, M., Prochaska, J. J., & Ramo, D. E. (2019). Sexual and gender minority young adults' smoking characteristics: Assessing differences by sexual orientation and gender identity. *Addictive Behaviors, 95*, 98–102. https://doi.org/10.1016/j.addbeh.2019.03.005

Walburn, J., Vedhara, K., Hankins, M., Rixon, L., & Weinman, J. (2009). Psychological stress and wound healing in humans: A systematic review and meta-analysis. *Journal of Psychosomatic Research, 67*(3), 253–271. https://doi.org/10.1016/j.jpsychores.2009.04.002

Walls, M. L., Gonzalez, J., Gladney, T., & Onello, E. (2015). Unconscious biases: Racial microaggressions in American Indian health care. *Journal of the American Board of Family Medicine, 28*(2), 231–239. https://doi.org/10.3122/jabfm.2015.02.140194

Wei, M., Wang, K. T., Heppner, P. P., & Du, Y. (2012). Ethnic and mainstream social connectedness, perceived racial discrimination, and posttraumatic stress symptoms. *Journal of Counseling Psychology, 59*, 486–493. https://doi.org/10.1037/a0028000

World Health Organization (2025) *Tobacco*. Retrieved August 6, 2025, from https://www.who.int/news-room/fact-sheets/detail/tobacco

Zautra, A. J. (2003). *Emotions, stress, and health*. Oxford University Press.

Zellner, D. A., Loaiza, S., Gonzalez, Z., Pita, J., Morales, J., Pecora, D., & Wolf, A. (2006). Food selection changes under stress. *Physiology & Behavior, 87*(4), 789–793. https://doi.org/10.1016/j.physbeh.2006.01.014

Zellner, D. A., Saito, S., & Gonzalez, J. (2007). The effect of stress on men's food selection. *Appetite, 49*(3), 696–699. https://doi.org/10.1016/j.appet.2007.06.013

9 Chronic diseases

Chapter contents

- The divide in chronic diseases between high-, middle- and low-income countries.
- Cardiovascular disease.
- CVD in different populations.
- Cancer.
- Cancer in different populations.
- Chronic obstructive pulmonary disease.
- Obesity.
- Obesogenic environment.
- Weight loss and culture.
- Consequences of obesity.
- Diabetes.
- DESMOND
- Diabetes in different populations.
- Looking forward

Chapter objectives

After reading this chapter, you should be able to answer the following questions:

- Discuss how the development of cardiovascular disease may be influenced by sex/gender sexual orientation, ethnicity and the enduring impacts of colonisation.
- Outline barriers to cancer screening experienced by people from ethnic minority groups, LGBTQI+ communities and people with disabilities.
- Describe and discuss factors influencing smoking behaviours and the barriers to quitting across diverse populations.
- Explain the concept of an obesogenic environment and how it relates to social determinants of health.
- Discuss the relationship between social determinants of health and the prevalence of type 2 diabetes mellitus.

In Chapter 2, we learned that global estimates of life expectancy had increased across all countries, but in 2023, there was still a marked differential between high-income countries (78.2 years) and low- and middle-income countries (LMICs), with a life expectancy of around 45–55 years in the central belt of the African continent (see Figure 9.1).

DOI: 10.4324/9781003423157-9

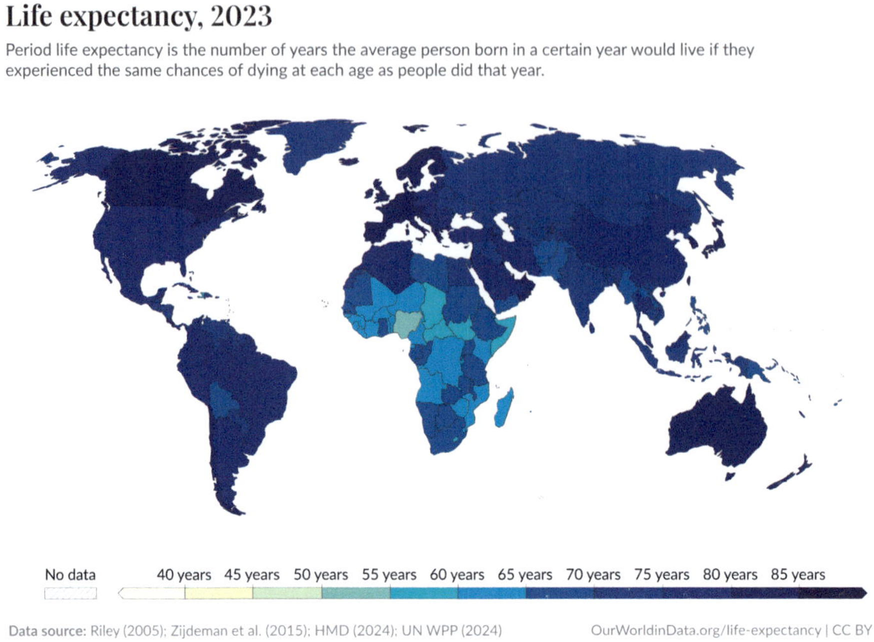

Figure 9.1
World map of life expectancy 2023

Source: Dattani et al. (2023)

The divide in chronic diseases between high-, middle- and low-income countries

People are living longer, but many of them have developed chronic diseases, which are influenced by lifestyle factors and behaviours. According to the Institute for Health Metrics and Evaluation (IHME) (2024), hypertension, smoking, high fasting blood glucose levels and air pollution are putting people at increased risk of developing chronic diseases, which contribute to poor quality of life and mortality. In 2021, cardiovascular disease (CVD), cancer, chronic respiratory diseases and diabetes-related kidney disease caused approximately 80% of premature deaths across the globe (WHO, 2024a). Data from the World Heart Federation (2023) showed that CVD, which includes coronary heart disease, hypertension and stroke, accounted for a third of global deaths. While advances in knowledge, technology and medicines have contributed to reductions in CVD deaths across high-income countries (HICs), most premature CVD-related deaths now occur in low- and middle-income countries WHO (2025a), with Central Asia, Eastern and Central Europe reporting the highest rates of mortality (Di Cesare et al., 2024). In low- and middle-income countries, the limited availability of care and treatments for CVD means that if and when people are diagnosed, it tends to be later in the disease trajectory, which is often associated with poorer health outcomes. In high-income countries (HICs), inequities are evident in the diagnosis and treatment of CVD across gender and ethnicity (IHME, 2020). In the European Union (EU), men generally have higher CVD mortality rates than women, in contrast, LMICs of North Africa, the Middle East region and Sub-Saharan Africa show higher CVD mortality rates for women

(Di Cesare et al., 2024). Countries that spend more of their economic wealth, that is their Gross Domestic Product (GDP) on healthcare, have lower mortality rates due to CVD (World Heart Federation, 2023). Research findings generally agree that people of lower socioeconomic status (SES), who have lower incomes, have an increased risk of CVD and lower life expectancies than their wealthier counterparts (de Mestral & Stringhini, 2017; Gerber et al., 2008). It should be noted that research into chronic disease often conflates gender with biological sex. Using the terms women/men rather than females/males seems to be the preferred terminology in public health communication, as it is seen as more patient/person-centred. However it is important to be aware that physiological sex differences and gendered social determinants can independently affect disease outcomes.

Cardiovascular disease

In Chapter 4, we learned about the physiological aspects of CVD, which describe diseases that affect the blood vessels and heart. Terminologies vary across studies, some use the broader term CVD, while others focus on specific named conditions, such as coronary artery disease (CAD), typified by arterial narrowing due to the build-up of plaque (atherosclerosis). Coronary heart disease (CHD), which includes damage to the heart muscle as a consequence of a heart attack, whereas ischaemic heart disease (IHD) is a broader term that covers both CAD and CHD, denoting reduced blood flow to the heart muscle. Where possible in this chapter, evidence will be reported in relation to the specific conditions referred to by researchers.

In the past, most research that tried to understand factors that predisposed people to develop CHD had focused on **Eurocentric populations** (Yusuf et al., 2001), this led researchers to explore risk factors between different countries across the globe. A large case-control study examined potentially modifiable (Rosengren et al., 2004) and psychosocial risk factors (Yusuf et al., 2004) associated with acute heart attacks across 52 countries in Africa, Asia, Australia, Europe, the Middle East, North and South America. People were selected as being in the 'cases' group if they had been admitted to hospital with symptoms and clinical signs of a heart attack and were within a 24 hours of symptom onset. Age- and sex-matched participants in the 'control' group had no history of heart disease or chest pain when engaging in physical activity. Results indicated that across all countries, men were more likely to have a heart attack nine years earlier than women; people living in the Middle East and South Asia tended to experience heart attacks at an earlier age (51 and 53 years, respectively) compared with those in China, Western Europe and Hong Kong (63 years).

Findings from the 2021 Global Burden of Disease (IHME, 2024) placed stroke as the second non-communicable worldwide cause of death. Most strokes are ischaemic in nature, with most occurring in HICs, but in LMICs, the unavailability of preventative, acute treatments and rehabilitation services means that stroke results in a higher disease burden and mortality.

Non-modifiable risk factors for CVD

The number of reported heart attacks escalated from 2.7 million in 2020 to 9.1 million in 2021 (WHO, 2024b), illustrating the extent of this global health issue. The main causes of CVD have been attributed to lifestyle behaviours, but there are also non-modifiable factors, such as a genetic predisposition to heart problems, which may be indicated by an immediate male relative who had a heart attack before the age of 55 or in the case of a female before the age of 65. Men who are over 50 years old are at greater risk of CVD than women. Ethnicity can be a risk factor for CVD, especially in people who are of South Asian and Sub-Saharan African descent (National Institute for Health and Care Excellence [NICE], 2025a). It should be noted that research into CVD often conflates sex and gender terminology, hence research presented here will switch between terminology as reflected in the research literature.

Modifiable risk factors for CVD

Many of the risk factors that are common to CVD include smoking, consuming an unhealthy diet, sedentary behaviour, hypertension, being overweight or obese, drinking too much alcohol, especially binge drinking, high fasting blood glucose levels, excess low-density lipoprotein (LDL) cholesterol and type 2 diabetes mellitus (T2DM). More recently, climate change (increased ambient temperature) and air pollution (Feigin et al., 2025) have been added to that list, while not directly within an individual's control, they are still considered to be collectively modifiable on a global scale.

The impacts of these factors on health can be measured and monitored; blood pressure and blood tests can be used to help calculate risk factors for CHD and stroke. Blood is examined for levels of **triglycerides** (a type of fat), the ability to metabolise glucose (sugar) and cholesterol levels. It is important to note that not all cholesterol is bad, two types of cholesterol are considered in CHD, low- and high-density lipoprotein (LDL and HDL). **LDL** is the 'bad' type of cholesterol, which is deposited on artery walls and leads to the development of atherosclerosis. **HDL** or 'good' cholesterol helps to transport blood cholesterol to the liver and is excreted. Another risk factor for CHD, hypertension, strokes, T2DM and cancer is being overweight or obese. Of those who have CHD around 80% are obese (BMI ≥ 30) or overweight (BMI ≥ 25 and ≤ 30) and obesity is an independent risk factor for CHD (Ades & Savage, 2017).

Smoking

The Framingham Heart Study (FHS), which started in 1948, is frequently cited as the first major longitudinal investigation into CVD. This helped identify the association between smoking, high cholesterol, hypertension and CHD (Dawber et al., 1957). The seminal study by Doll and Hill (1950) cautioned that smoking could reduce life expectancy and was detrimental to cardiovascular health; shortly after, the 1964 Surgeon General's Report highlighted that one-third of all CHD deaths were linked to smoking. Sixty years on, smoking is still a leading cause of preventable mortality in the US, contributing to the development of atherosclerosis, CHD, lung diseases and certain cancers (Office of the Surgeon General & Office on Smoking and Heath, 2024). The WHO (2021a) estimated that 20% of CHD deaths were directly related to smoking and that even second-hand smoke (breathing in exhaled smoke and smoke from the burning cigarette) also increased the risk of heart disease. Across the globe, various countries have put in place tobacco control and prevention polices, such as the introduction of higher taxes on tobacco, free interventions to help people quit smoking, the inclusion of health warnings on products containing tobacco, a ban on promoting or advertising tobacco and the introduction of smoking bans in public buildings. The aims of such measures are to educate people on the health risks of smoking and reduce smoking-related illnesses (WHO, 2021b), while they have helped drive reductions in smoking, people still smoke.

Physical activity

A lack of physical activity is a modifiable risk factor for CVD. Physical activity is different to exercise, the former is usually defined as any muscular bodily movement that uses energy, for example, walking, housework, using the stairs, working in the garden and it can be light or vigorous. Exercise is planned and structured, usually undertaken on a regular basis and includes running, football, weightlifting, swimming, etc., with the aim to improve physical fitness. Early research by Morris et al. (1953) showed a difference in the rate of CHD between bus drivers and bus conductors, which was attributed to physical activity and occupational stress. Drivers were mostly sedentary, subjected to the stress of negotiating traffic and had higher rates of CHD, whereas conductors had less stressful jobs, played more active roles, climbing stairs on double-decker buses and walked around the bus during their shifts to collect fares. Since these early findings, many thousands of research studies have highlighted the deleterious effects of sedentary behaviour across a range of diseases. Despite health organisations and governments emphasising the detrimental impacts of sedentary behaviour on health (WHO, 2021c), it remains a stubborn feature in many individuals' lives (Fletcher et al., 2018).

Having a mainly sedentary lifestyle can increase the risk of CVD by around 15% (Biswas et al., 2015). However, a more recent meta-analysis found that people who had high levels of sedentary behaviour (e.g. watching TV, sitting and working at a desk) were at a 30% greater risk of CVD compared to those who had some level of physically active lifestyles. For every hour spent sitting, the risk of CVD increased by around 5%; however, this can be negated if people take part in a similar duration of activities, such as standing and moving around the office or home (Onagbiye et al., 2024).

In the US, Patel et al. (2022) reported that some ethnic groups were less likely to be physically active than others. Using cross-sectional data from the National Health Interview Survey (2006–2015) and after adjusting for sociodemographic differences, Black, Asian and Hispanic adults were less likely to engage in adequate physical activity than White Americans. The Active Lives Adult Survey in England (Sport England, 2024) showed that around 25% of people in England were sedentary, with people of White British origin being more active (67%) compared to their Chinese (58%), Black (56%) and Asian (55%) counterparts. Many factors contribute to sedentary behaviour, a systematic review found time, lack of motivation, family responsibilities, cultural expectations, safety and socioeconomic status were barriers to taking part in physical activity (Batalha et al., 2025) for ethnic minority women across 12 different countries. Similar findings were identified for South Asian immigrants, with language being an added barrier to taking part in group activities (Maricar et al., 2024).

The WHO (2020) guidelines on physical activity for people living with disabilities advocate that any type and amount of physical activity is better than doing nothing. These guidelines emphasise the need for this population to become less sedentary but recognised that many barriers existed to stop people with disabilities from becoming more physically active (Bull et al., 2020). Physical activity is viewed as being safe for adults living with a disability but they may need to seek advice from healthcare professionals to ascertain what is the best type of physical activity and intensity that is suited to individual needs.

Diet and CVD

Dietary behaviours can help reduce or modify the risk of CVD by limiting alcohol intake, especially binge drinking, and making dietary changes that help in leading to weight reduction (WHO, 2020). Diets that are rich in vegetables, fruit, nuts, wholegrains, lean animal meat and fish, along with minimal intakes of processed foods, refined carbohydrates and sweetened drinks, are viewed as beneficial for heart health (Arnett et al., 2019). Even though people may want to follow a healthy diet, French et al. (2019) found that low-income households tend to have diets that are deficient in nutritional quality compared to higher income households. Low-income families tend to purchase more sugary drinks and frozen desserts compared to higher-income families and lower amounts of fresh fruit and vegetables. In Chapter 8, we found out that there was a link between daily hassles and food choices, people with higher levels of stress are more inclined to eat high sugar and fat snacks and decrease their intake of fruits and vegetables (O'Connor et al., 2008). This can result in increased LDL cholesterol, thereby promoting atherosclerosis and abdominal fat, all of which increase the risk of CVD.

Psychological correlates of CVD

In 2024, the average working life expected of a European adult was around 37 years (Eurostat, 2024). Work can often be a source of stress, especially for those in low status jobs and clerical work has been associated with a higher chance of early onset of atherosclerosis in women (Gallo et al., 2003). Jobs with **high demand and low control** or a mismatch between education level and job status (under- or overqualified) can cause psychological stress. Likewise, temporary employment or being on a **zero hours contract** can lead to stress due to financial insecurity. While these factors may not lead to heart problems in people at low risk for CVD, they can increase the likelihood of heart disease in those at high risk (Ogunmoroti et al., 2024). Over a 6-year period, Kamarck et al. (2012) assessed perceptions of **job control** and demands of daily life, such as feeling rushed and having to engage in multiple tasks and the development of atherosclerosis in the carotid arteries of healthy adults. They found that increased job demands were associated with increased atherosclerosis and blood pressure.

In the previous chapter, we explored the link between the Type A behaviour pattern (TABP) and the risk of CAD (Friedman & Rosenman, 1959). Subsequent research identified hostility, which is a persistent attitude, as the key aspect of the TABP most strongly associated with the development of heart disease (Siegman & Smith, 1994). Being reactive to stress, distrustful, suspicious, antagonistic and resentful of others and being overly angry or aggressive appears to be a central aspect of hostility. When placed under an experimental stressful situation of being harassed, people scoring high on hostility (assessed by the 50-item Cook-Medley Hostility Scale; [CMHS]; Cook & Medley (1954) showed greater increases in blood pressure and cortisol than people who were low on hostility (Suarez et al., 1998). However, this research was conducted with healthy participants and studies with patients found no significant association between hostility and deaths due to heart disease (Barefoot et al., 1989a). This led to a re-examination of the CMHS to remove items that did not measure hostility (Barefoot et al., 1989b) and the development of the Abbreviated Cook-Medley (ACM) scale. Higher scores on the ACM scale were predictive of daily reductions in blood supply to the heart, especially in women (Helmers et al., 1993).

People with a hostile attitude are more likely to experience episodes of anger. Further examination of the anger component of the TABP separated it into two aspects, 'anger-in' (suppressed anger) and 'anger-out' (expressed anger). The latter has been linked with greater cardiovascular reactivity, which may contribute to heart disease (Siegman & Snow, 1997). In people with a family history of CVD, the anger-in component has been linked with increased blood pressure (Vögele & Steptoe, 1993). However, in a more recent study (Shimbo et al., 2024), young adults were asked to recall experiences over an 8-minute period that were associated with feeling angry, sad, anxious or no emotion. The anger group showed reduced ability in blood vessel dilation, which is linked to increased blood pressure. This suggests that the acute affects of anger-in may increase the risks of having a heart attack. Given that people do tend to recall and ruminate about events that result in negative emotional experiences, Shimbo et al. (2024) suggested that repeated anger experiences may build up over time, contributing to the development of atherosclerosis. Teaching people to manage current anger and anger associated with past experiences may be useful for those who are at increased risk of heart disease. It should be noted that this study only included young adults who were healthy and had no risk factors or history of CVD.

Evidence linking TABP and CVD has been called into question, as depression (Gan et al., 2014), social isolation and loneliness can also contribute to the development and progression of this disease (Yang et al., 2025). In addition, unhealthy lifestyle factors, such as smoking, poor diet, sedentary behaviour, sleep problems and obesity, have a role to play in morbidity and mortality of CAD (Livingstone et al., 2021).

Social determinants of health

The US government formally recognised disease and mortality disparities between racial and ethnic groups in 1985 (Heckler, 1985) and has tried to assess why such inequities exist, despite this, the health divide in the US persists today. The non-medical risk factors that can have negative or positive implications for health include income, access to healthy foods, level of education, the neighbourhoods that people live in, their place of birth, housing, occupation, access to healthcare, social inclusion, historical oppression and discrimination. The WHO (n.d.-a) stressed the importance of these factors in determining health and disease outcomes by referring to them as social determinants of health (SDOH).

Poverty and educational level are significant predictors for CVD, irrespective of race or ethnicity (Sells et al., 2023). Having a lower level of education is linked with lower health literacy and an increased number of risk factors for CVD mortality (Mackenbach et al., 2000). People without a college level education tend to have higher rates of unemployment or work in lowly paid occupations and both factors are associated with living in poorer neighbourhoods, not being able to afford a healthy diet and healthcare. Within the US, Black, Asian, Hispanic and Indigenous groups tend to have lower incomes, receive lower pay for the same work and have a higher probability of being unemployed compared to their White non-Hispanic counterparts (Bureau of Labor Statistics, 2023). Evidence shows that those on low incomes have higher rates of CHD than those with higher incomes (Abdalla et al., 2020).

Compared with other groups, Black, Hispanic and urban dwelling Indigenous Peoples tend to live in poorer neighbourhoods that lack green spaces and safe areas to walk (Wen et al., 2013). These neighbourhoods have a higher incidence of violence (Sprung et al., 2019), which can contribute to prolonged stress and have detrimental consequences for health. Poorer neighbourhoods have limited transport links, which can be a structural barrier to accessing healthcare (Syed et al., 2013), contributing to delayed diagnosis, treatment, access to medication and ongoing healthcare.

Poorer neighbourhoods tend to have higher levels of air pollution, which has been associated with reduced life expectancy, increased mortality due to CHD (Lelieveld et al., 2020), hospitalisation, strokes and heart attacks (Al-Kindi et al., 2020; Rajagopalan & Landrigan, 2021). There is a positive association between chronic exposure to air pollution and the likelihood of developing atherosclerosis (Jacobs et al., 2011) and chronic obstructive pulmonary disease (COPD). Furthermore, air pollution particles PM2.5 (particles in the air that are inhaled deep into the lungs; they come from a variety of sources including vehicle emissions, wild fires and industrial pollutants) have been implicated in reducing the beneficial impact of HDL cholesterol in the body and increase **C-reactive protein** (Ossoli et al., 2023), which may lead to low-grade inflammation that plays a key role in the development of atherosclerosis and increased hypertension (Cai et al., 2016).

CVD in different populations

Sex/Gender and CVD

Traditionally, CHD was viewed as a 'man's disease' (Vogel et al., 2021), as the sex hormone oestrogen was thought to protect women from developing the disease. While women do have a lower prevalence of CHD during their reproductive years, once they reach the menopause (see Box 9.1), any cardiac advantage they had reduces (Maas et al., 2021). However, over their lifespan, women may experience premature or early menopause (before 40 years old), a diagnosis of hypertension and/or diabetes during pregnancy (gestational diabetes, which often goes away after the baby is born), which are risk factors for CHD. Post-menopause, women share the same CHD risks as men in terms of increasing blood pressure, cholesterol and triglycerides, but women may also experience increases in weight and accumulation of abdominal fat (Kamińska et al., 2023; Toth et al., 2000). Higher body mass index (BMI) is more common in women (Kroll et al., 2020), but it is unclear whether this is due to the general ageing process or it is specifically linked with the menopause. Chichlowska et al. (2008) found that a group of risk factors for CHD which includes difficulty metabolising sugar, high cholesterol, hypertension and central adiposity, referred to as **metabolic syndrome**, was more prevalent in women who had lower incomes, lower educational levels and in those living in disadvantaged neighbourhoods. This illustrates that factors other than physiology play a role in the risk of developing CHD and other chronic diseases.

BOX. 9.1
WHAT IS THE MENOPAUSE?

The menopause is a time that signals the end of a women's reproductive years. It is marked by complete cessation of menstrual periods due to reduction in the hormones oestrogen and progesterone, which regulate mensuration and fertility. This is a normal part of the ageing process, which occurs around the age of 45–55 years.

The British Heart Foundation (2025) reported that women in the UK have a CHD rate that is twice that of breast cancer. One in every three deaths in women in the US is caused by heart disease, compared to one in 39 deaths being due to breast cancer (American Heart Association, 2024), yet women take breast cancer much more seriously and fear it more than heart disease (Berry et al., 2016). It is becoming increasingly clear that women's CHD experiences, treatment and rehabilitation needs do not mirror those of men (Tayal et al., 2024). Due to societal perceptions that CHD is a 'man's disease', symptoms of CHD in women may be overlooked by healthcare professionals and by women themselves (Kunadian, 2024). This may, in part, be explained by the fact that most diagnostic, treatment and rehabilitative research has been conducted on men and results extrapolated to women (Tobb et al., 2022). CHD healthcare practices may still unintentionally discriminate against females, as the 'traditional' or 'well known' heart attack symptoms, such as chest pain, left arm pain and sweating reported by males, are not always the same for females. Symptoms reported by females (see Figure 9.2) tend to be more diffuse, they can include neck, jaw, upper back, abdominal, left hand, arm and/or shoulder pain, nausea and shortness of breath (Schulte & Mayrovitz, 2023). Healthcare professionals tend to attribute women's chest pain to non-cardiac causes, such as anxiety, stress, stomach and/or musculoskeletal problems (Sawan et al., 2023). Misdiagnosis may reduce women's chances of receiving early investigations and interventions (Vogel et al., 2021), resulting in longer hospital stays and poorer outcomes, including increased mortality (Khan et al., 2018; Sawan et al., 2023; Stehli et al., 2019). While women's awareness and knowledge about CHD have improved since the 1990s, Mosca et al. (2013) found they still have limited awareness of nontraditional heart attack symptoms, with knowledge gaps particularly pronounced in those from ethnic minority groups and younger people. Women have a 25% greater risk of developing CVD if they smoke (Huxley & Woodward, 2011) and a 44% greater risk if they have diabetes (Peters et al., 2014). Yet in

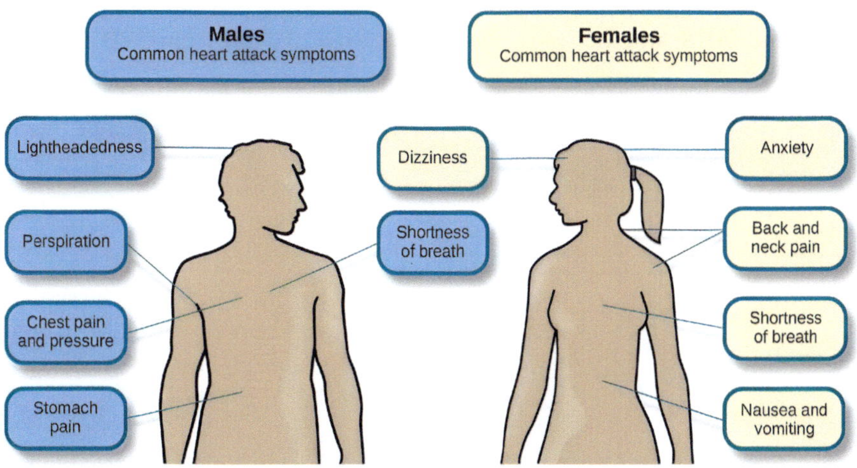

Figure 9.2
Symptoms of a heart attack in male and female patients

Source: Spielman et al. (2020)[1]

primary care settings, women continue to be underassessed for their cardiovascular risks in comparison to men (Hyun et al., 2017; Hyun et al., 2019). The underdiagnosis and treatment of women's cardiovascular symptoms have been recognised by British Cardiovascular Societies, which produced a consensus document specific to the diagnosis and treatment of CHD for women, in this they call for more emphasis on heart care for women (Tayal et al., 2024).

Other risk factors for CVD in women include lower SES, being subjected to intimate partner violence, having higher rates of depression, anxiety, poorer health literacy about CHD (Vogel et al., 2021) and increased stress associated with caregiving roles and responsibilities (Connelly et al., 2021). O'Neil et al. (2018) reported that even from a young age, gendered influences of sport and physical activity are encouraged more in teenage boys than girls (Kaestner & Xu, 2010; Lampinen et al., 2017; Lau et al., 2007); this can act as a social determinant for increased sedentary behaviour predisposing young girls and women to the development of CVD and obesity.

Similar to research into CHD, most studies on stroke have been conducted with men. While the incidence of stroke across the globe in 2021 was higher in men (52.5%) than women (47.4%; Feigin et al., 2025), women are more likely to have poorer stroke outcomes and higher mortality (Gasbarrino et al., 2022). The lifetime risk of stroke varies across and within countries and in the US, women have a 20% lifetime risk of stroke, which is 5% higher than men (Seshadri et al., 2006), with hypertension being the main contributing factor (Centers for Disease Control and Prevention, [CDC], 2020). In addition, women's risk of stroke may be increased by some contraceptive medications that make clot formation more likely and this can be exacerbated if the woman smokes (CDC, 2024a).

Ethnicity and CVD

Ethnicity classifications vary between countries, which makes it difficult to make direct comparisons across different studies or populations. In the US, the prevalence of heart disease is highest in non-Hispanic Black American men (see Table 9.1), who have hypertension rates that are among the highest in the world (Ferdinand, 2018) and they have over twice the risk of dying from CVD compared

Table 9.1 Percentage of deaths due to heart disease by race or ethnic group in the US, 2021

Race or ethnic group	Percentage of deaths
Black (non-Hispanic)	22.6
Asian	18.6
Native Hawaiian or Other Pacific Islander	18.3
White (non-Hispanic)	18.0
American Indian or Alaskan Native	15.5
Hispanic	11.9
All groups	17.4

Source: https://www.cdc.gov/heart-disease/data-research/facts-stats/index.html

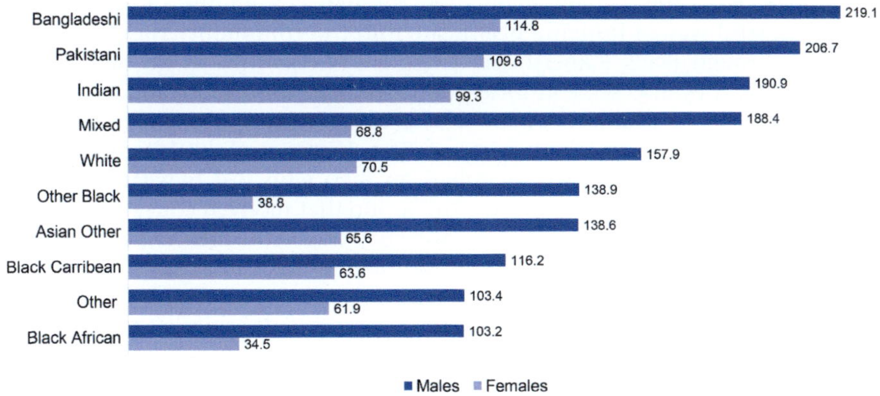

Figure 9.3
Deaths due to CHD by ethnicity in England and Wales (2017–2019), per 100 thousand

Source: ONS (2021) Mortality from leading causes of death

to White adults (CDC, 2024b). Data from England and Wales show that deaths due to CHD were higher among men from Bangladeshi, Pakistani and Indian origin (Office for National Statistics [ONS], 2023; see Figure 9.3), which may be linked to more sedentary behaviours, a tendency to store fat around the abdominal area, insulin resistance and a higher prevalence of T2DM compared to the national average (ONS, 2023). In contrast to US data, men from Black groups in the UK were less likely to die from CHD than White British men.

Ethnic minority groups within the US often face disparities in accessing healthcare, with cost being a major barrier for many (Fang et al., 2014). This contributes to lower access to CVD assessment for risk prevention, missed diagnoses and treatments, leading to worse long-term CVD outcomes (Hannan et al., 2016). For example, among people who self-reported having hypertension, 15% of White, 20% of Black and 27% of Hispanic adults did not have consistent access to care provided by a family doctor (Fang et al., 2014). In a study of over 1,100 hospitals across the US, White patients who lived in deprived areas were 24% more likely to receive coronary artery bypass surgery compared to their Black counterparts (Popescu et al., 2010). Furthermore, healthcare professionals have been found to exhibit **unconscious and conscious bias** towards patients from ethnic minorities. Breathett et al. (2019) reported that doctors tend to assume that Black patients will be less adherent to medication and treatment advice, which can lead to White patients being offered more advanced interventions for CHD. Doctors tend to behave in a more dominant manner towards those from African American descent, showing less empathy and patient-centred care compared to interactions with White patients (Johnson et al., 2004). To ensure that culturally sensitive care is provided to all, health professional training needs to address conscious and unconscious bias through education about systemic racism, cultural awareness and barriers to care that can create and perpetuate health disparities.

In America, attempts to reduce hypertension in non-Hispanic Black men have been hampered by a reluctance of this section of the population to engage in **pharmacological trials** in healthcare settings. This may be due to historical distrust, which is based upon unethical health experiments on African American people in the US (see Chapter 3). Researchers have tried to establish other ways to connect with this patient population through community outreach trials. One successful way of bringing healthcare into the community was established in 2006 through Black Barbershops. These are not just places for hair cutting and shaving, they also serve as focal points for men to socialise and are 'culturally safe' places to promote health and disease screening (Luque et al., 2014; Releford et al., 2010). In a barbershop setting, Victor et al. (2018) conducted a research study with Black African American men who had hypertension. The men were randomly allocated to a control group that received educational material on hypertension from barbers who also encouraged the men to make lifestyle changes to diet, physical activity and visit their doctor. The intervention group received the same educational material and advice from barbers, but in addition, they were encouraged to meet with specifically trained pharmacists in the barber shops who checked their blood pressure and if required changed their prescribed hypertensive medication. After six months, the group who received the intervention showed a significantly greater reduction in blood pressure (27.0 mmHg) compared to the control group (9.3 mmHg). This provided evidence that combining health promotion by barbers and medication management by pharmacists, as part of a community health outreach programme, was an effective way to help Black African American men reduce their blood pressure. This approach has been endorsed in a more recent study, as a cost-effective way of managing hypertension and reducing CVD in this population (Bryant et al., 2021). The Black Barbershop health programme is a more nuanced and culturally acceptable way of reaching Back African American men compared to traditional healthcare delivery and has been instrumental in helping to reduce health disparities by screening over 30,000 men across the US for hypertension and diabetes (Black Barbershop Health Outreach Program, 2020).

Statistics in the US show that there are ethnic disparities in the risk of having a stroke, with African Americans at the highest risk, but women seem to be more susceptible than men (Tsao et al., 2023). The main contributors to stroke in African American women included hypertension and being obese (CDC, 2023; National Center for Health Statistics; n.d.; Ostchega et al., 2020). Hispanic women are also at a greater risk of stroke than White women, which may be explained by the former having higher rates of T2DM (CDC, 2023), coupled with hypertension and obesity. In a national audit of adverse stroke outcomes within the United Kingdom (UK), Fluck et al. (2023) reported that men and women from ethnic minority groups tend to experience stroke around five years earlier than the White population and were two to four times more likely to have worse outcomes in terms of disability and mortality. The only major pre-stroke difference between the two groups was the prevalence of T2DM, which was two times higher in the ethnic minority group. Most patients in this audit were from South Asian ethnic groups, but no analysis was undertaken to compare stroke risk or outcomes between the various minority ethnic groups.

Indigenous Peoples and CVD

Indigenous Peoples of Canada have 1.5 times greater prevalence of CVD compared to their non-Indigenous White counterparts (US Department of Health and Human Services, 2021). This disparity has been attributed to Indigenous Peoples' tendency to live in rural areas that require long distance travel to obtain healthcare, socioeconomic factors, distrust of non-Indigenous healthcare providers/systems, lower educational levels and low health literacy about CVD (Anand et al., 2019). Similar to ethnic minority groups, Indigenous patients experience barriers to receiving equitable care compared to their non-Indigenous counterparts (Okwuosa et al., 2016). Previous negative experiences with healthcare services and professionals have created barriers for Indigenous People when seeking healthcare (Cameron et al., 2014) and this is compounded by the tendency for healthcare professionals to ignore the importance of Indigenous medicine and cultural practices (Horrill et al., 2018). Access to healthcare can also be hampered by problems recruiting and retaining healthcare staff in areas that Indigenous populations live. Indigenous representatives have highlighted the need for healthcare systems that are culturally sensitive to the populations that they serve. In addressing this need, Harrop et al. (2024) worked with an Indigenous health liaison officer to develop a culturally informed intervention for Aboriginal and Torres Islander patients in Australia who had acute CVD symptoms. In addition to standard care, the health liaison officer assisted with cultural support, education advocacy and care coordination. This helped patients and families to navigate the healthcare system from admission to discharge and community care. The authors reported that unplanned hospital readmissions, deaths, acute heart attacks and unplanned **invasive cardiac procedures** to **revascularise** the heart were lower for Indigenous patients who received culturally informed care compared to a retrospective cohort of Indigenous patients who received standard care.

Similar to people from other minority ethnic groups, Indigenous populations have multiple risk factors for stroke. Within Australia, not only do Aboriginal and Torres Strait Islander Peoples have twice the incidence of stroke compared to non-Indigenous Australians (Balabanski et al., 2024), they also tend to experience strokes 10–15 years earlier than the non-Indigenous population (Balabanski et al., 2018; Santos et al., 2022; Tiedeman et al., 2019). A similar finding has been reported in the US, with strokes occurring at a younger age within American Indian and Alaskan Native populations compared to White or Black Americans (Harris et al., 2015). It is thought that such health disparities may be linked to factors such as intergeneration impacts of colonisation, social determinants of health and negative healthcare bias towards Indigenous Peoples (Churchwell et al., 2020). In a narrative review that examined stroke treatments across the world, Santos et al. (2021) reported that within Australia, Canada and the US, Indigenous People who had experienced an acute stroke were less likely to receive thrombolysis or endovascular thrombectomy (removal of a blood clot from a blood vessel) compared to the non-Indigenous population.

LGBTQI+ individuals and CVD

Studies have shown that LGBTQI+ (lesbian, gay and bisexual, with the use of plus to indicate other gender and sexual identities not already listed) populations share some of the same risk factors for CHD as their cisgender counterparts. This includes smoking, excessive alcohol consumption, sedentary behaviour and unhealthy diet, resulting in the development of hypertension and atherosclerosis (Caceres et al., 2019). Rates of CVD are higher in LGBTQI+ groups compared to the cisgender and heterosexual population, with transgender men having double the risk of having a heart attack compared to cisgender men and nearly five times more likely than cisgender women (Alzahrani et al., 2019). Many LGBTQI+ adults experience sexual and gender minority discrimination, along with internalised and external stigma, which leads to activation of the sympathetic nervous system

(SAM) and hypothalamic-pituitary-adrenal-axis (HPA). This can generate low-grade inflammation that is detrimental to heart health (Sherman et al., 2022). LGBTQI+ populations experience multiple types of stress across the lifespan, for example, 12–18-year-olds were more likely to experience stress relating to bullying, engagement in risky sexual behaviours and many have been forced to leave home (Robinson et al., 2013) compared to their heterosexual peers. LGBTQI+ adults over the age of 50 are more likely to have experienced lifetime discrimination and avoided healthcare interactions or concealed their identities due to concerns about discrimination from healthcare professionals. The additional stress that people from LGBTQI+ groups experience may be an important driver of increased morbidity (Caceres et al., 2020). Individuals who are in a constant state of alertness, who are anxious or who constantly monitor their surroundings for potential threats are more likely to experience health detrimental impacts associated with the impact of prolonged stress. LGBTQI+ individuals may experience additional stress because of internalised expectations of rejection and concealing their identity from family members, co-workers and healthcare professionals (Meyer, 2003). It is of concern that around one-third of sexual and gender minority adults have experienced unfair and/or disrespectful treatment from healthcare professionals (Montero et al., 2024). At best this may be due to unconscious bias, which is symptomatic of minimal or no training in relation to healthcare needs of LGBTQI+ populations (Caceres et al., 2020).

In attempting to review the literature on cardiovascular events, including stroke in LGBTQI+ populations, Naik et al. (2020) reported that gender reaffirming oestrogen therapy may be involved in clot formation leading to stroke and heart attacks in transgender women. For transgender men, higher cholesterol levels associated with testosterone therapy may expose them to higher cardiovascular risks. Despite these risks being well known, 79% of healthcare professionals did not consider minority gender status as a factor when assessing cardiovascular risk in LGBTQI+ individuals. However, this may also have been affected by LGBTQI+ patients being reticent to share their gender orientation with healthcare professionals. Diaz and Rosendale (2023) examined hospital records to determine if there were any differences or commonalities in CVD risk factors and outcomes between sexual and gender minority (SGM) and non-SGM patients. SMG patients had additional risk factors for stroke, which included HIV status (human immunodeficiency virus), syphilis and **hepatitis C** (a blood-borne liver infection that can cause serious liver damage). Patients from SGM groups tended to experience stroke at an early age and have higher stroke recurrence.

Disabilities and CVD

People with learning disabilities are at higher risk of CVD, which has been attributed to having a higher prevalence of hypertension (Wyszyńska et al., 2020), higher cholesterol levels, a higher likelihood of being obese and having diabetes (Lin et al., 2010). This may be compounded by less-than-optimal access to healthcare (Engen et al., 2019), which is concerning, as a cohort study found that people with learning disabilities had a 24% higher likelihood of developing CVD and at a younger age compared to the general population (Wang et al., 2023). In addition to health inequities, Mitra et al. (2022) highlighted that the healthcare needs of people with learning disabilities are not well understood and they attract less health research interest compared to the general population. Having a physical disability may place people at greater risk of developing obesity, high cholesterol and diabetes (Wu et al., 2021, 2023), which are risk factors for developing CVD. It is thought that mobility limitations imposed by physical disabilities may contribute to CVD, as people who sit more may have a higher likelihood of developing hypertension (Dempsey et al., 2018) and that the risk may be greater for women (Wu et al., 2024). In a four-year longitudinal cohort study, Adebisi et al. (2025) compared blood pressures of people with and without physical disabilities, they found significantly greater rates of hypertension in people who had physical disabilities. The authors concluded that disability status needs to be considered as a future predictor of cardiovascular risk.

Stroke can cause a range of disabilities that can have minor and major impacts on quality of life. The treatment and rehabilitation of stroke have attracted quite a lot of research, but few studies have investigated the potential link between pre-existing physical disabilities and stroke risk. Yang et al. (2023) examined a database of health information in South Korea and found that the incidence of stroke was higher in people with disabilities, especially in those with severe disabilities related to heart and kidney disease and in people who had communication difficulties. On average, people with disabilities experienced stroke around 20 years earlier than those without disabilities. In addition, people with disabilities and **dementia** often experience disproportionate delays in diagnosis and access to treatment compared to those without a disability (Denny et al., 2024; Ganesh et al., 2022).

Understanding the risk factors for CVD has facilitated health promotion initiatives, along with medical interventions to reduce disease progression and mortality rates, despite this CVD persists as the leading global cause of mortality (Gibbons et al., 2021). Discrimination and socioeconomic disadvantage contribute to health inequities and heighten the risk of CVD in minoritised groups, but evidence is emerging that other factors, such as environmental pollution (air, soil, water and chemicals) and social isolation, are implicated (Bhatnagar, 2017; Cosselman et al., 2015). Climate change in the form of more frequent and prolonged heat waves has been linked with CHD mortality (Münzel et al., 2023), which can be exacerbated by air pollution (Xu et al., 2023). Excessive rainfall can cause leeching of soil pesticides, microplastics and heavy metals into drinking water, with the latter being strongly associated with unfavourable cardiac outcomes (Münzel et al., 2022). It is not possible to take a purely global approach to try and reduce deaths due to CVDs, as there are variations in risk factors and lifestyles across countries and economic regions. However, there are some notable polices that can be implemented to help reduce CVD, which include tobacco control to try and prevent and curb smoking behaviours, dietary and physical activity interventions, stress management, the use of drugs to try and reduce the most common causes of CVD, such as hypertension and high LDL, and sufficient funding for healthcare to help improve cardiovascular health. Coupled with these factors is the need to enhance data collection on CVDs in LMICs, so that country-specific risks can be identified, targeted and monitored to reduce global health inequities to reduce morbidity and mortality from CVDs.

Cancer

Across the globe in 2022, the WHO (n.d.-b) reported that cancer was the second leading cause of disease and estimated that one in six people died from cancer. The top three cancers diagnosed in men are lung, prostate and colorectal; in women, breast cancer was the most common, followed by lung and colorectal. Certain cancers have a genetic element, which increases the cancer risk, but lifestyle factors also have a role to play. Approximately 30–50% of cancer deaths could be prevented if more people engaged in health preventative measures, such as attending cancer screening, eating a diet rich in fruit and vegetables, engaging in more physical activity, not smoking, reducing alcohol consumption, avoiding weight gain, practising safe sex, getting vaccinated against the **human papillomavirus** (HPV), using sun screen and avoidance of air pollution. Research indicates that people are not very good at estimating the risk to health associated with lifestyle behaviours, such as smoking, excessive sun exposure and unhealthy diets. The main reason for this is the perceived indirect link between these behaviours and cancer, as disease may not become apparent for 30, 40 or even 50 years. In addition, not everyone who engages in these behaviours goes on to develop cancer, such individual differences can help influence behaviour and that is why cancer education is so important.

Cancer prevention

There are three main approaches to cancer prevention, which are primary, secondary and tertiary in nature. In primary prevention, the focus is on stopping cancer from occurring in the first place by trying to minimise the chance of a person being exposed to anything that is known to cause or contribute to the development of cancer. This can involve the promotion of vaccinations, such as HPV, to reduce the chance of developing cervical cancer and vaccination against hepatitis, which can lead to liver cancer. Education is a central part of primary prevention in relation to the dangers of smoking, getting sunburnt, eating a healthy diet and avoiding processed meats and engaging in safe sex. The UK has three free national cancer screening programmes; they target breast, cervical and colorectal cancers. Cancer screening is a secondary cancer prevention strategy to detect disease at an asymptomatic or very early stage. This stage also includes public health messaging about being aware of the early symptoms of certain cancers, such as blood in poo or pee, finding unexplained lumps, looking out for new skin moles or changes to existing moles. Tertiary prevention is concerned with preventing further development of disease and suffering in those who already have a cancer diagnosis. This can involve rehabilitation strategies to help people live better with and beyond cancer by helping them with symptom management and trying to stop cancer from spreading. For people who are in cancer remission (when cancer symptoms have gone and scans or tests show that the individual is currently free from disease, but it does not mean that the cancer is cured), tertiary prevention also includes surveillance to detect cancer recurrence.

Cancer in different populations

Ethnicity and cancer

The incidence of cancer varies across ethnic groups (Vaccarella et al., 2019), but veracity of data can be hampered by limitations in accurate recording of ethnicity or the absence of such data. Within the UK, the incidence of cancer is higher in the White British population, especially for malignant melanoma, lung, oesophageal and bladder cancers. These differences are thought to be due to higher rates of smoking and exposure to ultraviolet radiation from the sun and sunbeds compared to other ethnicities. Certain ethnic groups have a genetic predisposition to developing certain cancers, for example in England, the incidence of prostate cancer in Black men is twice that of their White counterparts and myeloma (blood cancer) three times as high (Delon et al., 2022). Differences in other cancers may be influenced by access to and uptake of cancer screening invitations. Barriers to screening can include language, culture and/or religious factors (Campbell et al., 2020), which can lead to cancers being diagnosed at a later stage, contributing to poorer health outcomes.

Within the UK, people who have a cervix and aged between 25 and 49 years are invited for **cervical screening** on a 3-year basis and those between 50 and 64 years are invited every five years. The uptake of cervical screening in England (2023–2024) was 68.8%, down slightly from the previous year (National Health Service [NHS]; 2024). There are a range of barriers that impact screening for cervical cancer; these include embarrassment, discomfort, memories of pain from previous experiences, the experiences of others, not wanting to know if cancer is present and not being aware of the need for or importance of screening. In addition, the location or timing of screening appointments may be inconvenient due to other commitments, such as work, looking after children and/or caring responsibilities.

In 2021, the Office for Health Improvement and Disparities (OHID) reported a differential of 11% between screening uptake in women aged 25–49 years living in areas of high deprivation (64.5%) compared to people living in wealthier areas (75.7%). Precise statistics relating to the uptake of cancer screening across different ethnic groups in the UK is scant, mainly due to ethnicity not being routinely or accurately recorded. Proxy measures of ethnicity have been used, such as area-based statistics on ethnicity (von Wagner et al., 2011) or by using software to match family names to religious and linguistic groupings. Screening rates for cervical cancer are lower for women who come from ethnic minority backgrounds and who have lower levels of education (Public Health England, 2017). Abdullahi et al. (2009) found that women from Somalia who were living in London (UK) lacked knowledge about cervical screening, had fears about testing, which were based on a lack of knowledge and prior negative experiences that included language difficulties. A subsequent study by Marlow et al. (2015) revealed that ethnic minority and White British women living in London also had unmet educational needs about cervical cancer and found the terminology of cervical screening and smear tests confusing. Cadman et al. (2015) explained that while most Hindu women in their study knew that the role of cervical screening was to detect abnormal cells, many of them perceived screening as only being for women who were having sexual intercourse outside of marriage, thus attending screening and receiving a diagnosis of cervical cancer would result in shame. Consistent with previous findings, a previously negative experience of screening was a barrier to subsequent attendance. Additionally, some women did not see the need for cervical screening, unless they had symptoms (Marlow et al., 2015), highlighting misconceptions surrounding the rationale for cancer screening, which is to detect the disease prior to symptoms occurring.

Within London, Renshaw et al. (2010) found attendance for **breast screening** was lower for Black and Asian women compared to their White counterparts; however, this study also used geographical location as a proxy measure of ethnicity. A study in Scotland was able to link **secondary data** on ethnicity and religion that had been self-reported in the 2001 Census in Scotland with data on breast screening. This provided evidence that women from minority ethnic groups had a lower uptake of breast screening than their White counterparts (Bansal et al., 2012). More specifically, the lowest uptake of screening was found in Pakistani women, followed by those from Bangladeshi descent. These findings were independent of deprivation, living in urban or rural areas, educational level or having a long-term illness. However, due to the use of secondary data, it was not possible to assess the impact of factors, such as knowledge or awareness of screening, perceived risk of breast cancer, language or cultural barriers in ethnic minority women. A subsequent study in London (Jack et al., 2014) explored more fine-grained categories of self-identified ethnicity. It found the highest uptake for first attendance for breast screening was in Mixed White and Asian women (75%), followed by those of White British (67%), Black Caribbean (63%), Indian (61%), Pakistani (52%) and Bangladeshi (43%) descent.

Campbell et al. (2020) used 2001 census data, linked to secondary data from the National Health Service in Scotland, the Scottish **Bowel Cancer Screening** Programme and the Scottish Cancer Registry database, to assess bowel cancer screening uptake across ethnic groups. Men from Indian, Pakistani and Bangladeshi backgrounds were more likely to decline screening compared to men from Chinese or White groups, with similar findings for women. In terms of religion, people who identified as Hindu, Muslim or Sikh were less likely to take up screening invitations when compared to people who self-identified as being from the Church of Scotland, Catholic or Jewish faith groups. These data are descriptive in nature, as such they do not provide any explanation for the differential findings in screening uptake. However, previous research indicates that barriers, such as lack of information, culture, type of screening and fear of finding cancer, may affect screening uptake. Some evidence points to the need for more tailored education for ethnic minority groups and for those living in areas of deprivation (Robb et al., 2009).

People with disabilities and cancer

A retrospective analysis of linked data from the Scottish Cancer Registry, the census and death certificates revealed that people with learning disabilities were more likely to die from cancer and at a younger age compared with the general population (Ward et al., 2024). In England, people with learning disabilities are 45% less likely to attend screening for cervical cancer (NHS Digital, 2016), 18% less likely to engage in bowel screening and 15% less likely to attend for breast screening (NHS Digital, 2022). However, within the UK, there are slight regional variations, women from Scotland with learning disabilities were also less likely than women with no learning disabilities to take part in screening for cervical (46%), breast (24%) and bowel (22%) cancers (McCowan et al., 2019). The exact reasons for the lower uptake of cervical screening in this population are not clear but may be dependent on how family members and/or carers view screening in relation to their own health beliefs and behaviours.

People with learning disabilities tend to have poorer outcomes from breast, lung and colon cancers. In a retrospective analysis, using UK-linked secondary data records, Heslop et al. (2022) found that almost half of cancers in people with learning disabilities were diagnosed at a late stage and 43% who had colon cancer died prior to reaching the age for screening. This suggests that earlier and tailored screening (Caton et al., 2012) may be required for this population, along with prompt onward referral. Similar to the general population, people with learning disabilities share risk factors for cancers, such as obesity and smoking. However, many people with learning disabilities often face communication problems in relation to cancer screening, treatment and care. While there are individual differences in ability to understand health information, healthcare professionals often make assumptions about a patient's **capacity**, only communicating with family members or the support worker, rather than conveying information directly to the patient. Having to depend on support workers or family members may result in information being 'filtered' to protect the individual from a diagnosis of cancer, explanation of possible treatments, side effects and prognosis. Support workers may lack confidence, understanding or the skills to have emotionally sensitive conversations about cancer with someone who has a learning disability (Witham & Haigh, 2018), which may culminate in unmet informational needs (Tuffrey-Wijne & Davies, 2007). Families may try to shield the patient from any information about cancer that has the potential to cause distress (Flynn et al., 2015); hence, people with learning disabilities may not be empowered with sufficient information to make decisions about their own treatment (Tuffrey-Wijne et al., 2009).

For people with physical disabilities accessing cancer screening services and attending for treatment may be a challenge due to mobility problems and transport. Wheelchair users may require healthcare staff to assist with accessibility needs, such as transferring from a wheelchair to an examination couch (Kett et al., 2020; Ross et al., 2019). Furthermore, people who are deaf may require professional sign language interpreters, who may not always be available. Research shows that health professionals do not always have sufficient information about the specific disability needs of patients, which can result in care and communication that is perceived by the patient as being uncaring and dehumanising (Peters & Cotton, 2016).

LGBTQI+ individuals and cancer

There is a scarcity of statistics on the incidence rates of cancer in people from LGBTQI+ groups, but they do smoke and consume more alcohol than their cisgender and heterosexual counterparts, which predisposes them to higher risks of developing some cancers (Daniel et al., 2015). However, data on the uptake of cancer screening by LGBTQI+ individuals are limited, as providers do not routinely collect data on sexual orientation and gender identity; in addition, patients may not self-identify due to previous negative experiences and fear of discrimination/stigma. Johnson et al. (2016) reported that transgender men, lesbian, bisexual and queer women are less like to engage in cervical cancer screening due to lack of knowledge about screening guidelines, low health literacy on the benefits of screening, low perceived susceptibility to this type of cancer, previous discriminatory experiences and a perceived lack of health professional cultural competence and sensitivity.

In order to provide patient-centred care, it is important than healthcare professionals have access to information and training to meet the needs of sexual and gender minority patients. Assumptions on the part of healthcare professionals regarding the sexual orientation and/or gender identity of patients may lead to negative experiences for patients attending for breast (Agénor et al., 2015) and **prostate cancer screening** (Hoyt et al., 2020) and any subsequent treatments (Kamen et al., 2019). When multiple marginalised identities intersect, care may be less than optimal for people who are Black and lesbian, compared to White, cisgender women (Poteat et al., 2021). Shires et al. (2025) found that Black sexual minority women of low socioeconomic status felt that they were provided with less information and their care was of lower quality than their White counterparts. Due to internalised racism and fear of stigma, gay and bisexual men in the US felt the need to conceal their sexual identities when undergoing screening for anal cancer (Acree et al., 2020). Research into cancer screening invitations, uptake, treatments and living beyond cancer is somewhat limited in transgender populations (Estupiñán Fdez de Mesa et al., 2025).

Indigenous Peoples and cancer

Global evidence indicates that Indigenous Peoples are at higher risk of developing cancer; they tend to be diagnosed at a later stage of disease, experience more treatment barriers and have poorer outcomes than non-Indigenous populations (Go et al., 2025). Reasons for these differentials include traditional cancer risk factors, such as smoking, unhealthy diets, sedentary behaviour, higher rates of obesity and high alcohol consumption, which intersect with social determinants of health (poverty, low health literacy, poor housing, rural location) and are compounded by the enduring impacts of colonisation.

Statistics on the uptake of cancer screening for Indigenous populations, even within high-income countries, remain incomplete (Moore et al., 2015). For example, Jemal et al. (2025) reported that breast cancer screening rates were lower for Indigenous populations compared to non-Indigenous populations by 8% in Canada, 9% in New Zealand, 13% in Australia and 15% in the US. However, survey years varied between countries, with some being as recent as 2024 and others based on data collected between 2007 and 2011. Screening rates can change over time due to public health campaigns, shifts in health policy due to governmental administrative changes and specific interventions targeting marginalised groups; hence, the data reported may not reflect current disparities.

For cervical screening, the gap between Indigenous People was only 1% lower than the general population within Canada, compared with much larger disparities in Australia (25%), New Zealand (9%) and the US (15%). However, the Canadian data were collected between 2007 and 2011 and appear to represent the most recent available dataset, as reported in the Burden of Cancer in Indigenous Peoples, as part of The Cancer Atlas for 2025 (Jemal et al., 2025). The lack of up-to-date data limits understanding of current trends, which are used to initiate and inform health promotion campaigns and programmes.

The presentation of older data may help perpetuate inequalities in cancer detection, treatment and outcomes. The Cancer Atlas (Jemal et al., 2025), drawing on 2007–2011 data for Canada, reported that colorectal screening rates were 12% higher among Indigenous Peoples, compared to the general population. This might suggest that screening invitations and uptake are working well within Indigenous populations and that targeted interventions are primarily needed for the rest of the population. However, recent data from the province of Alberta (Klassen et al., 2025) indicate that colorectal screening rates are, on average, 16% lower for Indigenous groups, similar to those in New Zealand (13%) and the US (14%), with a lower discrepancy in Australia (7%; Jemal et al., 2025). There is no country-wide integrated cancer care strategy for Indigenous People in Canada, care is fragmented and organised at federal, provincial and local levels, often with little consideration of the views and needs of Indigenous communities (Beckett et al., 2021). However, some progress has been made in cancer care for these communities, for example in the province of British Colombia (BC) culturally safe cancer care is being shaped through collaborative working with BC Cancer and the Metis Nation, led by the First Nations Health Authority, which has increased screening uptake (First Nations Health Authority, Métis Nation British Columbia, BC Association of Aboriginal Friendship Centres, & BC Cancer, 2017). In addition, Australia and New Zealand are trying to improve cancer care and screening for Indigenous populations through collaborative working and tailoring services for community needs (Seneviratne et al., 2015; Zorbas & Elston, 2016).

Chronic obstructive pulmonary disease

In 2021, chronic obstructive pulmonary disease (COPD) accounted for around 5% of all deaths across the world and it was ranked as the fourth most common cause of death. Most COPD deaths (70%) that occur in high- income countries are linked to tobacco smoking, but nearly all global deaths from COPD (90%) happen in low- and middle-income countries (WHO, 2024d). In Chapter 4, we found out that symptoms of COPD include difficulty breathing, shortness of breath and increased production of mucus. These symptoms can lead to fatigue, limit daily activities and have negative consequences for quality of life. Nine out of 10 cases of COPD are attributable to smoking (NHS, 2023), but people who have never smoked can develop COPD, because of passive smoking, exposure to chemicals and environmental pollutants.

The prevalence of COPD

Within the US in 2022, the prevalence of COPD in adults was 4.6%; White people had the highest self-reported prevalence (5.6%), followed by Black (4.1%) and Hispanic (2.3%) groups. Women had a higher prevalence (5%) compared to men (4.1%) and people over the age of 65 years had a prevalence of 9.7% (American Lung Association, n.d.). There are no statistics available on the prevalence of COPD that enable a direct comparison between Indigenous and non-Indigenous populations on a global basis. The prevalence of COPD within Indigenous Australians is 3% higher compared to the non-Indigenous population (Australian Institute of Health and Welfare, 2025). Various statistics are reported across Canada, with no overall country-wide statistics, but within the province of Alberta, COPD is between 1.5 and 2.4 times higher within the Indigenous population (Ospina et al., 2015). Statistics from New Zealand estimate that the prevalence of COPD in Māori people aged between 65 and 74 years is 7.7% higher than their non-Indigenous counterparts (Health Quality & Safety Commission, 2025). Within the US, the prevalence of COPD in American Indian/Alaskan Natives is around 4% higher than that of the non-Hispanic White population (Ford et al., 2013).

Smoking

People with COPD often experience stigma, blame and shame, as the condition is often perceived by others to be due to smoking; hence, COPD is considered as being self-inflicted (Jerpseth et al., 2021). The views of others may become internalised, with embarrassment and shame acting as a barrier to help-seeking from healthcare professionals (Harrison et al., 2015). The prevalence of COPD is 1.5 times higher and in some studies 3 times higher in people of low socioeconomic status. In addition, people on low incomes or who have low educational attainment tend to experience poorer COPD-related quality of life, access to specialist treatment and health outcomes (Pleasants et al., 2016).

Ethnicity and smoking

Within the US, the percentage of people who smoke varies across racial and ethnic groups. The Office of Disease Prevention and Health Promotion statistics (2021) show that smoking is higher for Indigenous Peoples (25.7%), followed by Black African Americans (14.6%), Whites (13.7%), Hispanics (8.1%), with Asians having the lowest level (8%). Higher smoking within Indigenous communities is not confined to the US. Smoking rates are twice as high among Australian Aboriginal and Torres Islanders and around 2.5 times higher for Indigenous populations in Canada and the Māori of New Zealand compared to their respective non-Indigenous populations (Romo-Stuppy & Maddox, 2023). The use of tobacco by Indigenous Peoples has a long history, which prior to colonisation was based on traditional ceremonial practices and offerings. However, colonial settlers introduced Indigenous Peoples to commercial tobacco and within the US, Canada and Australia, cigarette smoking is the main contributor to disease and premature death for these populations (CDC, 2025; Public Health Agency of Canada, 2018; Thurber et al., 2021).

LGBTQI+ individuals and smoking

People from LBGTQI+ communities are often subjected to minority stress from direct and indirect discrimination and internalised prejudice that can have negative consequences on self-esteem and self-worth; these effects may contribute to minority stress and increased smoking prevalence. McElroy et al. (2011) conducted one of the earliest studies that explored gender identity and smoking, which showed that transgender and gender-queer individuals had almost twice the prevalence of smoking (43%) compared to the cisgender population (27%). This finding has been confirmed by Buchting et al. (2017) and Vogel et al. (2019), with Buchting et al. (2017) adding that transgender females tend to smoke less than transgender males. In Australia, smoking prevalence is 40% higher in men who have sex with men compared to lesbian and/or bisexual women (Berger & Mooney-Somers, 2017). Praeger et al. (2019) found some slight differences in the smoking prevalence rates between bisexual women (26.4%), lesbians (23.7%) and heterosexual women (23.7%). While there have been some reductions in the smoking within gay and lesbian populations in the UK, it remains higher than that of the heterosexual population (Jackson et al., 2021). In line with previous findings, a cross-sectional survey conducted in England with LGB (lesbian, gay and bisexual) groups found that smoking prevalence was twice as likely in bisexual participants compared to heterosexual men and women. However, when age, socioeconomic factors (being single, from a low socioeconomic (SES), having a disability, no post-16 education and living in the North of England) were statistically controlled for, differences in smoking between LGB and heterosexual participants were no longer evident (Shahab et al., 2017).

Stopping smoking

Stopping smoking is beneficial to health, as it helps to lower the likelihood of developing CVD, COPD, lung cancer and premature death (NICE, 2025b). For people who have COPD, stopping smoking can help slow down disease progression (Anthonisen et al., 2002). There are a range of nicotine replacement products available to reduce withdrawal symptoms associated with stopping smoking, which include nicotine gum, patches, lozenges and electronic cigarettes (vapes); most of them are designed to deliver a metered dose of nicotine. These are seen as being viable ways of harm reduction from tar and other noxious chemicals within traditional cigarettes, but the safety of vapes is coming under greater scrutiny. Individual counselling and/or support groups may also be used as an adjunct to nicotine replacement therapy (NRT), psychological interventions based on cognitive behaviour therapy (CBT) (Kumar et al., 2025) or motivational interviewing (Soria et al., 2006). CBT can help identify and change people's thoughts and beliefs about smoking, identify environmental/contextual triggers for smoking and implement strategies to combat the urge to smoke. Goal setting may be used to help incentivise people to stop smoking and assist behaviour change through rewards. The specific methods used to stop smoking should be guided by the facilitator who is delivering the service and the individual's preference. Strategies for stopping smoking have varying rates of success, but higher success rates are usually found when two or more methods are combined (e.g. nicotine gum and behaviour change), compared to a single method (Stead et al., 2016). Low socioeconomic status, living in deprived neighbourhoods, poor social support and limited mechanisms for coping can have negative consequences for being able to stop smoking (Businelle et al., 2010). In addition, smoking cessation may contribute to stress, through concerns about weight gain, fear of failure, side effects of and becoming addicted to NRT.

To be successful, stop-smoking interventions may need to be gender specific. Dieleman et al. (2021) found key factors that hindered women from quitting smoking were internal, such as stress and emotional problems, which women felt could be helped by emotionally supportive counselling. For men, external factors were more important, such as the context and environment they were in and they preferred behaviour change techniques that focused on goal setting and incentivisation. People from LGBTQI+ communities may have fewer opportunities to avail of smoking cessation programmes, as fear of discrimination can reduce the likelihood of accessing healthcare services. Even though healthcare professionals routinely ask patients about smoking behaviours, they are less likely to follow this up with LGBTQI+ patients by providing information (Matthews et al., 2017). Stop-smoking interventions need to be informed by an understanding of the determinants of the behaviour (see Chapter 7), for example, Schwappach (2009) reported that gay men saw smoking as being a part what they called the 'gay scene'. It was a way of bonding with other gay men in bars, clubs, at events such as Gay Pride and social groups, whereas smoking cessation was viewed as being akin to leaving the 'gay scene' and becoming an 'outsider'. Smoking cessation interventions that tend to take a 'one size fits all' approach often ignore the minority stress experiences of marginalised groups that contribute to smoking behaviours (Li et al., 2024).

Inviting Indigenous patients to take part in smoking cessation programmes that are mainly designed for Western Eurocentric populations may hinder success, as relevance of information and methods of delivery may lack cultural sensitivity. A systematic review examined 73 studies of interventions to reduce the use of commercial tobacco by Indigenous populations; it found that education about the health harms of tobacco had a positive impact in reducing rates of smoking initiation, but no reduction in consumption was observed among smokers. Interventions were more likely to be successful if they were led by members of Indigenous communities in conjunction with non-Indigenous healthcare workers, offered as part of conventional healthcare provision, with culturally appropriate delivery that was guided by local Elders (Minichiello et al., 2016).

Predesigned 'universal' smoking cessation programmes that are implemented without sufficient attention to cultural awareness are likely to be ineffective. The design and content of interventions must consider the cultural needs of the target group and be delivered with cultural sensitivity (Lukowski et al., 2017). Moreover, it is important to disaggregate gender identity and sexual orientation, as the drivers of smoking can vary across identities and certain groups may require more tailored support to aid cessation. Sociodemographic factors may also intersect with gender identity, sexual orientation and belonging to a minoritised ethnic and/or Indigenous group, suggesting that intersectionality needs to be considered in both content and delivery of interventions.

Obesity

Obesity is now considered to be a chronic disease that is typified by excess deposits of bodily fat that have negative consequences for health. Across the world in 1990 approximately 7% of people over the age of 18 were categorised as obese, but by 2022, this had more than doubled to 16% (WHO, 2025b). In the past, men generally had a lower prevalence of obesity than women, but data from the WHO (2025b) indicate that this gap has closed with just as many men being diagnosed as obese. Even in low-income countries, the prevalence of obesity is showing an upward trend, especially in the wealthy highly educated population compared to high-income countries, where obesity is more common in low socioeconomic groups (Dinsa et al., 2012).

Ethnicity, body mass index, waist-to-hip ratio and ethnocentric norms

Currently, within the UK, a BMI of 30 kg/m^2 (see Chapter 4) is the point where the National Health Service (NHS) recommends that people should receive an intervention to prevent T2DM; however, this BMI cutoff point is for White Eurocentric populations. Evidence shows that people of Chinese, Japanese, Korean and Indian descent tend to have higher amounts of body fat at lower BMIs and this body fat tends to accumulate around the abdomen (Deurenberg 2002). In investigating this further, Caleyachetty et al. (2021) used data from over 1 million electronic healthcare records of patients in England to examine the links between BMI levels, risk of T2DM and ethnicity. They found that people from South Asian descent were at risk of developing T2DM at a much lower BMI (23.9 kg/m^2) compared to their White counterparts (30 kg/m^2), likewise for Black (28 kg/m^2), Chinese (26.9 kg/m^2) and Arab (26.6 kg/m^2) groups. From this, Caleyachetty et al. recommended the implementation of lower BMI cutoff rates when initiating interventions to reduce the risk of T2DM for some ethnic groups (see Figure 9.4).

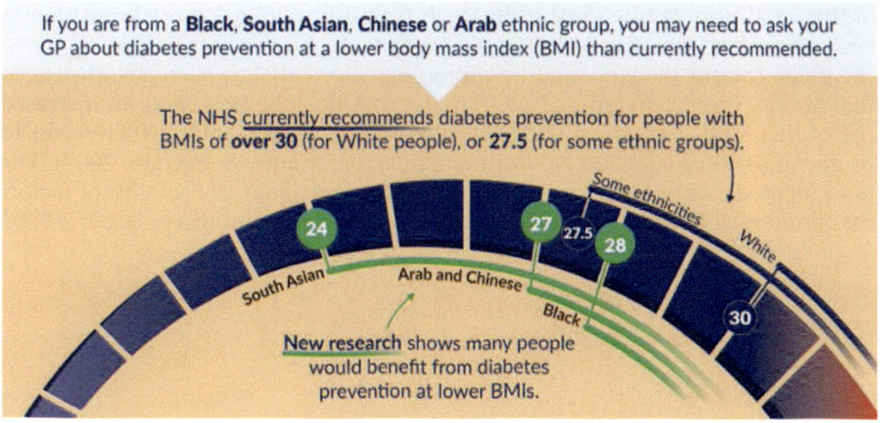

Figure 9.4
Body mass index, risk of diabetes and ethnicity

Source: National Institute for Health and Care Research (2022).

We learned in Chapter 4 that using BMI on its own as a measure of obesity was limited as it did not distinguish been lean muscle mass, fat or where fat is stored. It has been reported that waist-to-hip ratio (WHR) provides a crude estimation of fat distribution for use in clinic practice (Onat et al., 2004). Like BMI, healthcare professionals had been using WHR norms based on Western patients, but the WHO (2008) determined that the Eurocentric WHR cutoff points used to determine the risk of CHD were not universally valid across all ethnic groups. Furthermore, in the US, Xu et al. (2022) found the location of fat storage varied across different ethnic groups (Black, White, Hispanic and Asians) who had similar waist circumferences or BMIs. White people had greater tendency towards **visceral fat** storage, whereas accumulations of **subcutaneous fat** were more likely in Black people. This is an important distinction, as visceral rather than subcutaneous fat provides a better indication of cardiovascular risk (Emamat et al., 2024; Kang & Neeland, 2023) and may be used to identify ethnic groups who are at higher risk of CHD and T2DM. Combining measures, such as BMI, waist circumference and WHR, may help in identifying those at the highest risk of developing cardiovascular problems (Egeland et al., 2016). This may permit timely interventions, such as dietary changes and reductions in sedentary behaviour to prevent or reduce CVD. However, it must be noted that precise measurements of visceral fat require medical scanning, which is costly and not readily available to all. Nevertheless, it is essential that healthcare professionals ensure that when determining risk of CHD using BMI, WHR and/or waist circumference, that they do not impose Eurocentric norms on other ethnic groups, as merely adopting a 'one size fits' all approach will only perpetuate structural health inequities.

Obesogenic environment

In Chapter 4, we found out that obesity is not as simple as ingesting more calories than are used as fuel by the body. There is no single cause of obesity and experts agree that there are numerous synergic factors that are fuelling the rise of this condition. While some individuals have a physiological predisposition to becoming obese (Trayhurn, 2007), the pace at which obesity is increasing across the globe cannot be explained by physiology alone. It has been acknowledged that obesity has a generational pattern, if a parent is obese, there is an increased risk of their child becoming obese (Webber-Ritchey et al., 2023), which seems to be due to psychosocial and environmental factors (Canoy & Buchan, 2007). The term 'obesogenic environment' has been used to explain the totality of factors that promote and drive the global increase in obesity (Swinburn & Egger, 2002).

BOX 9.1
CRITICAL THINKING

Do you eat because you are hungry or because it is time to eat (e.g. breakfast, lunch or dinner time)? Do you eat because you enjoy the taste, texture or satisfying feeling of having eaten? What types of food do you snack on if you are bored or stressed?

Calorie-dense and ultra-processed foods

The amount of food that we eat is important, but especially in developed countries, as access to calorie-dense processed and ultra-processed foods can drive hedonic hunger, food cravings and weight gain (Wardle, 2007). Affordability of food is a salient issue for many families and cheaper foods tend to be calorifically high in sugars and fats, but nutritionally low in minerals and vitamins. The way in which we eat has changed, greater availability of convenience chilled and heat foods and the relatively higher cost of fresh fruit and vegetables means that families may make less healthy choices to manage their food budgets. In addition, the rise in fast-food outlets and associated advertising has been accompanied by a corresponding increase in ultra-processed food consumption.

Sedentary behaviour

For some people, their working day and leisure time are spent sitting (Fox & Hillsdon, 2007). Sedentary behaviour is a major contributor to obesity in adults and children, especially as technology has exacerbated the sedentary nature of everyday life. Take, for example, something as simple as turning on the television or changing the channel; before remote control devices, changing channels meant that the individual had to physically get out of their seat, now this is done without moving. While this may seem to be a minor activity, it does serve to highlight how we are becoming more sedentary; greater reliance on technology means that we can shop online, order takeaway food to be delivered, access library books and send e-mails, rather than posting letters. In the past, all these tasks would have involved being physically active to some degree. Children and adults spend more time watching TV, streaming TV programmes and playing computer games than in the past. Paradoxically, people engaging in multiple hours of 'TV bingeing', while snacking on high fat, sugar and salty foods may profess to not having the time to engage in physical activity (Tambalis et al., 2020). We have also become more sedentary due to changes in our ways of working, with technology and machinery replacing manual jobs. Even since the COVID-19 pandemic, there are more opportunities to remain sedentary due to online meetings and online food shopping.

Residential planning

Residential planning has an important role to play in physical activity, as walkable streets, cycle paths and open spaces can encourage active lifestyles. A reduction in open spaces and fear of walking in areas that do not have street lighting contribute to reduced physical activity (Cerin et al., 2017) and safety concerns are often a barrier to physical activity in women. Within the UK, people of Bangladeshi, Pakistani, Black Caribbean and Black African descent and many people who are already obese tend to live in obesogenic environments, characterised by areas of deprivation that have high levels of crime, less social support, greater access to processed foods in convenience stores and more fast-food outlets (Higgins, 2022). Recent research suggests air pollution from industrial and transport sources may contribute to obesity, the exact mechanism of this is unclear, but pollutants may cause inflammation, disrupt hormonal systems and lead to metabolic problems (Shi et al., 2022).

Weight loss and culture

Interventions to tackle obesity usually comprise dietary and physical activity advice, which places responsibility on the individual to take control of their health. Such an approach does not accord with Indigenous approaches to health, or holistically address obesogenic factors related to colonisation. In New Zealand, the rate of obesity among Māori groups is almost twice that of the non-Indigenous population. In trying to ascertain Māori perspectives on obesity, Bell et al. (2017) conducted one-to-one interviews with participants who had a BMI $\geq 30kg/m^2$. Similar to non-Indigenous People, Māori participants were aware of the role of diet and inactivity in promoting and sustaining obesity and the ensuring negative impact on health but did not consider these as the most important factors influencing their weight control. For these participants, hedonic eating was used as a way of coping with the intergenerational impacts of colonisation. Connections with others and to the land and nature are central to the wellbeing of Indigenous People. Land dispossession and relocation to urban areas have caused a disconnect with spiritual ancestors, culminating in loneliness and prolonged stress, which can manifest in hedonic eating, sedentary behaviour and obesity (Lewis et al., 2021). Some Indigenous patients have reported that their interactions with healthcare professionals mainly consisted of dietary advice, reducing sedentary activity and the setting of weight reduction targets. Patients often felt shamed by healthcare professionals for not reaching weight targets and reported such encounters as culturally toxic (Warbrick et al., 2019). Western informed weight management programmes that just emphasise diet and physical activity may be doomed to failure when used with Indigenous populations as there is a need to acknowledge the ongoing and detrimental impacts of colonisation and paternalistic healthcare advice. Thus culturally informed interventions are required to address Indigenous specific needs and take a strengths-based approach to intervention development (Gee et al., 2022; Schafte & Bruna, 2023).

Consequences of obesity

There are a range of physical and psychological consequences associated with obesity, some of these have already been discussed in this chapter, e.g. CVD, T2DM and some types of cancer. T2DM is 6 times more common in people who are obese compared to the normal weight population and people who have abdominal obesity are more likely to develop metabolic syndrome, making them susceptible to CVD. Approximately 4%–8% of gallbladder, pancreatic, endometrial, kidney, liver and oesophageal cancers are associated with obesity. In addition, people who are obese and have other types of cancer are more likely to have adverse outcomes from cancer treatments, an increased probability of cancer recurrence and a 17% greater chance of dying, in comparison to their non-obese peers Pati et al. (2023). Obesity has been linked with poor health-related quality of life, joint and back pain and premature death. These obesity-related conditions are not just a cause of pain and suffering for the individual, they may also have detrimental consequences for family life. Obesity can result in higher levels of general sickness and time off work that have financial implications for the person, family, employer and resource burdens for healthcare services (Office for Economic Co-operation and Development, 2019).

In addition to having physical health risks, obesity can have negative psychological consequences and contribute to stress. People who are obese tend to have poor self-image, self-esteem and low self-confidence. This is often perpetuated by Western stereotypic notions of slimness being the most soughtafter body shape, that being obese is undesirable and associated with shame. People do not make a conscious decision to become obese, but in many societies, obesity is attributed by others as the individual's fault, they are seen as being unable or unwilling to control their eating, viewed as being lazy and lacking the will power to engage in physical activity (Tomiyama, 2014). These stigmatising attitudes can be internalised, resulting in low confidence, self-esteem, self-loathing, stress and poor mental health. The resultant coping strategy may be comfort eating of foods that are high in sugar and fat, which can become a vicious circle (Lee et al., 2021). Most public health messaging about obesity places responsibility on the individual to control calorie intake and increase physical activity, offering weightloss medications and surgical options to those patients who are unable to lose weight (Bray et al., 2016), seemingly ignoring the impact of the obesogenic environment.

Diabetes

The International Diabetes Federation (IDF) (2025) estimate that around the globe 11.1% of people have diabetes, with 90% of all cases being T2DM. In 2024, based on the World Bank Income criteria classification, the prevalence of diabetes was 12.4% in high-income countries, compared to 6.1% in low-income countries and older adults (75–79 years) had the highest prevalence of diabetes (IDF, 2025). T2DM puts people at greater risk of having a heart attack (73%), stroke (54%) and a 25% chance of developing serious vision problems that can lead to blindness, compared to non-diabetic peers (IDF, 2025). Due to the insidious nature of T2DM, it may go unrecognised for quite sometime, placing individuals at risk of developing serious, but silent complications (IDF, 2025).

Risk factors for T2DM

The risk of developing T2DM is higher if there is a family history of diabetes, but more so if a parent had T2DM and obesity (Abbasi et al., 2011). T2DM usually manifests later in life, with the main independent risk factors being central obesity, elevated LDL cholesterol, hypertension and impaired glucose intolerance (Kyrou et al., 2020). An individual who has metabolic syndrome is 3.5 to 5 times more likely to develop T2DM compared to someone without the cluster (Ford et al., 2008). The most consistent modifiable risk factor for T2DM is being overweight or obese, with central and visceral adiposity being linked to insulin resistance and metabolic syndrome (Kyrou et al., 2018). Increasing rates of obesity and T2DM have led to the term 'diabesity' being used (Astrup & Finer, 2000). While diagnosis of T2DM is higher for men, women's risk of developing the condition varies over their lifetime, due to changes in sex hormones, and when they do develop T2DM, they are more likely to face a greater risk of CVD complications. In a European study, O'Sullivan et al. (2024) found that migrant women, especially those from the Middle East, North Africa and South Asia who had lower educational levels, had a fourfold greater risk of developing T2DM compared to highly educated nonmigrant women.

Dietary factors and sedentary behaviour are modifiable risk factors for T2DM that contribute to obesity and metabolic syndrome. Even in people who have a healthy BMI, high consumption of sugary drinks, foods, alcohol, processed meats and grains are linked with higher risks of developing T2DM. In contrast, diets high in fruit, vegetables, wholegrains, poultry, fish and whole grains reduce the risks of developing T2DM (Ley et al., 2014).

DESMOND

Within the UK, the Diabetes Education and Self-Management for Ongoing and Newly Diagnosed (DESMOND) programme is a freely available educational package for patients who have been diagnosed with T2DM. It helps to educate people about T2DM and lifestyle changes that they can make to successfully manage their condition (Davies et al., 2008). DESMOND can be delivered in group sessions, it provides peer support and there is an online version that patients can work through on their own, at a pace that suits their learning needs. The programme started in the early 2000s, was developed within the NHS and is used quite widely across the UK. DESMOND has been tailored to suit people from different cultural backgrounds who may have different dietary habits, languages other than English (Stone et al., 2008), along with health and illness beliefs that differ according to the culture it was initially developed for. The adaptations to meal planning and diet consider dietary needs common to people from South Asian and African Caribbean communities; it considers fasting in relation to Ramadan (Daly et al., 2014) and other religious dietary needs. The cultural changes to the programmes were informed by community involvement with service users, which ensured that content was relevant, culturally appropriate and sensitive to community needs. Additional adaptations have been made to DESMOND to support people with visual impairments and learning disabilities.

Diabetes in different populations

Ethnicity and diabetes

Certain ethnic groups (Chinese, Japanese, South Asian) appear to have a greater genetic predisposition to developing T2DM, especially if they have **abdominal obesity** (Meeks et al., 2016). In the UK, individuals of Black African or Caribbean descent or from Bangladeshi, Indian or Pakistani backgrounds are between 3 and 5 times more likely to develop T2DM and tend to be diagnosed around 10 to 12 years earlier than White British individuals (Goff, 2019). Similarly, non-White ethnic populations residing in Europe show an increased prevalence of T2DM compared with White European ethnic groups (Meeks et al., 2016). Farmaki et al. (2022) reported that first-generation African, Asian and Caribbean migrants to the UK had a 20% high rate of T2DM than the second generation, with lower socioeconomic status thought to have contributed to the higher rates of T2DM observed among the first generation. An examination of risk of T2DM, ethnicity and socioeconomic status reported that 64% of cases of diabetes were linked to low socioeconomic status. The intersection of ethnicity and socioeconomic status meant that Asian patients from deprived areas were 9 times more likely to develop diabetes compared to their White counterparts in the least deprived areas.

Socioeconomic status and diabetes

In a longitudinal study of adults, conducted over 7.5 years in England, Stringhini et al. (2016) found that people of low SES had twice the risk of T2DM than the high SES group, with lifestyle factors being the major factor. People of lower SES were more likely to have a higher BMI, be sedentary and smoke. In a review of literature that examined the association between SES, obesity and T2DM, Volaco et al. (2018) reported that central obesity, a higher intake of fatty and sugary foods, lower fruit and vegetable intake were associated with being in a low SES group. In addition, being sedentary, living in areas of neighbourhood deprivation, which included less safe environments and lack of spaces for exercise, were more commonly found in people of low SES.

Low socioeconomic status (SES), which may be indicative of low educational level and income, has shown a constantly higher risk of developing T2DM and disease-related complications. Valentelyte et al. (2025) explored the links between socioeconomic factors and age on the prevalence of diabetes using data collected via the Healthy Ireland Survey from 2015 to 2023. Socioeconomic status was defined by educational level and area-based deprivation. As expected, older adults (13%) had a higher prevalence of diabetes in comparison to those under 40 (1%) years old. Diabetes was nearly three times more prevalent for those living in areas of deprivation (6%) compared to people in wealthier areas (2.2%). More striking was the finding that those with the lowest levels of education had almost five times the prevalence of diabetes compared to those who were more highly educated. These findings underscore the ongoing association between low socioeconomic status, lower education levels and higher diabetes prevalence in Ireland. This echoes similar patterns observed in relation to deprivation in England (Office for Health Improvement and Disparities, 2025), the US (Chen et al., 2023) and for people with lower educational levels in most European countries (Sidahmed et al., 2025).

Indigenous Peoples and diabetes

The prevalence of diabetes among Aboriginal and Torres Strait Islanders is 3 times higher than in the non-Indigenous population (Australian Institute of Health and Wellbeing, n.d.). Similar disparities are found in Canada with diabetes rates 3 to 4 times greater among Indigenous Peoples (Waapihk Research, 2024) and around 4 times higher for the Māori (Health New Zealand, 2025). In the US the disparity is smaller, with prevalence 1.5 times higher among Indigenous Americans (American Diabetes Association n.d.). Explanations for the higher prevalence of diabetes within Indigenous populations include the loss of traditional hunting and gathering food practices, land and ways of living, which have had negative influences on diet and sedentary behaviours. In addition, poverty has prohibited access to healthy foods, meaning that highly nutritious diets that were traditionally high in protein, low in fats and refined sugars have been replaced with Western high fat, high sugar, processed diets. Prior to colonisation, Indigenous Peoples were largely self-sufficient, hunting, growing and gathering food that was prepared from raw and unprocessed ingredients, with no convenience or fast foods. These dietary changes combined with a sedentary lifestyle have contributed to greater obesity (Compher, 2006) and prevalence of T2DM. The types of interventions developed for non-Indigenous populations often lack cultural specificity, they emphasise control of T2DM in relation to blood tests, weight measurement, advice about eating a healthy diet and becoming more physically active. The relevance of this approach may be unclear to Indigenous People, who view health as including spiritual, emotional, physical and mental wellbeing (Crowshoe, 2005). A community-based intervention for Indigenous People (Prima Indians) in the US compared two lifestyle interventions over a 12-month period. One intervention (Prima Pride) involved activities that were based on history and unstructured cultural activities, delivered by local speakers; the other group (Prima Action) included structured physical activity and dietary interventions. Both interventions lead to reductions in sedentary behaviours. Pride participants showed reductions in waist circumference and intake of starchy foods, even though no specific dietary advice had been provided, whereas the blood glucose, weight and blood pressure increased in the Action group (Narayan et al., 1998). The authors concluded that interventions, which include self-directed traditional, unstructured and culturally relevant information, may be more suited to Prima Indigenous populations compared to Western informed interventions that are designed to target specific risk factors, such as eating a heathy diet and reducing sedentary behaviour.

A systematic review examined the designs of interventions that were effective in supporting Indigenous Peoples across Australia, New Zealand and the US to manage T2DM. It identified seven key interventional features that could enhance glucose control within these populations (Chopra et al., 2022). Barriers to healthcare for Indigenous Peoples include season work, which often takes individuals away from their usual area of residence, it was suggested that relocating health services to workplaces may improve adherence. Community involvement as equal partners in intervention planning ensures the integration of Indigenous knowledge, values, self-determination and cultural safety. Community health workers play a key role by explaining health information and transporting patients in rural areas to medical appointments and markets where they can access fresh foods. Individualised education helps in the self-management of diabetes, empowering Indigenous People at an individual and community level to actively manage their own health. Free checkups to monitor blood glucose and any other diabetes-related conditions, along with continuity of care with trusted healthcare professionals, can help T2DM management. Short interventions of around three months can keep participants engaged and have lasting changes, but a duration of change beyond one year is unclear. Group-based interventions may enhance intervention engagement reflecting the collective nature of wellbeing within Indigenous communities.

Due to the legacy of colonialism, paternalistic care and systemic racism, interventions based on Eurocentric models of care may be viewed with mistrust by Indigenous Peoples. These models tend to emphasise individual responsibility for health, which neglects Indigenous values of community and the four aspects of wellbeing. Indigenous interventions for T2DM need to be co-designed, integrate traditional knowledge and be culturally safe (Crowshoe et al., 2018). In addition, non-Indigenous healthcare professionals need to acknowledge the effects of intergeneration trauma due to colonisation and the perpetuation of socioeconomic inequities, which have negative impacts on T2DM outcomes.

LGBTQI+ individuals and diabetes

Some LGBTQI+ communities are at greater risk of T2DM than others. The prevalence of T2DM is significantly higher in bisexual men compared to heterosexual and gay men, with the latter having the lowest prevalence (Newlin Lew et al., 2018). Lesbian and bisexual women have greater risks of T2DM and are more likely to be diagnosed at a younger age than their heterosexual counterparts (Corliss et al., 2018). This is thought to be due to lesbian and bisexual women having higher rates of obesity (Caceres et al., 2019; Garland-Forshee et al., 2014), alcohol consumption and smoking (Gonzales et al., 2016). Islam et al. (2022) found that the prevalence of T2DM was 30% higher in transgender women compared to their cisgender counterparts. These findings indicate that people from sexual and gender minority groups could benefit from prevention screening for metabolic health, along with early intervention to try and ward off the development of T2DM. However, transgender individuals tend to be a hard-to-reach population, as they avoid healthcare interactions because of anticipated and real discrimination, along with fear of mistreatment Correll-King et al., 2025).

In Chapter 1, we learned that the intersection of multiple identities may be associated with privilege or oppression, the latter can result in discrimination (Meyer, 2003). Minority stress in the form of harassment, discrimination and violence has negative impacts on health outcomes in LGBTQI+ populations (Institute of Medicine, 2011), which can be magnified by the intersection of multiple minority statuses, such as ethnicity and having a disability. The prolonged physiological effects of stress response (Cohen et al., 2012; Xue et al., 2015), coupled with deleterious coping, such as smoking, inactivity, having a poor diet and binge drinking (American Psychological Association, 2017), suggest that standard T2DM interventions may need to be more tailored to meet the needs of LGBTQI+ individuals to include coping with the detrimental impacts of minority stress (Corliss et al., 2018).

People with disabilities and diabetes

People with learning disabilities, similar to those with no disabilities, may not pick up on the symptoms of T2DM, added to this, the nature of their disability may result in an inability or difficulty with self-management (Bryant et al., 2018). Diabetes is nearly 7 times more likely in people with learning disabilities and occurs at a younger age compared with the general population. Additionally, the intersection of being from Black or South Asian backgrounds increases this risk (Baksh et al., 2025). T2DM risk factors for people with learning disabilities include obesity, being sedentary, taking **anti-psychotic medication** (prescribed for people who have severe mental illnesses, such as schizophrenia, bipolar disorder and/or challenging behaviours, such as aggression of self-harming) and eating a high fat diet (Bryant et al., 2018) In addition, having hypertension and a mild as opposed to profound learning disability have been associated with T2DM (Vancampfort et al., 2022). Bryant et al. (2018) conducted a cross-sectional study using clinical data on glucose control (HbA1c), blood pressure, risk of CVD, cholesterol and interviews to ascertain medication adherence and diabetes self-care in adults with mild to moderate learning disabilities. They found that glucose control was similar to that in the non-learning disability population, with around 20% of participants having higher than recommended **HbA1c**. Many of the patients with learning disabilities were overweight or obese, 33% had problems with medication adherence and there were gaps in routine monitoring of blood pressure and obesity by GPs. Lifestyle behaviours of these patients showed that diets were high in fat and sugar and physical activity was low, suggesting that lifestyle is an area for targeted intervention in people with learning disabilities. Furthermore barriers to regular health monitoring by GPs need to be addressed.

Individuals who have physical disabilities, especially those with limited mobility due to spinal cord injuries (SCIs), are at higher risk of T2DM, especially as they get older (Hoekstra et al., 2024). This may be due to the SCI resulting in reduced physical activity, contributing to muscle loss and increased abdominal fat (Gater et al., 2021). An alternative explanation comes from the impact an SCI has on the autonomic nervous system, which is thought to affect the body's ability to regulate blood glucose (Smith & Yarar-Fisher, 2016). Research had suggested that people with SCIs that affected all four limbs (tetraplegia) had a greater risk of T2DM compared to those where two limbs (paraplegia) were affected; however, a more recent research study has been unable to substantiate this finding (Hoekstra et al., 2024). A Korean study noted that people who had traumatic limb amputations due to accidents or injury had an 11% higher risk of developing T2DM, especially if the amputation occurred high up the leg or at the hip (Yoo et al., 2025). Similar to people with SCI, those with limb loss that affected their mobility tended to have sedentary lifestyles, which contributed to accumulations of abdominal fat. After amputation increased smoking, alcohol consumption and unhealthy eating also contributed to weight gain and the potential to develop T2DM. It seems that the physiological effects of amputation may interfere with blood glucose control and insulin resistance, and these effects can be more marked when people engage in unhealthy lifestyle behaviours. Thus, people who experience SCIs or who have lower limb amputations may benefit from educational information as part of their post-surgical journey to highlight the risks of developing of T2DM.

Poverty, ethnicity, gender, education level, disability and being from an Indigenous group can compound the risk of developing T2DM and negatively impact an individual's ability to engage in preventative health behaviours and/or successfully manage the condition. All too often, provision of education and advice on lifestyle management overlook intersecting social determinants of health in those most affected by T2DM diabetes-related health inequities.

Looking forward

The biomedical approach to disease is concerned with investigation and diagnosis of patient symptoms and subsequent treatment. This approach works extremely well for infectious diseases that are caused by bacteria, treated with antibiotics and for simple bone fractures that are X-rayed and immobilised for a specific time period. The same cannot be said for chronic diseases, which are unlikely to be solely managed by a biomedical approach. While medication, medical and/or surgical intervention may be required, psychosocial and cultural aspects of the disease are extremely important. The accumulated evidence about chronic diseases indicates that rather than just providing treatments and interventions, a proactive approach is necessary to prevent diseases or identify them early in the disease trajectory, through health promotion and disease prevention activities. These can include screening at an asymptomatic stage and educational interventions that are targeted at stopping or preventing uptake of unhealthy lifestyle behaviours (Riekert et al., 2013).

The risk factors for many chronic diseases can be modified through behaviour change, but social determinants of health, such as differential educational levels, socioeconomic status, healthcare barriers, lack of neighbourhood safety and poor environmental living conditions, can contribute to poorer health outcomes. Addressing socioeconomic disadvantage and culturally insensitive services that impact engagement with preventative healthcare is essential. Cultural awareness and sensitivity are improving, but we must involve Indigenous, ethnic, LGBTQI+ and disabled communities as partners in research and health intervention development, while recognising that intersectional identities can compound health disadvantage. Inclusive, culturally tailored healthcare that responds to diverse lived experiences is crucial, without it, health disparities will only continue flourish.

Chapter Summary

Discuss how belonging to a minoritsed or Indigenous group may influence the development of cardiovascular disease

Social inequity, discrimination and stress all influence the development of cardiovascular disease (CVD). Minority stress experienced by people from LGBTQI+ communities and Indigenous Peoples can lead to deleterious health behaviours, such as smoking, excess alcohol consumption and unhealthy dietary choices. Social determinants of health, such as income, education, neighbourhood conditions, access to healthcare and lower health literacy, are associated with a higher prevalence of CVD, especially for minoritised groups. In addition, women may experience greater barriers to diagnosis and treatment of heart disease compared to men.

Outline barriers to cancer screening experienced by people from ethnic minority groups, LGBTQI+ communities and people with disabilities

Low health literacy, language barriers, a lack of culturally appropriate information, discrimination, religious beliefs and limited cultural safety can all act as barriers to cancer screening for people from ethnic minority groups. LGBTQI+ individuals may avoid screening due to a fear of discrimination, assumptions from healthcare professionals regarding cisgender and heterosexual identities and a lack of inclusive information about screening procedures. People with learning disabilities may not receive information in suitable formats to make informed choices about screening and may have to rely on others to make screening choices for them. Transport challenges and accessibility issues at clinics are barriers that restrict screening opportunities for people with physical disabilities.

Describe and discuss factors influencing smoking behaviours and the barriers to quitting across diverse populations

Smoking is more common in people who are on low incomes, those living in deprived neighbourhoods, LGBTQI+, Indigenous communities and some ethnic minority groups. For many of these individuals, smoking is a coping mechanism for managing chronic stress, discrimination and microaggressions. Smoking behaviour can also be intergenerational and associated with peer group pressure. A range of smoking cessation products are available, but cost and fear of becoming addicted to nicotine replacement substances can be barriers to use. For LGBTQI+ individuals, fear of discrimination can be a barrier to seeking help from health professionals and for Indigenous Peoples, the legacy of colonisation and limited access to culturally sensitive care can reduce the likelihood of quitting.

Explain the concept of an obesogenic environment and how it relates to social determinants of health

An obesogenic environment is one that promotes unhealthy eating and sedentary behaviours, increasing the likelihood of obesity. Many low-income neighbourhoods are characterised by easy-to-access high fat, high sugar, ultra-processed foods, fast-food outlets, convenience stores and a lack of fresh nutritious foods. In addition, these neighbourhoods may lack adequate safe paths and green spaces to engage in physical activity, which makes it more difficult to maintain a healthy weight.

Discuss the relationship between social determinants of health and the prevalence of type 2 diabetes mellitus

Type 2 diabetes (T2DM) is strongly linked to lower income and educational levels and low health literacy about the condition. Living in low-income neighbourhoods, with limited access to fresh nutritious foods, safe spaces and green areas for physical activity, are also important factors. Being overweight or obese is an independent risk factor for T2DM, but some groups have a greater susceptibility to T2DM, which can be magnified by factors such as cultural norms regarding diet, a lack of culturally safe healthcare and appropriate diabetes education and intervention programmes.

Keywords

Eurocentric populations: Having a perspective that considers European cultural values, experiences and knowledge as being the norm, overlooking or viewing other cultures and world views less favourably.

Triglycerides: A type of fat found in the blood and high levels of it are linked with heart disease.

LDL cholesterol: Considered as the 'bad' type of cholesterol that contributes to atherosclerosis.

HDL cholesterol: Considered as the 'good' type of cholesterol that is protective against heart disease.

High demand and low control job: Working under higher pressure (psychological or physical), but having little to no decision-making ability, which can contribute to stress.

Zero hours contract: A work contract with no guaranteed hours, workers are only paid for the hours they work, which can lead to financial worries and stress.

Job control: The amount of autonomy a person has over when and how they work.

C-reactive protein: A marker in the blood that provides an indication of inflammation and can be associated with increased cardiovascular risk.

Metabolic syndrome: A cluster of conditions that include abdominal fat, hypertension and high LDL cholesterol.

Unconscious bias: Discriminatory attitudes, behaviours and/or prejudice towards others that the person is unaware of.

Conscious bias: Deliberate discriminatory attitudes, behaviours and/or prejudicet towards others.

Pharmacological trials: Research studies used to test the safety or efficacy of medications in humans.

Hepatitis C: A viral infection that causes liver inflammation, which can lead to cancer.

Dementia: A group of progressive diseases that affect memory and everyday tasks.

Herpes papillomavirus: A sexually transmitted infection, some types can increase the risk of cervical, head and neck cancers.

Cervical screening: A test to detect cervical cancer at an asymptomatic stage, which involves a cervical smear test.

Breast screening: Involves the use of a special x-ray (mammogram) to detect breast cancer at an asymptomatic stage.

Secondary data: Data that have already been collected by someone else as part of a large dataset that can be used at a later date for research purposes.

Bowel screening: A test to detect bowel cancer at an asymptomatic stage, usually involves the collection of a very small sample of poo that is tested for hidden blood.

Capacity: An individual's ability to understand, retain and consider information to make an informed decision about healthcare.

Prostate cancer screening: A test used to detect prostate cancer usually involves a blood test and rectal examination.
Visceral fat: Fat that is stored around the internal organs and is associated with an increased risk of heart disease.
Subcutaneous fat: Fat that is stored just underneath the skin, which is less harmful than visceral fat.
Abdominal obesity: An excess of fat around the waistline, which is linked with obesity, increased cardiovascular disease and T2DM.
Anti-psychotic medication: Prescribed drugs used to treat symptoms associated with severe mental health conditions.
HbA1c: A blood test that provides an average measure of blood glucose over the previous two or three months.

Key Readings

Baez, A. S., Ortiz-Whittingham, L. R., Tarfa, H., Osei Baah, F., Thompson, K., Baumer, Y., & Powell-Wiley, T. M. (2023). Social determinants of health, health disparities, and adiposity. *Progress in Cardiovascular Diseases*, *78*, 17–26. https://doi.org/10.1016/j.pcad.2023.04.011

Estupiñán Fdez de Mesa, M., Marcu, A., Ream, E., & Whitaker, K. L. (2025). Understanding and tackling cancer inequities: What opportunities does intersectionality offer researchers, policymakers, and providers? A scoping review. *Journal of Psychosocial Oncology*, *43*(1), 105–132. https://doi.org/10.1080/07347332.2024.2361642

Hill-Briggs, F., & Fitzpatric, S. L. (2023). Overview of social determinants of health in the development of diabetes. *Diabetes Care*, *46*(9), 1590–1598. https://doi.org/10.2337/dci23-0001

Tuffrey-Wijne, I., & Davies, J. (2007). This is my story: I've got cancer. *British Journal of Learning Disabilities*, *35*, 7–11. https://doi.org/10.1111/j.1468-3156.2006.00421.x

Reflective Questions

1 Consider how social determinants, such as ethnicity, gender, socioeconomic status or disability, may influence the prevalence and health outcomes in one chronic disease of your choosing.
2 How might ethnicity, gender, disability or LGBTQI+ status affect an individual's access to cancer screening, diagnosis, and treatment?
3 How might BMI, waist circumference and waist-to-hip ratio differ in accurately assessing health risks for diverse populations?
4 How do obesogenic environments and hedonic eating influence individual and population-level obesity?
5 Why might T2DM prevalence and outcomes differ across ethnic groups, Indigenous populations, LGBTQI+ communities and in people with disabilities?

Note

1 Access for free at https://openstax.org/details/books/psychology-2e

References

Abbasi, A., Corpeleijn, E., van der Schouw, Y. T., Stolk, R. P., Spijkerman, A. M., van der A, D. L., Navis, G., Bakker, S. J., & Beulens, J. W. (2011). Maternal and paternal transmission of type 2 diabetes: Influence of diet, lifestyle and adiposity. *Journal of Internal Medicine, 270*(4), 388–396. https://doi.org/10.1111/j.1365-2796.2011.02347.x

Abdalla, S. M., Yu, S., & Galea, S. (2020). Trends in cardiovascular disease prevalence by income level in the United States. *JAMA Network Open, 3*(9), e2018150. https://doi.org/10.1001/jamanetworkopen.2020.18150

Abdullahi, A., Copping, J., Kessel, A., Luck, M., & Bonell, C. (2009). Cervical screening: Perceptions and barriers to uptake among Somali women in Camden. *Public Health, 123*(10), 680–685. https://doi.org/10.1016/j.puhe.2009.09.011

Acree, M. E., McNulty, M., Blocker, O., Schneider, J., & Williams, H. S. (2020). Shared decision-making around anal cancer screening among black bisexual and gay men in the USA. *Culture, Health & Sexuality, 22*(2), 201–216. https://doi.org/10.1080/13691058.2019.1581897

Adebisi, Y. A., Alshahrani, N. Z., Ogunkola, I. O., & Lucero-Prisno, D. E. 3rd (2025). Physical disability and risk of incident hypertension: A prospective cohort analysis. *Journal of Human Hypertension.* https://doi.org/10.1038/s41371-025-01061-1. Advance online publication.

Ades, P. A., & Savage, P. D. (2017). Obesity in coronary heart disease: An unaddressed behavioral risk factor. *Preventive Medicine, 104*, 117–119. https://doi.org/10.1016/j.ypmed.2017.04.013

Agénor, M., Bailey, Z., Krieger, N., Austin, S. B., & Gottlieb, B. R. (2015). Exploring the cervical cancer screening experiences of Black lesbian, bisexual, and queer women: The role of patient-provider communication. *Women & Health, 55*(6), 717–736. https://doi.org/10.1080/03630242.2015.1039182

Al-Kindi, S. G., Brook, R. D., Biswal, S., & Rajagopalan, S. (2020). Environmental determinants of cardiovascular disease: Lessons learned from air pollution. *Nature Reviews Cardiology, 17*(10), 656–672. https://doi.org/10.1038/s41569-020-0371-2

Alliance for Healthy Hearts and Minds First Nations Research Group (2019). Explaining the variability in cardiovascular risk factors among First Nations communities in Canada: A population-based study. *The Lancet. Planetary Health, 3*(12), e511–e520. https://doi.org/10.1016/S2542-5196(19)30237-2

Alzahrani, T., Nguyen, T., Ryan, A., Dwairy, A., McCaffrey, J., Yunus, R., Forgione, J., Krepp, J., Nagy, C., Mazhari, R., & Reiner, J. (2019). Cardiovascular disease risk factors and myocardial infarction in the transgender population. *Circulation: Cardiovascular Quality and Outcomes, 12*(4), e005597. https://doi.org/10.1161/CIRCOUTCOMES.119.005597

American Diabetes Association (n.d). Statistics about diabetes. Retrieved September 28, 2025, from https://diabetes.org/about-diabetes/statistics/about-diabetes

American Heart Association (2024). *Go Red for women: Common myths about heart disease.* Retrieved November 26, 2024, from https://www.goredforwomen.org/en/about-heart-disease-in-women/facts/common-myths-about-heart-disease

American Lung Association (n.d.). *COPD trends Brief: Prevalence.* Retrieved September 26, 2025, from https://www.lung.org/research/trends-in-lung-disease/copd-trends-brief/copd-prevalence

American Psychological Association (2017). *Stress and health disparities: Contexts, mechanisms, and interventions among racial/ethnic minority and low socioeconomic status populations.* Retrieved September 25, 2025, from: https://www.apa.org/pi/health-equity/resources/stress-report.pdf

Anand, S. S., Abonyi, S., Arbour, L., Balasubramanian, K., Brook, J., Castleden, H., Chrisjohn, V., Cornelius, I., Davis, A. D., Desai, D., de Souza, R. J., Friedrich,

M. G., Harris, S., Irvine, J., L'Hommecourt, J., Littlechild, R., Mayotte, L., McIntosh, S., Morrison, J., Ster, R. T. ... Canadian Alliance for Healthy Hearts and Minds First Nations Research Group (2019). Explaining the variability in cardiovascular risk factors among First Nations communities in Canada: A population-based study. *The Lancet. Planetary Health, 3*(12), e511–e520. https://doi.org/10.1016/S2542-5196(19)30237-2

Anthonisen, N. R., Connett, J. E., & Murray, R. P. (2002). Smoking and lung function of lung health study participants after 11 years. *American Journal of Respiratory and Critical Care Medicine, 166*(5), 675–679. https://doi.org/10.1164/rccm.2112096

Arnett, D. K., Blumenthal, R. S., Albert, M. A., Buroker, A. B., Goldberger, Z. D., Hahn, E. J., Himmelfarb, C. D., Khera, A., Lloyd-Jones, D., McEvoy, J. W., Michos, E. D., Miedema, M. D., Muñoz, D., Smith, S. C. Jr, Virani, S. S., Williams, K. A. Sr, Yeboah, J., & Ziaeian, B. (2019). 2019 ACC/AHA Guideline on the primary prevention of cardiovascular disease: Executive summary: A report of the American College of Cardiology/American Heart Association Task Force on Clinical Practice Guidelines. *Circulation, 140*(11), e563–e595. https://doi.org/10.1161/CIR.0000000000000677

Astrup, A., & Finer, N. (2000). Redefining type 2 diabetes: 'diabesity' or 'obesity dependent diabetes mellitus'? *Obesity Reviews, 1*(2), 57–59. https://doi.org/10.1046/j.1467-789x.2000.00013.x

Australian Institute of Health and Wellbeing (n.d.). *Health status and outcomes: Diabetes*. Retrieved September 28, 2025, from https://www.indigenoushpf.gov.au/measures/1-09-diabetes?utm_source

Australian Institute of Health and Welfare (2025). *Aboriginal and Torres Strait Islander Health Performance Framework: Summary report June 2025*. AIHW: Australian Government. Retrieved September 26, 2025, from https://www.indigenoushpf.gov.au/Report-overview/Overview/Summary-report

Baksh, R. A., Pape, S. E., Chan, L. F., Sheehan, R., White, A., Chauhan, U., Gulliford, M. C., & Strydom, A. (2025). Type 2 diabetes mellitus in people with intellectual disabilities: Examining incidence, risk factors, quality of care and related complications. A population-based matched cohort study. *Diabetes Research and Clinical Practice, 222*, 112090. https://doi.org/10.1016/j.diabres.2025.112090

Balabanski, A. H., Newbury, J., Leyden, J. M., Arima, H., Anderson, C. S., Castle, S., Cranefield, J., Paterson, T., Thrift, A. G., Katzenellenbogen, J., Brown, A., & Kleinig, T. J. (2018). Excess stroke incidence in young Aboriginal people in South Australia: Pooled results from two population-based studies. *International Journal of Stroke, 13*(8), 811–814. https://doi.org/10.1177/1747493018778113

Balabanski, A. H., Dos Santos, A., Woods, J. A., Mutimer, C. A., Thrift, A. G., Kleinig, T. J., Suchy-Dicey, A. M., Siri, S. R. A., Boden-Albala, B., Krishnamurthi, R. V., Feigin, V. L., Buchwald, D., Ranta, A., Mienna, C. S., Zavaleta-Cortijo, C., Churilov, L., Burchill, L., Zion, D., Longstreth, W. T. Jr, Tirschwell, D. L., & Katzenellenbogen, J. M. (2024). Incidence of stroke in Indigenous populations of countries with a very high human development index: A systematic review. *Neurology, 102*(5), e209138. https://doi.org/10.1212/WNL.0000000000209138

Bansal, N., Bhopal, R. S., Steiner, M. F., Brewster, D. H.; Scottish Health and Ethnicity Linkage Study (2012). Major ethnic group differences in breast cancer screening uptake in Scotland are not extinguished by adjustment for indices of geographical residence, area deprivation, long-term illness and education. *British Journal of Cancer, 106*(8), 1361–1366. https://doi.org/10.1038/bjc.2012.83

Barefoot, J. C., Peterson, B. L., Harrell, F. E. Jr, Hlatky, M. A., Pryor, D. B., Haney, T. L., Blumenthal, J. A., Siegler, I. C., & Williams, R. B. Jr (1989a). Type A behavior and survival: A follow-up study of 1,467 patients with coronary artery disease. *The American Journal of Cardiology, 64*(8), 427–432. https://doi.org/10.1016/0002-9149(89)90416-5

Barefoot, J. C., Dodge, K. A., Peterson, B. L., Dahlstrom, W. G., &, & Williams, R. B., Jr (1989b). The Cook-Medley hostility scale: Item content and ability to predict survival. *Psychosomatic Medicine, 51*(1), 46–57. https://doi.org/10.1097/00006842-198901000-00005

Batalha, A. P. D. B., Marcal, I. R., Main, E., & Ghisi, G. L. M. (2025). Barriers to physical activity in women from ethnic minority groups: A systematic review. *BMC Women's Health, 25*(1), 330. https://doi.org/10.1186/s12905-025-03877-y

Beckett, M., Cole, K., White, M., Chan, J., McVicar, J., Rodin, D., Clemons, M., & Bourque, J. M. (2021). Decolonizing cancer care in Canada. *Journal of Cancer Policy, 30*, 100309. https://doi.org/10.1016/j.jcpo.2021.100309

Bell, R., Smith, C., Hale, L., Kira, G., & Tumilty, S. (2017). Understanding obesity in the context of an Indigenous population: A qualitative study. *Obesity Research & Clinical Practice, 11*(5), 558–566. https://doi.org/10.1016/j.orcp.2017.04.006

Berger, I., & Mooney-Somers, J. (2017). Smoking cessation programs for lesbian, gay, bisexual, transgender, and intersex people: A content-based systematic review. *Nicotine & Tobacco Research, 19*(12), 1408–1417. https://doi.org/10.1093/ntr/ntw216

Berry, T. R., Stearns, J. A., Courneya, K. S., McGannon, K. R., Norris, C. M., Rodgers, W. M., & Spence, J. C. (2016). Women's perceptions of heart disease and breast cancer and the association with media representations of the diseases. *Journal of Public Health, 38*(4), e496–e503. https://doi.org/10.1093/pubmed/fdv177

Bhatnagar, A. (2017). Environmental determinants of cardiovascular disease. *Circulation Research, 121*(2), 162–180. https://doi.org/10.1161/CIRCRESAHA.117.306458

Biswas, A., Oh, P. I., Faulkner, G. E., Bajaj, R. R., Silver, M. A., Mitchell, M. S., & Alter, D. A. (2015). Sedentary time and its association with risk for disease incidence, mortality, and hospitalization in adults: A systematic review and meta-analysis. *Annals of Internal Medicine, 162*(2), 123–132. https://doi.org/10.7326/M14-1651

Black Barbershop Health Outreach Program. (2020). Retrieved January 4, 2025, from https://www.blackbarbershop.org/

Bryant, L. D., Russell, A. M., Walwyn, R. E. A., Farrin, A. J., Wright-Hughes, A., Graham, E. H., Nagi, D., Stansfield, A., Birtwistle, J., Meer, S., Ajjan, R. A., & House, A. O. (2018). Characterizing adults with Type 2 diabetes mellitus and intellectual disability: Outcomes of a case-finding study. *Diabetic Medicine, 35*(3), 352–359. https://doi.org/10.1111/dme.13510

Bray, G. A., Frühbeck, G., Ryan, D. H., & Wilding, J. P. (2016). Management of obesity. *Lancet, 387*(10031), 1947–1956. https://doi.org/10.1016/S0140-6736(16)00271-3

Breathett, K., Yee, E., Pool, N., Hebdon, M., Crist, J. D., Knapp, S., Larsen, A., Solola, S., Luy, L., Herrera-Theut, K., Zabala, L., Stone, J., McEwen, M. M., Calhoun, E., & Sweitzer, N. K. (2019). Does race influence decision making for advanced heart failure therapies? *Journal of the American Heart Association, 8*(22), e013592. https://doi.org/10.1161/JAHA.119.013592

British Heart Foundation (2025) *UK fact sheet*. Retrieved September 22, 2025, from https://www.bhf.org.uk/-/media/files/for-professionals/research/heart-statistics/bhf-cvd-statistics-uk-factsheet.pdf

Bryant, K. B., Moran, A. E., Kazi, D. S., Zhang, Y., Penko, J., Ruiz-Negrón, N., Coxson, P., Blyler, C. A., Lynch, K., Cohen, L. P., Tajeu, G. S., Fontil, V., Moy, N. B., Ebinger, J. E., Rader, F., Bibbins-Domingo, K., & Bellows, B. K. (2021). Cost-effectiveness of hypertension treatment by pharmacists in black barbershops. *Circulation, 143*(24), 2384–2394. https://doi.org/10.1161/CIRCULATIONAHA.120.051683

Buchting, F. O., Emory, K. T., Scout, Kim, Y., Fagan, P., Vera, L. E., & Emery, S. (2017). Transgender use of cigarettes, cigars, and e-cigarettes in a national study. *American Journal of Preventive Medicine, 53*(1), e1–e7. https://doi.org/10.1016/j.amepre.2016.11.022

Bull, F. C., Al-Ansari, S. S., Biddle, S., Borodulin, K., Buman, M. P., Cardon, G., Carty, C., Chaput, J. P., Chastin, S., Chou, R., Dempsey, P. C., DiPietro, L., Ekelund, U., Firth, J., Friedenreich, C. M., Garcia, L., Gichu, M., Jago, R., Katzmarzyk, P. T., Lambert, E., & Willumsen, J. F. (2020). World Health Organization 2020 guidelines on physical activity and sedentary behaviour. *British Journal of Sports Medicine, 54*(24), 1451–1462. https://doi.org/10.1136/bjsports-2020-102955

Businelle, M. S., Kendzor, D. E., Reitzel, L. R., Costello, T. J., Cofta-Woerpel, L., Li, Y., Mazas, C. A., Vidrine, J. I., Cinciripini, P. M., Greisinger, A. J., & Wetter, D. W. (2010). Mechanisms linking socioeconomic status to smoking cessation: A structural equation modeling approach. *Health Psychology, 29*(3), 262–273. https://doi.org/10.1037/a0019285

Caceres, B. A., Makarem, N., Hickey, K. T., & Hughes, T. L. (2019). Cardiovascular disease disparities in sexual minority adults: An examination of the Behavioral Risk Factor Surveillance System (2014-2016). *American Journal of Health Promotion, 33*(4), 576–585. https://doi.org/10.1177/0890117118810246

Caceres, B. A., Streed, C. G. Jr, Corliss, H. L., Lloyd-Jones, D. M., Matthews, P. A., Mukherjee, M., Poteat, T., Rosendale, N., Ross, L. M.; American Heart Association Council on Cardiovascular and Stroke Nursing; Council on Hypertension; Council on Lifestyle and Cardiometabolic Health; Council on Peripheral Vascular Disease; and Stroke Council (2020). Assessing and addressing cardiovascular health in LGBTQ adults: A scientific statement from the American Heart Association. *Circulation, 142*(19), e321–e332. https://doi.org/10.1161/CIR.0000000000000914

Cadman, L., Ashdown-Barr, L., Waller, J., & Szarewski, A. (2015). Attitudes towards cytology and human papillomavirus self-sample collection for cervical screening among Hindu women in London, UK: A mixed methods study. *The Journal of Family Planning and Reproductive Healthcare, 41*(1), 38–47. https://doi.org/10.1136/jfprhc-2013-100705

Cai, Y., Zhang, B., Ke, W., Feng, B., Lin, H., Xiao, J., Zeng, W., Li, X., Tao, J., Yang, Z., Ma, W., & Liu, T. (2016). Associations of short-term and long-term exposure to ambient air pollutants with hypertension: A systematic review and meta-analysis. *Hypertension, 68*(1), 62–70. https://doi.org/10.1161/HYPERTENSIONAHA.116.07218

Caleyachetty, R., Barber, T. M., Mohammed, N. I., Cappuccio, F. P., Hardy, R., Mathur, R., Banerjee, A., & Gill, P. (2021). Ethnicity-specific BMI cutoffs for obesity based on type 2 diabetes risk in England: A population-based cohort study. *The Lancet Diabetes & Endocrinology, 9*(7), 419–426. https://doi.org/10.1016/S2213-8587(21)00088-7

Campbell, C., Douglas, A., Williams, L., Cezard, G., Brewster, D. H., Buchanan, D., Robb, K., Stanners, G., Weller, D., Steele, R. J., Steiner, M., & Bhopal, R. (2020). Are there ethnic and religious variations in uptake of bowel cancer screening? A retrospective cohort study among 1.7 million people in Scotland. *BMJ Open, 10*(10), e037011. https://doi.org/10.1136/bmjopen-2020-037011

Cancer UK. (n.d.) *About Cancer*. Retrieved February 10, 2025, from https://www.cancerresearchuk.org/about-cancer/what-is-cancer/how-cancer-starts/types-of-cancer

Canoy, D., & Buchan, I. (2007). Challenges in obesity epidemiology. *Obesity Reviews, 8*(1), 1–11. https://doi.org/10.1111/j.1467-789X.2007.00310.x

Cameron, B. L., Carmargo Plazas, M. P., Salas, A. S., Bourque Bearskin, R. L., & Hungler, K. (2014). Understanding inequalities in access to health care services for aboriginal people: A call for nursing action. *Advances in Nursing Science, 37*(3), E1–E16. https://doi.org/10.1097/ANS.0000000000000039

Caton, S., Chadwick, D., Chapman, M., Turnbull, S., Mitchell, D., & Stansfield, J. (2012). Healthy lifestyles for adults with intellectual disability: Knowledge, barriers, and facilitators. *Journal of Intellectual & Developmental disability, 37*(3), 248–259. https://doi.org/10.3109/13668250.2012.703645

Centers for Disease Control and Prevention (2020). *Hypertension prevalence among adults aged 18 and over: United States, 2017–2018* (NCHS Data Brief No. 364).

National Center for Health Statistics. Retrieved September 25, 2025, from https://www.cdc.gov/nchs/products/databriefs/db364.htm

Centers for Disease Control and Prevention. (2023). *National diabetes statistics report: Estimates of diabetes and its burden in the United States*. Retrieved September 25, 2025, from https://stacks.cdc.gov/view/cdc/148231

Centers for Disease Control and Prevention (2024a). *About women and stroke*. Retrieved September 24, 2025, from https://www.cdc.gov/stroke/about/women-and-stroke.html

Centers for Disease Control and Prevention (2024b). *Heart disease facts*. Retrieved November 25, 2024, from https://www.cdc.gov/heart-disease/data-research/facts-stats/index.html

Centers for Disease Control and Prevention (2025). *Tobacco campaign, American Indian and Alaskan Natives People. Know the facts*. Retrieved February 3, 2025, from https://www.cdc.gov/tobacco/campaign/tips/groups/american-indian-alaska-native.html

Cerin, E., Nathan, A., van Cauwenberg, J., Barnett, D. W., Barnett, A.; Council on Environment and Physical Activity (CEPA) – Older Adults working group (2017). The neighbourhood physical environment and active travel in older adults: A systematic review and meta-analysis. *The International Journal of Behavioral nutrition and physical activity, 14*(1), 15. https://doi.org/10.1186/s12966-017-0471-5

Chen, Y., Zhou, X., Bullard, K. M., Zhang, P., Imperatore, G., & Rolka, D. B. (2023). Income-related inequalities in diagnosed diabetes prevalence among US adults, 2001-2018. *PloS One, 18*(4), e0283450. https://doi.org/10.1371/journal.pone.0283450

Chichlowska, K. L., Rose, K. M., Diez-Roux, A. V., Golden, S. H., McNeill, A. M., & Heiss, G. (2008). Individual and neighborhood socioeconomic status characteristics and prevalence of metabolic syndrome: The Atherosclerosis Risk in Communities (ARIC) Study. *Psychosomatic Medicine, 70*(9), 986–992. https://doi.org/10.1097/PSY.0b013e318183a491

Chopra, S., Lahiff, T. J., Franklin, R., Brown, A., & Rasalam, R. (2022). Effective primary care management of type 2 diabetes for indigenous populations: A systematic review. *PloS One, 17*(11), e0276396. https://doi.org/10.1371/journal.pone.0276396

Churchwell, K., Elkind, M. S. V., Benjamin, R. M., Carson, A. P., Chang, E. K., Lawrence, W., Mills, A., Odom, T. M., Rodriguez, C. J., Rodriguez, F., Sanchez, E., Sharrief, A. Z., Sims, M., Williams, O.; American Heart Association (2020). Call to action: Structural racism as a fundamental driver of health disparities: A Presidential advisory from the American Heart Association. *Circulation, 142*(24), e454–e468. https://doi.org/10.1161/CIR.0000000000000936

Cohen, S., Janicki-Deverts, D., Doyle, W. J., Miller, G. E., Frank, E., Rabin, B. S., & Turner, R. B. (2012). Chronic stress, glucocorticoid receptor resistance, inflammation, and disease risk. *Proceedings of the National Academy of Sciences, 109*(16), 5995–5999. https://doi.org/10.1073/pnas.1118355109

Compher, C. (2006). The nutrition transition in American Indians. *Journal of Transcultural Nursing, 17*(3), 217–223. https://doi.org/10.1177/1043659606288376

Connelly, P. J., Azizi, Z., Alipour, P., Delles, C., Pilote, L., & Raparelli, V. (2021). The importance of gender to understand sex differences in cardiovascular disease. *The Canadian Journal of Cardiology, 37*(5), 699–710. https://doi.org/10.1016/j.cjca.2021.02.005

Cook, W. W., & Medley, D. M. (1954). Proposed hostility and pharisaic-virtue scales for the MMPI. *Journal of Applied Psychology, 38*(6), 414–418. https://doi.org/10.1037/h0060667

Correll-King, W. M., Dusic, E. J., Suen, D., Gamarel, K. E., Shook, A. G., & Restar, A. J. (2025). Healthcare avoidance and delay among trans adults: Associations with mental and behavioral health outcomes. *American Journal of Preventive Medicine, 68*(4), 726–734. https://doi.org/10.1016/j.amepre.2024.12.018

Cosselman, K. E., Navas-Acien, A., & Kaufman, J. D. (2015). Environmental factors in cardiovascular disease. *Nature Reviews Cardiology, 12*(11), 627–642. https://doi.org/10.1038/nrcardio.2015.152

Crowshoe, C. (2005). *Sacred ways of life: Traditional knowledge.* First Nations Centre, National Aboriginal Health Organization. Retrieved September 28, 2025, from https://ruor.uottawa.ca/server/api/core/bitstreams/36033399-56f7-4fbb-b252-1f094f6d69b1/content

Crowshoe, L., Dannenbaum, D., Green, M., Henderson, R., Hayward, M. N., Toth, E.; Diabetes Canada Clinical Practice Guidelines Expert Committee (2018). Type 2 diabetes and Indigenous Peoples. *Canadian Journal of Diabetes, 42*(1), S296–S306. https://doi.org/10.1016/j.jcjd.2017.10.022

Corliss, H. L., VanKim, N. A., Jun, H. J., Austin, S. B., Hong, B., Wang, M., & Hu, F. B. (2018). Risk of type 2 diabetes among lesbian, bisexual, and heterosexual women: Findings from the Nurses' Health Study II. *Diabetes Care, 41*(7), 1448–1454. https://doi.org/10.2337/dc17-2656

Daly, H., Byrne, J., Martin-Stacey, L., Mandalia, P., Carey, M., Hadjiconstantinou, M., Hassanein, M., Mehar, S., Khunti, K., & Davies, M. (2014). 'A Safer Ramadan': Developing an integrated approach to support safer fasting and feasting for people with type 2 diabetes. *Practical Diabetes, 31*, 292–297. https://doi.org/10.1002/pdi.1889

Daniel, H., Butkus, R., & Health and Public Policy Committee of American College of Physicians (2015). Lesbian, gay, bisexual, and transgender health disparities: Executive summary of a policy position paper from the American College of Physicians. *Annals of Internal Medicine, 163*(2), 135–137. https://doi.org/10.7326/M14-2482

Dattani, S., Rodés-Guirao, L., Ritchie, H., Ortiz-Ospina, E., & Roser, M. (2023). *Life Expectancy*. Data adapted from Human Mortality Database, United Nations, Zijdeman et al., James C. Riley. Retrieved February 21, 2025, from https://archive.ourworldindata.org/20260304-094028/grapher/life-expectancy.html

Davies, M. J., Heller, S., Skinner, T. C., Campbell, M. J., Carey, M. E., Cradock, S., Dallosso, H. M., Daly, H., Doherty, Y., Eaton, S., Fox, C., Oliver, L., Rantell, K., Rayman, G., & Khunti, K.; Diabetes Education and Self Management for Ongoing and Newly Diagnosed Collaborative (2008). Effectiveness of the diabetes education and self management for ongoing and newly diagnosed (DESMOND) programme for people with newly diagnosed type 2 diabetes: Cluster randomised controlled trial. *British Medical Journal, 336*(7642), 491–495. https://doi.org/10.1136/bmj.39474.922025.BE

Dawber, T. R., Moore, F. E., & Mann, G. V. (1957). Coronary heart disease in the Framingham study. *American Journal of Public Health and the Nation's Health, 47* (2) 4–24. https://doi.org/10.2105/ajph.47.4_pt_2.4

Delon, C., Brown, K. F., Payne, N. W. S., Kotrotsios, Y., Vernon, S., & Shelton, J. (2022). Differences in cancer incidence by broad ethnic group in England, 2013–2017. *British Journal of Cancer, 126*(12), 1765–1773. https://doi.org/10.1038/s41416-022-01718-5

de Mestral, C., & Stringhini, S. (2017). Socioeconomic status and cardiovascular disease: An update. *Current Cardiology Reports, 19*(11), 115. https://doi.org/10.1007/s11886-017-0917-z

Dempsey, P. C., Larsen, R. N., Dunstan, D. W., Owen, N., & Kingwell, B. A. (2018). Sitting less and moving more: Implications for hypertension. *Hypertension, 72*(5), 1037–1046. https://doi.org/10.1161/HYPERTENSIONAHA.118.11190

Denny, M. C., Rosendale, N., Gonzales, N. R., Leslie-Mazwi, T. M., & Middleton, S. (2024). Addressing disparities in acute stroke management and prognosis.

Journal of the American Heart Association, 13(7), e031313. https://doi.org/10.1161/JAHA.123.031313

Deurenberg, P., Deurenberg-Yap, M., & Guricci, S. (2002). Asians are different from Caucasians and from each other in their body mass index/body fat per cent relationship. *Obesity Reviews, 3*(3), 141–146. http://doi.org/10.1046/j.1467-789x.2002.00065.x

Diaz, M. A., & Rosendale, N. (2023). Exploring stroke risk factors and outcomes in sexual and gender minority people. *Neurology. Clinical Practice, 13*(1), e200106. https://doi.org/10.1212/CPJ.0000000000200106

Di Cesare, M., Perel, P., Taylor, S., Kabudula, C., Bixby, H., Gaziano, T. A., McGhie, D. V., Mwangi, J., Pervan, B., Narula, J., Pineiro, D., & Pinto, F. J. (2024). The heart of the world. *Global Heart, 19*(1), 11. https://doi.org/10.5334/gh.1288

Dieleman, L. A., van Peet, P. G., & Vos, H. M. M. (2021). Gender differences within the barriers to smoking cessation and the preferences for interventions in primary care a qualitative study using focus groups in the Hague, the Netherlands. *British Medical Journal Open, 11*(1), e042623. https://doi.org/10.1136/bmjopen-2020-042623

Dinsa, G. D., Goryakin, Y., Fumagalli, E., & Suhrcke, M. (2012). Obesity and socioeconomic status in developing countries: A systematic review. *Obesity, 13*(11), 1067–1079. https://doi.org/10.1111/j.1467-789X.2012.01017.x

Doll, R., & Hill, A. B. (1950). Smoking and carcinoma of the lung; preliminary report. *British Medical Journal, 2*(4682), 739–748. https://doi.org/10.1136/bmj.2.4682.739

Egeland, G. M., Igland, J., Vollset, S. E., Sulo, G., Eide, G. E., & Tell, G. S. (2016). High population attributable fractions of myocardial infarction associated with waist-hip ratio. *Obesity, 24*(5), 1162–1169. https://doi.org/10.1002/oby.21452

Emamat, H., Jamshidi, A., Farhadi, A., Ghalandari, H., Ghasemi, M., & Tangestani, H. (2024). The association between the visceral to subcutaneous abdominal fat ratio and the risk of cardiovascular diseases: A systematic review. *BMC Public Health, 24*(1), 1827. https://doi.org/10.1186/s12889-024-19358-0

Engen, M., Rømer, M., & Jørgensen, A. S. (2019). Public care for people with intellectual disability in Denmark-Ideals, policy and practice. *Scandinavian Journal of Disability Research, 21*(1), 228–37. https://doi.org/10.16993/sjdr.582

Estupiñán Fdez de Mesa, M., Marcu, A., Ream, E., & Whitaker, K. L. (2025). Understanding and tackling cancer inequities: What opportunities does intersectionality offer researchers, policymakers, and providers? A scoping review. *Journal of Psychosocial Oncology, 43*(1), 105–132. https://doi.org/10.1080/07347332.2024.2361642

Eurostat (2024). *Duration of working life – statistics*. Retrieved September 2, 2025, from https://ec.europa.eu/eurostat/statistics-explained/index.php?title=Duration_of_working_life_-_statistics

Fang, J., Yang, Q., Ayala, C., & Loustalot, F. (2014). Disparities in access to care among US adults with self-reported hypertension. *American Journal of Hypertension, 27*(11), 1377–1386. https://doi.org/10.1093/ajh/hpu061

Farmaki, A. E., Garfield, V., Eastwood, S. V., Farmer, R. E., Mathur, R., Giannakopoulou, O., Patalay, P., Kuchenbaecker, K., Sattar, N., Hughes, A., Bhaskaran, K., Smeeth, L., & Chaturvedi, N. (2022). Type 2 diabetes risks and determinants in second-generation migrants and mixed ethnicity people of South Asian and African Caribbean descent in the UK. *Diabetologia, 65*(1), 113–127. https://doi.org/10.1007/s00125-021-05580-7

Ferdinand, K. C. (2018). Novel interventions in addressing racial disparities in blood pressure control: Potential utilisation of barbershops in Black Men. *Circulation, 138*(4), 339–341. https://doi.org/10.1161/CIRCULATIONAHA.118.034869

Feigin, V. L., Brainin, M., Norrving, B., Martins, S. O., Pandian, J., Lindsay, P., F Grupper, M., & Rautalin, I. (2025). World Stroke Organization: Global stroke fact sheet 2025. *International Journal of Stroke, 20*(2), 132–144. https://doi.org/10.1177/17474930241308142

First Nations Health Authority, Métis Nation British Columbia, BC Association of Aboriginal Friendship Centres, & BC Cancer. (2017). *Improving Indigenous cancer journeys in BC: A road map*. http://www.fnha.ca/wellnessContent/Wellness/improving-indigenous-cancer-journeys-in-bc.pdf

Fletcher, G. F., Landolfo, C., Niebauer, J., Ozemek, C., Arena, R., & Lavie, C. J. (2018). Promoting physical activity and exercise: JACC Health Promotion Series. *Journal of the American College of Cardiology, 72*(14), 1622–1639. https://doi.org/10.1016/j.jacc.2018.08.2141

Fluck, D., Fry, C. H., Gulli, G., Affley, B., Robin, J., Kakar, P., Sharma, P., & Han, T. S. (2023). Adverse stroke outcomes amongst UK ethnic minorities: A multi-centre registry-based cohort study of acute stroke. *Neurological Sciences, 44*(6), 2071–2080. https://doi.org/10.1007/s10072-023-06640-z

Flynn, S., Hulbert-Williams, L., Bramwell, R., Stevens-Gill, D., & Hulbert-Williams, N. (2015). Caring for cancer patients with an intellectual disability: Attitudes and care perceptions of UK oncology nurses. *European Journal of Oncology Nursing, 19*(5), 568–574. https://doi.org/10.1016/j.ejon.2015.03.002

Ford, E. S., Li, C., & Sattar, N. (2008). Metabolic syndrome and incident diabetes: Current state of the evidence. *Diabetes Care, 31*(9), 1898–1904. https://doi.org/10.2337/dc08-0423

Ford, E. S., Croft, J. B., Mannino, D. M., Wheaton, A. G., Zhang, X., & Giles, W. H. (2013). *COPD surveillance–United States, 1999-2011. Chest, 144*(1), 284–305. https://doi.org/10.1378/chest.13-0809

Fox, K. R., & Hillsdon, M. (2007). Physical activity and obesity. *Obesity Reviews, 8*(1), 115–121. https://doi.org/10.1111/j.1467-789X.2007.00329.x

French, S. A., Tangney, C. C., Crane, M. M., Wang, Y., & Appelhans, B. M. (2019). Nutrition quality of food purchases varies by household income: The SHoPPER study. *BMC Public Health, 19*(1), 231. https://doi.org/10.1186/s12889-019-6546-2

Friedman, M., & Rosenman, R. H. (1959). Association of specific overt behavior pattern with blood and cardiovascular findings; blood cholesterol level, blood clotting time, incidence of arcus senilis, and clinical coronary artery disease. *Journal of the American Medical Association, 169*(12), 1286–1296. https://doi.org/10.1001/jama.1959.03000290012005

Gallo, L. C., Troxel, W. M., Matthews, K. A., Jansen-McWilliams, L., Kuller, L. H., & Sutton-Tyrrell, K. (2003). Occupation and subclinical carotid artery disease in women: Are clerical workers at greater risk? *Health Psychology, 22*(1), 19–29. https://doi.org/10.1037/0278-6133.22.1.19

Garland-Forshee, R. Y., Fiala, S. C., Ngo, D. L., & Moseley, K. (2014). Sexual orientation and sex differences in adult chronic conditions, health risk factors, and protective health practices, Oregon, 2005-2008. *Preventing Chronic Disease, 11*, E136. https://doi.org/10.5888/pcd11.140126

Gan, Y., Gong, Y., Tong, X., Sun, H., Cong, Y., Dong, X., Wang, Y., Xu, X., Yin, X., Deng, J., Li, L., Cao, S., & Lu, Z. (2014). Depression and the risk of coronary heart disease: A meta-analysis of prospective cohort studies. *BMC Psychiatry, 14*, 371. https://doi.org/10.1186/s12888-014-0371-z

Ganesh, A., Fraser, J. F., Gordon Perue, G. L., Amin-Hanjani, S., Leslie-Mazwi, T. M., Greenberg, S. M., Couillard, P., Asdaghi, N., Goyal, M.; American Heart Association Stroke Council (2022). Endovascular treatment and thrombolysis for acute ischemic stroke in patients with premorbid disability or dementia: A scientific statement from the American Heart Association/American Stroke Association. *Stroke, 53*(5), e204–e217. https://doi.org/10.1161/STR.0000000000000406

Gasbarrino, K., Di Iorio, D., & Daskalopoulou, S. S. (2022). Importance of sex and gender in ischaemic stroke and carotid atherosclerotic disease. *European Heart Journal, 43*(6), 460–473. https://doi.org/10.1093/eurheartj/ehab756

Gater, D. R. Jr, Farkas, G. J., & Tiozzo, E. (2021). Pathophysiology of neurogenic obesity after spinal cord injury. *Topics in Spinal Cord Injury Rehabilitation, 27*(1), 1–10. https://doi.org/10.46292/sci20-00067

Gee, G., Sheridan, S., Charles, L., Dayne, L., Joyce, L., Stevens, J., Paradies, Y., Hulbert, C., Haslam, N., Thorpe, R., Thorpe, L., Thorpe, A., Stewart, P., Austin, L., Lyons, L., Belfrage, M., Warber, R., Paxton, A., & Thompson, L. (2022). The her tribe and his tribe Aboriginal-designed empowerment programs. *International Journal of Environmental Research and Public Health, 19*(4), 2381. https://doi.org/10.3390/ijerph19042381

Gerber, Y., Weston, S. A., Killian, J. M., Therneau, T. M., Jacobsen, S. J., & Roger, V. L. (2008). Neighborhood income and individual education: Effect on survival after myocardial infarction. *Mayo Clinic Proceedings, 83*(6), 663–669. https://doi.org/10.4065/83.6.663

Gibbons, G. H., Seidman, C. E., & Topol, E. J. (2021). Conquering atherosclerotic cardiovascular disease - 50 years of progress. *The New England Journal of Medicine, 384*(9), 785–788. https://doi.org/10.1056/NEJMp2033115

Go, A. E., Guinaran, R. C., & Dee, E. C. (2025). Closing the cancer care gap: Cancer disparities among Indigenous peoples globally. *The Lancet regional health. Western Pacific, 57*, 101543. https://doi.org/10.1016/j.lanwpc.2025.101543

Goff, L. M. (2019). Ethnicity and Type 2 diabetes in the UK. *Diabetic Medicine, 36*(8), 927–938. https://doi.org/10.1111/dme.13895

Gonzales, G., Przedworski, J., & Henning-Smith, C. (2016). Comparison of health and health risk factors between lesbian, gay, and bisexual adults and heterosexual adults in the United States: Results from the National Health Interview Survey. *JAMA Internal Medicine, 176*(9), 1344–1351. https://doi.org/10.1001/jamainternmed.2016.3432

Hannan, E. L., Racz, M. J., Walford, G., Jacobs, A. K., Stamato, N. J., Gesten, F., Berger, P. B., Sharma, S., & King, S. B. 3rd (2016). Disparities in the use of drug-eluting coronary stents by race, ethnicity, payer, and hospital. *The Canadian Journal of Cardiology, 32*(8), 987.e25–987.e9.87E31. https://doi.org/10.1016/j.cjca.2016.01.012

Harris, R., Nelson, L. A., Muller, C., & Buchwald, D. (2015). Stroke in American Indians and Alaska Natives: A systematic review. *American Journal of Public Health, 105*(8), e16–e26. https://doi.org/10.2105/AJPH.2015.302698

Harrison, S. L., Robertson, N., Apps, L., C Steiner, M., Morgan, M. D., & Singh, S. J. (2015). "We are not worthy" - understanding why patients decline pulmonary rehabilitation following an acute exacerbation of COPD. *Disability and Rehabilitation, 37*(9), 750–756. https://doi.org/10.3109/09638288.2014.939770

Harrop, D. L., Bryce, V., Kitchener, T., Grugan, S., Renouf, S., Mitchell, S., Hasking, G., Pauza, D., Richards, G., Ng, A. C. T., & Wang, W. Y. S. (2024). Effects of a culturally informed model of care for Aboriginal and Torres Strait Islander patients with acute coronary syndrome in a tertiary hospital in Australia: A pre-post, quasi-experimental, interventional study. *The Lancet. Global health, 12*(4), e623–e630. https://doi.org/10.1016/S2214-109X(23)00601-0

Health New Zealand (2025). *Virtual diabetes register and web tool*. Retrieved September 28, 2025, from https://www.tewhatuora.govt.nz/for-health-professionals/data-and-statistics/diabetes/virtual-diabetes-register-web-tool

Health Quality & Safety Commission (2025). Chronic obstructive pulmonary disease in people aged 45 and over. Retrieved 26 September, 2015, from https://www.hqsc.govt.nz/our-data/atlas-of-healthcare-variation/chronic-obstructive-pulmonary-disease/?utm_source

Heckler, M. M. (1985). *The Heckler Report. Report of the Secretary's Task Force on Black and minority health*. Department of Health and Human Services, Office of Minority Health. Retrieved December 19, from, http://archive.org/stream/reportofsecretar00usde#page/n1/mode/2up

Helmers, K. F., Krantz, D. S., Howell, R. H., Klein, J., Bairey, C. N., & Rozanski, A. (1993). Hostility and myocardial ischemia in coronary artery disease patients: Evaluation by gender and ischemic index. *Psychosomatic Medicine, 55*(1), 29–36. https://doi.org/10.1097/00006842-199301000-00006

Heslop, P., Cook, A., Sullivan, B., Calkin, R., Pollard, J., & Byrne, V. (2022). Cancer in deceased adults with intellectual disabilities: English population-based study using linked data from three sources. *British Medical Journal Open, 12*(3), e056974. https://doi.org/10.1136/bmjopen-2021-056974

Higgins, V. (2022). Ethnic density and area-deprivation effects on central obesity among ethnic minority people in England - A cross-sectional, multilevel analysis. *Frontiers in Epidemiology, 2*, 1000155. https://doi.org/10.3389/fepid.2022.1000155

Hoekstra, S., Trbovich, M., Koek, W., Mader, M., & Salehi, M. (2024). The effect of level of injury on diabetes incidence and mortality after spinal cord injury - a longitudinal cohort study. *Spinal Cord, 62*(4), 164–169. https://doi.org/10.1038/s41393-024-00961-2

Horrill, T., McMillan, D. E., Schultz, A. S. H., & Thompson, G. (2018). Understanding access to healthcare among Indigenous peoples: A comparative analysis of biomedical and postcolonial perspectives. *Nursing Inquiry, 25*(3), e12237. https://doi.org/10.1111/nin.12237

Hoyt, M. A., Frost, D. M., Cohn, E., Millar, B. M., Diefenbach, M. A., & Revenson, T. A. (2020). Gay men's experiences with prostate cancer: Implications for future research. *Journal of Health Psychology, 25*(3), 298–310. https://doi.org/10.1177/1359105317711491

Huxley, R. R., & Woodward, M. (2011). Cigarette smoking as a risk factor for coronary heart disease in women compared with men: A systematic review and meta-analysis of prospective cohort studies. *Lancet, 378*(9799), 1297–1305. https://doi.org/10.1016/S0140-6736(11)60781-2

Hyun, K. K., Redfern, J., Patel, A., Peiris, D., Brieger, D., Sullivan, D., Harris, M., Usherwood, T., MacMahon, S., Lyford, M., & Woodward, M. (2017). Gender inequalities in cardiovascular risk factor assessment and management in primary healthcare. *Heart, 103*(7), 492–498. https://doi.org/10.1136/heartjnl-2016-310216

Hyun, K. K., Millett, E. R. C., Redfern, J., Brieger, D., Peters, S. A. E., & Woodward, M. (2019). Sex differences in the assessment of cardiovascular risk in primary health care: A systematic review. *Heart, Lung & Circulation, 28*(10), 1535–1548. https://doi.org/10.1016/j.hlc.2019.04.005

Institute for Health Metrics and Evaluation (IHME). (2020). *Global Burden of Disease compare data visualization*. Retrieved February 10, 2024, from https://vizhub.healthdata.org/gbd-compare/

Institute for Health Metrics and Evaluation (IHME). (2024). *Global Burden of Disease 2021: Findings from the GBD 2021 study*. Retrieved February 10, 2024, from https://www.healthdata.org/research-analysis/library/global-burden-disease-2021-findings-gbd-2021-study

Institute of Medicine (US) Committee on lesbian, gay, bisexual, and transgender health issues and research gaps and opportunities. (2011). *The health of lesbian, gay, bisexual, and transgender people: Building a foundation for better understanding*. Retrieved November 18, 2024, from https://nap.nationalacademies.org/read/13128/chapter/1

Islam, N., Nash, R., Zhang, Q., Panagiotakopoulos, L., Daley, T., Bhasin, S., Getahun, D., Sonya Haw, J., McCracken, C., Silverberg, M. J., Tangpricha, V., Vupputuri, S., & Goodman, M. (2022). Is there a link between hormone use and diabetes incidence in transgender people? Data from the STRONG Cohort. *The Journal of Clinical Endocrinology and Metabolism, 107*(4), e1549–e1557. https://doi.org/10.1210/clinem/dgab832

International Diabetes Federation (IDF). (2025). *IDF diabetes atlas* (11th ed.). Retrieved November 12, 2025, from https://diabetesatlas.org/resources/idf-diabetes-atlas-2025

Jack, R. H., Møller, H., Robson, T., & Davies, E. A. (2014). Breast cancer screening uptake among women from different ethnic groups in London: A population-based cohort study. *British Medical Journal Open, 14*(4), e005586. https://doi.org/10.1136/bmjopen-2014-005586

Jacobs, L., Emmerechts, J., Hoylaerts, M. F., Mathieu, C., Hoet, P. H., Nemery, B., & Nawrot, T. S. (2011). Traffic air pollution and oxidized LDL. *PloS One, 6*(1), e16200. https://doi.org/10.1371/journal.pone.0016200

Jackson, S. E., Brown, J., Grabovac, I., Cheeseman, H., Osborne, C., & Shahab, L. (2021). Smoking and quitting behavior by sexual orientation: A cross-sectional survey of adults in England. *Nicotine & Tobacco, 23*(1), 124–134. https://doi.org/10.1093/ntr/ntaa042

Jemal, A., Sung, H., Kelly, K., Soerjomataram, I., & Bray, F. (Eds.). (2025). *The cancer atlas* (4th ed.). Atlanta, GA: American Cancer Society. Retrieved September 25, 2025, from https://canceratlas.cancer.org/wp-content/uploads/2025/08/ACS_Atlas_Book_Spreads.pdf

Jerpseth, H., Knutsen, I. R., Jensen, K. T., & Halvorsen, K. (2021). Mirror of shame: Patients experiences of late-stage COPD. A qualitative study. *Journal of Clinical Nursing, 30*(19–20), 2854–2862. https://doi.org/10.1111/jocn.15792

Johnson, M. J., Nemeth, L. S., Mueller, M., Eliason, M. J., & Stuart, G. W. (2016). Qualitative study of cervical cancer screening among lesbian and bisexual women and transgender men. *Cancer Nursing, 39*(6), 455–463. https://doi.org/10.1097/NCC.0000000000000338

Johnson, R. L., Roter, D., Powe, N. R., & Cooper, L. A. (2004). Patient race/ethnicity and quality of patient-physician communication during medical visits. *American Journal of Public Health, 94*(12), 2084–2090. https://doi.org/10.2105/ajph.94.12.2084

Kaestner, R., & Xu, X. (2010). Title IX, girls' sports participation, and adult female physical activity and weight. *Evaluation Review, 34*(1), 52–78. https://doi.org/10.1177/0193841X09353539

Kamen, C. S., Alpert, A., Margolies, L., Griggs, J. J., Darbes, L., Smith-Stoner, M., Lytle, M., Poteat, T., Scout, N., & Norton, S. A. (2019). "Treat us with dignity": A qualitative study of the experiences and recommendations of lesbian, gay, bisexual, transgender, and queer (LGBTQ) patients with cancer. *Supportive Care in Cancer, 27*(7), 2525–2532. https://doi.org/10.1007/s00520-018-4535-0

Kamarck, T. W., Shiffman, S., Sutton-Tyrrell, K., Muldoon, M. F., & Tepper, P. (2012). Daily psychological demands are associated with 6-year progression of carotid artery atherosclerosis: The Pittsburgh Healthy Heart Project. *Psychosomatic Medicine, 74*(4), 432–439. https://doi.org/10.1097/PSY.0b013e3182572599

Kamińska, M. S., Schneider-Matyka, D., Rachubińska, K., Panczyk, M., Grochans, E., & Cybulska, A. M. (2023). Menopause predisposes women to increased risk of cardiovascular disease. *Journal of Clinical Medicine, 12*(22), 7058. https://doi.org/10.3390/jcm12227058

Kang, P. S., & Neeland, I. J. (2023). Body fat distribution, diabetes mellitus, and cardiovascular disease: An update. *Current Cardiology Reports, 25*(11), 1555–1564. https://doi.org/10.1007/s11886-023-01969-5

Kett, M., Cole, E., & Turner, J. (2020). Disability, mobility and transport in low- and middle-income countries: A thematic review. *Sustainability, 12*(2), 589. https://doi.org/10.3390/su12020589

Khan, E., Brieger, D., Amerena, J., Atherton, J. J., Chew, D. P., Farshid, A., Ilton, M., Juergens, C. P., Kangaharan, N., Rajaratnam, R., Sweeny, A., Walters, D. L., & Chow, C. K. (2018). Differences in management and outcomes for men and women with ST-elevation myocardial infarction. *The Medical Journal of Australia, 209*(3), 118–123. https://doi.org/10.5694/mja17.01109

Klassen, D., Cheung, W. Y., Letendre, A., Bill, L., Healy, B. A., Rahul, C. R., Kopciuk, K. A., & Yang, H. (2025). Assessing colorectal cancer screening and outcomes among First Nations people in Alberta. *Journal of the Canadian Association of Gastroenterology, 8*(3), 103–111. https://doi.org/10.1093/jcag/gwaf004

Koh, Y., Stehli, J., Martin, C., Brennan, A., Dinh, D. T., Lefkovits, J., & Zaman, S. (2019). Does sex predict quality of life after acute coronary syndromes: An Australian, state-wide, multicentre prospective cohort study. *British Medical Journal Open, 9*(12), e034034. https://doi.org/10.1136/bmjopen-2019-034034

Kroll, D. S., Feldman, D. E., Biesecker, C. L., McPherson, K. L., Manza, P., Joseph, P. V., Volkow, N. D., & Wang, G. J. (2020). Neuroimaging of sex/gender differences in obesity: A review of structure, function, and neurotransmission. *Nutrients, 12*(7), 1942. https://doi.org/10.3390/nu12071942

Kumar, R., Malhotra, P., As, V., Beniwal, K., & Charan, G. S. (2025). Effect of cognitive behavior therapy on abstinence among healthy smokers: A systematic review and meta-analysis of randomized controlled trials. *Osong Public Health and Research Perspectives, 16*(3), 223–235. https://doi.org/10.24171/j.phrp.2025.0019

Kunadian, V. (2024). Advancing the access to cardiovascular diagnosis and treatment among women with cardiovascular disease: A joint British Cardiovascular Societies' consensus document. *Heart, 110*(22), e4. https://doi.org/10.1136/heartjnl-2024-324625

Kyrou, I., Randeva, H. S., Tsigos, C., Kaltsas, G., & Weickert, M. O. (2018). Clinical problems caused by obesity. In K. R. Feingold, B. Anawalt, A. Boyce, G. Chrousos, K. Dungan, A. Grossman, J. Hershman, G. Kaltsas, C. Koch, P. Kopp, M. Korbonits, R. McLachlan, J. Morley, M. New, P. Perreault, J. Purnell, R. Rebar, F. Singer, D. L. Trence, A. Vinik, & D. P. Wilson (Eds.)., *Endotext.* MDText.com, Inc. Retrieved September 27, 2025, from https://www.ncbi.nlm.nih.gov/books/NBK278973/

Kyrou, I., Tsigos, C., Mavrogianni, C., Cardon, G., Van Stappen, V., Latomme, J., Kivelä, J., Wikström, K., Tsochev, K., Nanasi, A., Semanova, C., Mateo-Gallego, R., Lamiquiz-Moneo, I., Dafoulas, G., Timpel, P., Schwarz, P. E. H., Iotova, V., Tankova, T., Makrilakis, K., Manios, Y. ... Feel4Diabetes-study Group (2020). Sociodemographic and lifestyle-related risk factors for identifying vulnerable groups for type 2 diabetes: A narrative review with emphasis on data from Europe. *BMC Endocrine Disorders, 20*(1), 134. https://doi.org/10.1186/s12902-019-0463-3

Lampinen, E. K., Eloranta, A. M., Haapala, E. A., Lindi, V., Väistö, J., Lintu, N., Karjalainen, P., Kukkonen-Harjula, K., Laaksonen, D., & Lakka, T. A. (2017). Physical activity, sedentary behaviour, and socioeconomic status among Finnish girls and boys aged 6-8 years. *European Journal of Sport Science, 17*(4), 462–472. https://doi.org/10.1080/17461391.2017.1294619

Lau, P. W., Lee, A., & Ransdell, L. (2007). Parenting style and cultural influences on overweight children's attraction to physical activity. *Obesity, 15*(9), 2293–2302. https://doi.org/10.1038/oby.2007.272

Lee, K. M., Hunger, J. M., & Tomiyama, A. J. (2021). Weight stigma and health behaviors: Evidence from the Eating in America Study. *International Journal of Obesity, 45*(7), 1499–1509. https://doi.org/10.1038/s41366-021-00814-5

Lelieveld, J., Pozzer, A., Pöschl, U., Fnais, M., Haines, A., & Münzel, T. (2020). Loss of life expectancy from air pollution compared to other risk factors: A worldwide perspective. *Cardiovascular Research, 116,* 1910–1907. https://doi.org/10.1093/cvr/cvaa025

Lewis, M. E., Volpert-Esmond, H. I., Deen, J. F., Modde, E., & Warne, D. (2021). Stress and cardiometabolic disease risk for Indigenous Populations throughout the lifespan. *International Journal of Environmental Research and Public Health, 18*(4), 1821. https://doi.org/10.3390/ijerph18041821

Ley, S. H., Hamdy, O., Mohan, V., & Hu, F. B. (2014). Prevention and management of type 2 diabetes: Dietary components and nutritional strategies. *Lancet, 383*(9933), 999–2007. https://doi.org/10.1016/S0140-6736(14)60613-9

Li, M., Chau, K., Calabresi, K., Wang, Y., Wang, J., Fritz, J., & Tseng, T. S. (2024). The effect of minority stress processes on smoking for lesbian, gay, bisexual, transgender, and queer individuals: A systematic review. *LGBT Health, 11*(8), 583–605. https://doi.org/10.1089/lgbt.2022.0323

Lin, P. Y., Lin, L. P., & Lin, J. D. (2010). Hypertension, hyperglycemia, and hyperlipemia among adolescents with intellectual disabilities. *Research in Developmental Disabilities, 31*(2), 545–550. https://doi.org/10.1016/j.ridd.2009.12.002

Livingstone, K. M., Abbott, G., Ward, J., & Bowe, S. J. (2021). Unhealthy lifestyle, genetics and risk of cardiovascular disease and mortality in 76,958 individuals from the UK Biobank Cohort Study. *Nutrients, 13*(12), 4283. https://doi.org/10.3390/nu13124283

Lukowski, A. V., Morris, C., Young, S. E., & Tinkelman, D. (2017). Characteristics of LGBT Quitline callers across 14 States. *Journal of Smoking Cessation, 12*(4), 183–189. https://doi.org/10.1017/jsc.2016.18

Luque, J. S., Ross, L., & Gwede, C. K. (2014). Qualitative systematic review of barber-administered health education, promotion, screening and outreach programs in African-American communities. *Journal of Community Health, 39*(1), 181–190. https://doi.org/10.1007/s10900-013-9744-3

Maas, A. H. E. M., Rosano, G., Cifkova, R., Chieffo, A., van Dijken, D., Hamoda, H., Kunadian, V., Laan, E., Lambrinoudaki, I., Maclaran, K., Panay, N., Stevenson, J. C., van Trotsenburg, M., & Collins, P. (2021). Cardiovascular health after menopause transition, pregnancy disorders, and other gynaecologic conditions: A consensus document from European cardiologists, gynaecologists, and endocrinologists. *European Heart Journal, 42*(10), 967–984. https://doi.org/10.1093/eurheartj/ehaa1044

Mackenbach, J. P., Cavelaars, A. E., Kunst, A. E., & Groenhof, F. (2000). Socioeconomic inequalities in cardiovascular disease mortality. An international study. *European Heart Journal, 21*(14), 1141–1151. https://doi.org/10.1053/euhj.1999.1990

Maricar, N., Khan, B., David, T., Hyrich, K. L., & Barton, A. (2024). Factors facilitating and hindering South Asian immigrant adults from engaging in exercise and physical activity - A qualitative systematic review. *BMC Public Health, 24*(1), 1342. https://doi.org/10.1186/s12889-024-18288-1

Marlow, L. A., Waller, J., & Wardle, J. (2015). Barriers to cervical cancer screening among ethnic minority women: A qualitative study. *The Journal of Family Planning and Reproductive Healthcare, 41*(4), 248–254. https://doi.org/10.1136/jfprhc-2014-101082

Matthews, A. K., Cesario, J., Ruiz, R., Ross, N., & King, A. (2017). A qualitative study of the barriers to and facilitators of smoking cessation among lesbian, gay, bisexual, and transgender smokers who are interested in quitting. *LGBT Health, 4*(1), 24–33. https://doi.org/10.1089/lgbt.2016.0059

McCowan, C., McSkimming, P., Papworth, R., Kotzur, M., McConnachie, A., Macdonald, S., Wyke, S., Crighton, E., Campbell, C., Weller, D., Steele, R. J. C., & Robb, K. A. (2019). Comparing uptake across breast, cervical and bowel screening at an individual level: A retrospective cohort study. *British Journal of Cancer, 121*(8), 710–714. https://doi.org/10.1038/s41416-019-0564-9

McElroy, J. A., Everett, K. D., & Zaniletti, I. (2011). An examination of smoking behavior and opinions about smoke-free environments in a large sample of sexual and gender minority community members. *Nicotine & Tobacco Research, 13*(6), 440–448. https://doi.org/10.1093/ntr/ntr021

Meeks, K. A., Freitas-Da-Silva, D., Adeyemo, A., Beune, E. J., Modesti, P. A., Stronks, K., Zafarmand, M. H., & Agyemang, C. (2016). Disparities in type 2 diabetes prevalence among ethnic minority groups resident in Europe: A systematic review and meta-analysis. *Internal and Emergency Medicine, 11*(3), 327–340. https://doi.org/10.1007/s11739-015-1302-9

Meyer, I. H. (2003). Prejudice, social stress, and mental health in lesbian, gay, and bisexual populations: Conceptual issues and research evidence. *Psychological Bulletin, 129*(5), 674–697. https://doi.org/10.1037/0033-2909.129.5.674

Minichiello, A., Lefkowitz, A. R., Firestone, M., Smylie, J. K., & Schwartz, R. (2016). Effective strategies to reduce commercial tobacco use in Indigenous communities globally: A systematic review. *BMC Public Health, 16,* 21. https://doi.org/10.1186/s12889-015-2645-x

Mitra, M., Long-Bellil, L., Moura, I., Miles, A., & Kaye, H. S. (2022). Advancing health equity and reducing health disparities for people with disabilities in the United States. *Health affairs (Project Hope), 41*(10), 1379–1386. https://doi.org/10.1377/hlthaff.2022.00499

Moore, S. P., Antoni, S., Colquhoun, A., Healy, B., Ellison-Loschmann, L., Potter, J. D., Garvey, G., & Bray, F. (2015). Cancer incidence in indigenous people in Australia, New Zealand, Canada, and the USA: A comparative population-based study. *The Lancet. Oncology, 16*(15), 1483–1492. https://doi.org/10.1016/S1470-2045(15)00232-6

Montero, A., Hamel, L., Artiga, S., & Dawson, L. (2024). LGBT adults' experiences with discrimination and health care disparities: Findings from the KFF survey of racism, discrimination and health. Retrieved September 23, 2025, from https://www.kff.org/racial-equity-and-health-policy/lgbt-adults-experiences-with-discrimination-and-health-care-disparities-findings-from-the-kff-survey-of-racism-discrimination-and-health/#58056b5a-162b-494b-a376-ca11faacc93c

Morris, J. N., Heady, J. A., Raffle, P. A., Roberts, C. G., & Parks, J. W. (1953). Coronary heart-disease and physical activity of work. *Lancet, 262*(6795), 1053–1057. https://doi.org/10.1016/s0140-6736(53)90665-5

Mosca, L., Hammond, G., Mochari-Greenberger, H., Towfighi, A., & Albert, M. A. (2013). Fifteen-year trends in awareness of heart disease in women: Results of a 2012 American Heart Association national survey. *Circulation, 127*(11), 1254–e29. https://doi.org/10.1161/CIR.0b013e318287cf2f

Münzel, T., Hahad, O., Sørensen, M., Lelieveld, J., Duerr, G. D., Nieuwenhuijsen, M., & Daiber, A. (2022). Environmental risk factors and cardiovascular diseases: A comprehensive expert review. *Cardiovascular Research, 118*(14), 2880–2902. https://doi.org/10.1093/cvr/cvab316

Münzel, T., Sørensen, M., Hahad, O., Nieuwenhuijsen, M., & Daiber, A. (2023). The contribution of the exposome to the burden of cardiovascular disease. *Nature Reviews Cardiology, 20,* 651–69. https://doi.org/10.1038/s41569-023-00873-3

Naik, S., Naik, S., Kutty, G., Tareen, T. K., Kolikonda, M., Remmel, K., & Liu, W. (2020). Cardiovascular events in LGBT (lesbian, gay, bisexual, transgender): An overlooked disparity and a call to action (2704). *Neurology, 94*(15). https://doi.org/10.1212/WNL.94.15_supplement.2704

Narayan, K. M., Hoskin, M., Kozak, D., Kriska, A. M., Hanson, R. L., Pettitt, D. J., Nagi, D. K., Bennett, P. H., & Knowler, W. C. (1998). Randomized clinical trial of lifestyle interventions in Pima Indians: A pilot study. *Diabetic Medicine, 15*(1), 66–72. https://doi.org/10.1002/(SICI)1096-9136(199801)15:1<66::AID-DIA515>3.0.CO;2-A

National Center for Health Statistics (n.d). *FastStats: Health of Black or African American non-Hispanic population.* U.S. Department of Health and Human Services. Retrieved September 24, 2025, from https://www.cdc.gov/nchs/fastats/black-health.htm

National Health Service Digital (2016). *Health and care of people with learning disabilities 2014-15.* Retrieved September 25, 2025, from http://webarchive.nationalarchives.gov.uk/ukgwa/20171011011112tf_/http://content.digital.nhs.uk/catalogue/PUB22607/Health-care-learning-disabilities-2014-15-summary.pdf

National Health Service Digital (2022). *Health and care of people with learning disabilities, experimental statistics 2021-2022: Cancer screening*. Retrieved September 25, 2025, from https://digital.nhs.uk/data-and-information/publications/statistical/health-and-care-of-people-with-learning-disabilities/experimental-statistics-2021-to-2022/cancer-screening

National Health Service (2023). *Causes chronic obstructive pulmonary disease*. Retrieved September 25, from, https://www.nhs.uk/conditions/chronic-obstructive-pulmonary-disease-copd/causes/?utm_source

National Health Service England (2024). *Cervical screening programme England, 2023 -2024*. Retrieved February 10, 2025, from https://digital.nhs.uk/data-and-information/publications/statistical/cervical-screening-annual/england-2023-24#chapter-index

National Institute for Health and Care Excellence (2025a). *CVD risk assessment and management: What are the risk factors?* Retrieved September 22, 2025, from https://www.nice.org.uk/guidance/ng238

National Institute for Health and Care Excellence (2025b). *Benefits of stopping smoking*. Retrieved September 26, 2025, from https://cks.nice.org.uk/topics/smoking-cessation/background-information/benefits-of-stopping-smoking/

National Institute for Health and Care Research (2022). Are you at risk of diabetes? Research finds prevention should start at a different BMI for each ethnic group. Retrieved February 25, 2024, from https://evidence.nihr.ac.uk/alert/diabetes-prevention-should-start-at-different-bmi-for-each-ethnic-group/

Newlin Lew, K., Dorsen, C., & Long, T. (2018). Prevalence of obesity, prediabetes, and diabetes in sexual minority men: Results from the 2014 Behavioral Risk Factor Surveillance System. *The Diabetes Educator, 44*(1), 83–93. https://doi.org/10.1177/0145721717749943

O'Connor, D. B., Jones, F., Conner, M., McMillan, B., & Ferguson, E. (2008). Effects of daily hassles and eating style on eating behavior. *Health Psychology, 27*(1), S20–S31. https://doi.org/10.1037/0278-6133.27.1.S20

Office of Disease Prevention and Health Promotion. (2021). *Reduce current cigarette smoking in adults - TU-02 (2020 data)*. Healthy People 2030. U.S. Department of Health and Human Services. Retrieved September 27, 2025, from https://health.gov/healthypeople/objectives-and-data/browse-objectives/tobacco-use/reduce-current-cigarette-smoking-adults-tu-02/data?disparities=on&from=2020&group=Race%2FEthnicity&tab=data-table&to=2020

Office for Economic Co-operation and Development (2019). *The heavy burden of obesity: The economics of prevention* (OECD Health Policy Studies). OECD Publishing. https://doi.org/10.1787/67450d67-en

Office for Health Improvement and Disparities. (2025). *Diabetes profile: Statistical commentary, March 2025*. Retrieved September 28, 2025, from https://www.gov.uk/government/statistics/diabetes-profile-update-march-2025/diabetes-profile-statistical-commentary-march-2025

Office for National Statistics. (2021). Mortality from leading causes of death by ethnic group, England and Wales: 2017-2019. Retrieved February 9, 2025, from https://www.ons.gov.uk/peoplepopulationandcommunity/birthsdeathsandmarriages/deaths/articles/mortalityfromleadingcausesofdeathbyethnicgroupenglandandwales/2012to2019#mortality-from-leading-causes-of-death-2012-to-2019

Office for National Statistics (2023). *Inequalities in mortality involving common physical health conditions, England: 21 March to 31 January 2023*. Retrieved November 27, 2024, from https://www.ons.gov.uk/peoplepopulationandcommunity/healthandsocialcare/healthinequalities/bulletins/inequalitiesinmortalityinvolvingcommonphysicalhealthconditionsengland/21march2021to31january2023

Office of the Surgeon General (US), & Office on Smoking and Health (US) (2004). *The health consequences of smoking: A report of the surgeon general*. Centers for Disease Control and Prevention (US). Retrieved September 27, 2025, from https://www.ncbi.nlm.nih.gov/books/NBK44695/pdf/Bookshelf_NBK44695.pdf

Ogunmoroti, O., Osibogun, O., Allen, N. B., Okunrintemi, V., Commodore-Mensah, Y., Shah, A. J., & Michos, E. D. (2024). Work-related stress is associated with unfavorable cardiovascular health: The multi-ethnic Study of atherosclerosis. *Journal of the American Heart Association, 13*(22), e035824. https://doi.org/10.1161/JAHA.124.035824

Okwuosa, I. S., Lewsey, S. C., Adesiyun, T., Blumenthal, R. S., & Yancy, C. W. (2016). Worldwide disparities in cardiovascular disease: Challenges and solutions. *International Journal of Cardiology, 202,* 433–440. https://doi.org/10.1016/j.ijcard.2015.08.172

Onagbiye, S., Guddemi, A., Baruwa, O. J., Alberti, F., Odone, A., Ricci, H., Gaeta, M., Schmid, D., & Ricci, C. (2024). Association of sedentary time with risk of cardiovascular diseases and cardiovascular mortality: A systematic review and meta-analysis of prospective cohort studies. *Preventive Medicine, 179,* 107812. https://doi.org/10.1016/j.ypmed.2023.107812

Onat, A., Avci, G. S., Barlan, M. M., Uyarel, H., Uzunlar, B., & Sansoy, V. (2004). Measures of abdominal obesity assessed for visceral adiposity and relation to coronary risk. *International Journal of Obesity and Related Metabolic, 28*(8), 1018–1025. https://doi.org/10.1038/sj.ijo.0802695

O'Neil, A., Scovelle, A. J., Milner, A. J., & Kavanagh, A. (2018). Gender/sex as a social determinant of cardiovascular risk. *Circulation, 137*(8), 854–864. https://doi.org/10.1161/CIRCULATIONAHA.117.028595

Ospina, M. B., Voaklander, D., Senthilselvan, A., Stickland, M. K., King, M., Harris, A. W., & Rowe, B. H. (2015). Incidence and prevalence of chronic obstructive pulmonary disease among aboriginal peoples in Alberta, Canada. *PloS One, 10*(4), e0123204. https://doi.org/10.1371/journal.pone.0123204

Ossoli, A., Cetti, F., & Gomaraschi, M. (2023). Air pollution: Another threat to HDL function. *International Journal of Molecular Sciences, 24*(1), 317. https://doi.org/10.3390/ijms24010317

Ostchega, Y., Fryar, C. D., Nwankwo, T., & Nguyen, D. T. (2020). Hypertension prevalence among adults aged 18 and over: United States, 2017–2018. *NCHS Data Brief,* (364), 1–8. https://www.cdc.gov/nchs/data/databriefs/db364-h.pdf

O'Sullivan, J. L., Alonso-Perez, E., Färber, F., Fuellen, G., Rudolf, H., Heisig, J. P., Kreyenfeld, M., & Gellert, P. (2024). Onset of Type 2 diabetes in adults aged 50 and older in Europe: An intersectional multilevel analysis of individual heterogeneity and discriminatory accuracy. *Diabetology & Metabolic Syndrome, 16*(1), 291. https://doi.org/10.1186/s13098-024-01533-3

Patel, N. A., Kianoush, S., Jia, X., Nambi, V., Koh, S., Patel, J., Saeed, A., Ahmed, A. I., Al-Mallah, M., Agarwala, A., Virani, S. S., & Al Rifai, M. (2022). Racial/ethnic disparities and determinants of sufficient physical activity levels. *Kansas Journal of Medicine, 15*(2), 267–272. https://doi.org/10.17161/kjm.vol15.17592

Pati, S., Irfan, W., Jameel, A., Ahmed, S., & Shahid, R. K. (2023). Obesity and cancer: A current overview of epidemiology, pathogenesis, outcomes, and management. *Cancers, 15*(2), 485. https://doi.org/10.3390/cancers15020485

Peters, K., & Cotton, A. (2016). Environmental, structural and process barriers in breast cancer screening for women with physical disability: A qualitative study. *Radiography,* 22 (93): e184–e189. https://doi.org/10.1016/j.radi.2016.03.005

Peters, S. A., Huxley, R. R., & Woodward, M. (2014). Diabetes as risk factor for incident coronary heart disease in women compared with men: A systematic review and meta-analysis of 64 cohorts including 858,507 individuals and 28,203 coronary events. *Diabetologia, 57*(8), 1542–1551. https://doi.org/10.1007/s00125-014-3260-6

Pleasants, R. A., Riley, I. L., & Mannino, D. M. (2016). Defining and targeting health disparities in chronic obstructive pulmonary disease. *International Journal of Chronic Obstructive Pulmonary Disease, 11*, 2475–2496. https://doi.org/10.2147/COPD.S79077

Popescu, I., Nallamothu, B. K., Vaughan-Sarrazin, M. S., & Cram, P. (2010). Racial differences in admissions to high-quality hospitals for coronary heart disease. *Archives of Internal Medicine, 170*(14), 1209–1215. https://doi.org/10.1001/archinternmed.2010.227

Poteat, T. C., Adams, M. A., Malone, J., Geffen, S., Greene, N., Nodzenski, M., Lockhart, A. G., Su, I. H., & Dean, L. T. (2021). Delays in breast cancer care by race and sexual orientation: Results from a national survey with diverse women in the United States. *Cancer, 127*(19), 3514–3522. https://doi.org/10.1002/cncr.33629

Praeger, R., Roxburgh, A., Passey, M., & Mooney-Somers, J. (2019). The prevalence and factors associated with smoking among lesbian and bisexual women: Analysis of the Australian National Drug Strategy Household Survey. *The International Journal on Drug Policy, 70*, 54–60. https://doi.org/10.1016/j.drugpo.2019.03.028

Public Health Agency of Canada. (2018). *Key health inequalities in Canada: A national portrait.* Retrieved September 27, 2025, from https://www.canada.ca/en/public-health/services/publications/science-research-data/inequalities-smoking-infographic.html

Public Health England (2017). *Health matters: Making cervical screening more accessible.* Retrieved September 24, 2025, from https://www.gov.uk/government/publications/health-matters-making-cervical-screening-more-accessible/health-matters-making-cervical-screening-more-accessible–2

Rajagopalan, S., & Landrigan, P. J. (2021). Pollution and the heart. *The New England Journal of Medicine, 385*(20), 1881–1892. https://doi.org/10.1056/NEJMra2030281

Releford, B. J., Frencher, S. K. Jr, & Yancey, A. K. (2010). Health promotion in barbershops: Balancing outreach and research in African American communities. *Ethnicity & Disease, 20*(2), 185–188.

Renshaw, C., Jack, R. H., Dixon, S., Møller, H., & Davis, E. A. (2010). Estimating attendance for breast cancer screening in ethnic groups in London. *BMC Public Health, 10*, 157. https://doi.org/10.1186/1471-2458-10-157

Riekert, K. A., Ockene, J. K., & Pbert, L. (Eds.). (2013). *The handbook of health behaviour change* (4th ed.). Springer Publishing Company.

Robb, K., Stubbings, S., Ramirez, A., Macleod, U., Austoker, J., Waller, J., Hiom, S., & Wardle, J. (2009). Public awareness of cancer in Britain: A population-based survey of adults. *British Journal of Cancer, 101*(S2), S18–S23. https://doi.org/10.1038/sj.bjc.6605386

Robinson, J. P., Espelage, D. L., & Rivers, I. (2013). Developmental trends in peer victimization and emotional distress in LGB and heterosexual youth. *Pediatrics, 131*(3), 423–430. https://doi.org/10.1542/peds.2012-2595

Romo-Stuppy, K., & Maddox, R. (2023). International day of the world's Indigenous Peoples. Action on smoking and health. Retrieved December 03, 2024, from https://ash.org/international-day-of-the-worlds-Indigenous-peoples-2023/

Rosengren, A., Hawken, S., Ounpuu, S., Sliwa, K., Zubaid, M., Almahmeed, W. A., Blackett, K. N., Sitthi-Amorn, C., Sato, H., Yusuf, S., & INTERHEART investigators (2004). Association of psychosocial risk factors with risk of acute myocardial infarction in 11119 cases and 13648 controls from 52 countries (the INTERHEART study): Case-control study. *Lancet, 364*(9438), 953–962. https://doi.org/10.1016/S0140-6736(04)17019-0

Ross, E., Maguire, A., & Donnelly, M. (2019). Disability as a predictor of breast cancer screening uptake: A population-based study of 57,328 women. *Journal of Medical Screening, 27*(4), 194–200. https://doi.org/10.1177/0969141319888553

Santos, A. D., Mohr, K., Jude, M., Simon, N. G., Parsons, M., Eades, S., Burchill, L., Davis, S., Donnan, G., Churliov, L., & Delcourt, C. (2022). Prospective analysis of stroke recognition, stroke risk factors, thrombolysis rates and outcomes in Indigenous Australians from a large rural referral hospital. *Internal Medicine Journal, 52*(3), 468–473. https://doi.org/10.1111/imj.15080

Santos, A. D., Balabanski, A. H., Katzenellenbogen, J. M., Thrift, A. G., Burchill, L., & Parsons, M. W. (2021). A narrative review of stroke incidence, risk factors and treatment in Indigenous Peoples of the world. *Vessel Plus, 5,* 21. https://doi.org/10.20517/2574-1209.2020.69

Sawan, M. A., Steinberg, R. S., Sayegh, M. N., Devlin, C., Behbahani-Nejad, O., & Wenger, N. K. (2023). Chest pain in women: Gender- and sex-based differences in the presentation and diagnosis of heart disease. *US Cardiology, 17,* e19. https://doi.org/10.15420/usc.2022.30

Schafte, K., & Bruna, S. (2023). The influence of intergenerational trauma on epigenetics and obesity in Indigenous populations - A scoping review. *Epigenetics, 18*(1), 2260218. https://doi.org/10.1080/15592294.2023.2260218

Schulte, K. J., & Mayrovitz, H. N. (2023). Myocardial infarction signs and symptoms: Females vs. males. *Cureus, 15*(4), e37522. https://doi.org/10.7759/cureus.37522

Schwappach, D. L. B. (2009). *Queer Quit:* Gay smokers' perspectives on a culturally specific smoking cessation service. *Health Expectations, 12,* 383–395. https://doi.org/10.1111/j.1369-7625.2009.00550.x

Sells, M. L., Blum, E., Perry, G. S., Eke, P., & Presley-Cantrell, L. (2023). Excess burden of poverty and hypertension, by race and ethnicity, on the prevalence of cardiovascular disease. *Preventing Chronic Disease, 20,* E109. https://doi.org/10.5888/pcd20.230065

Seneviratne, S., Campbell, I., Scott, N., Coles, C., & Lawrenson, R. (2015). Treatment delay for Māori women with breast cancer in New Zealand. *Ethnicity & Health, 20*(2), 178–193. https://doi.org/10.1080/13557858.2014.895976

Seshadri, S., Beiser, A., Kelly-Hayes, M., Kase, C. S., Au, R., Kannel, W. B., & Wolf, P. A. (2006). The lifetime risk of stroke: Estimates from the Framingham Study. *Stroke, 37*(2), 345–350. https://doi.org/10.1161/01.STR.0000199613.38911.b2

Shahab, L., Brown, J., Hagger-Johnson, G., Michie, S., Semlyen, J., & West, R. (2017). Sexual orientation identity and tobacco and hazardous alcohol use: Findings from a cross-sectional English population survey. *British Medical Journal Open, 7*(10), e015058. http://dx.doi.org/10.1136/bmjopen-2016-015058

Sherman, J., Dyar, C., McDaniel, J., Funderburg, N. T., Rose, K. M., Gorr, M., & Morgan, E. (2022). Sexual minorities are at elevated risk of cardiovascular disease from a younger age than heterosexuals. *Journal of Behavioral Medicine, 45*(4), 571–579. https://doi.org/10.1007/s10865-021-00269-z

Shi, X., Zheng, Y., Cui, H., Zhang, Y., & Jiang, M. (2022). Exposure to outdoor and indoor air pollution and risk of overweight and obesity across different life periods: A review. *Ecotoxicology and Environmental Safety, 242,* 113893. https://doi.org/10.1016/j.ecoenv.2022.113893

Shimbo, D., Cohen, M. T., McGoldrick, M., Ensari, I., Diaz, K. M., Fu, J., Duran, A. T., Zhao, S., Suls, J. M., Burg, M. M., & Chaplin, W. F. (2024). Translational research of the acute effects of negative emotions on vascular endothelial health: Findings from a randomized controlled study. *Journal of the American Heart Association, 13*(9), e032698. https://doi.org/10.1161/JAHA.123.032698

Shires, D. A., Kattari, L., Hosea, F., Hirsch, J., Mulvaney, M., Matthews, A. K., & Thompson, H. S. (2025). Healthcare experiences among Black and White sexual and gender minority cancer survivors: A qualitative study. *Journal of Cancer Survivorship, 19*(3), 779–788. https://doi.org/10.1007/s11764-023-01504-z

Sidahmed, S., Geyer, S., & Beller, J. (2025). Socioeconomic inequalities in diabetes prevalence in Europe. *SAGE Open,* 15(1). https://doi.org/10.1177/21582440251316478

Siegman, A. W., & Smith, T. W. (Eds.). (1994). *Anger, hostility, and the heart*. Lawrence Erlbaum Associates, Inc.

Siegman, A. W., & Snow, S. C. (1997). The outward expression of anger, the inward experience of anger and CVR: The role of vocal expression. *Journal of Behavioral Medicine, 20*(1), 29–45. https://doi.org/10.1023/a:1025535129121

Smith, D. L. Jr, & Yarar-Fisher, C. (2016). Contributors to metabolic disease risk following spinal cord injury. *Current Physical Medicine and Rehabilitation Reports, 4*(3), 190–199. https://doi.org/10.1007/s40141-016-0124-7

Soria, R., Legido, A., Escolano, C., López Yeste, A., & Montoya, J. (2006). A randomised controlled trial of motivational interviewing for smoking cessation. *The British Journal of General Practice, 56*(531), 768–774.

Spielman, R. M., Jenkins, W. J., Lovett, M. D., Aruguete, M., Bryant, L., Chappell, B., Dumper, K., Lacombe, A., Lazzara, J., McClain, T., Oswald, B. B., Perimutter, M., & Thomas, M. D. (2020). Stress and illness. In *Psychology 2e* (p. 14.3). OpenStax. Retrieved September 27, 2025, from https://openstax.org/books/psychology-2e/pages/14-3-stress-and-illness#CNX_Psych_14_03_Symptoms

Sport England. (2024). *Active Lives Adult Survey: November 2023–24* Retrieved September 24, 2025, from https://www.sportengland.org/research-and-data/data/active-lives/active-lives-data-tables

Sprung, M. R., Faulkner, L. M. D., Evans, M. K., Zonderman, A. B., & Waldstein, S. R. (2019). Neighborhood crime is differentially associated with cardiovascular risk factors as a function of race and sex. *Journal of Public Health Research, 8*(3), 1643. https://doi.org/10.4081/jphr.2019.1643

Stead, L. F., Koilpillai, P., Fanshawe, T. R., & Lancaster, T. (2016). Combined pharmacotherapy and behavioural interventions for smoking cessation. *The Cochrane Database of Systematic Reviews, 3*(3), CD008286. https://doi.org/10.1002/14651858.CD008286.pub3

Stehli, J., Martin, C., Brennan, A., Dinh, D. T., Lefkovits, J., & Zaman, S. (2019). Sex differences persist in time to presentation, revascularization, and mortality in myocardial infarction treated with percutaneous coronary intervention. *Journal of the American Heart Association, 8*(10), e012161. https://doi.org/10.1161/JAHA.119.012161

Stone, M. A., Patel, N., Daly, H., Martin-Stacey, L., Amin, S., Carey, M., Khunti, K., & Davies, M. J. (2008). Using qualitative research methods to inform the development of a modified version of a patient education module for non-English speakers with type 2 diabetes: Experience from an action research project in two South Asian populations in the UK. *Diversity in Health and Social Care, 5*(3), 7–15.

Stringhini, S., Zaninotto, P., Kumari, M., Kivimäki, M., & Batty, G. D. (2016). Lifecourse socioeconomic status and type 2 diabetes: The role of chronic inflammation in the English Longitudinal Study of Ageing. *Scientific Reports, 6*, 24780. https://doi.org/10.1038/srep24780

Suarez, E. C., Kuhn, C. M., Schanberg, S. M., Williams, R. B. Jr, & Zimmermann, E. A. (1998). Neuroendocrine, cardiovascular, and emotional responses of hostile men: The role of interpersonal challenge. *Psychosomatic Medicine, 60*(1), 78–88. https://doi.org/10.1097/00006842-199801000-00017

Swinburn, B., & Egger, G. (2002). Preventive strategies against weight gain and obesity. *Obesity Reviews, 3*(4), 289–301. https://doi.org/10.1046/j.1467-789x.2002.00082.x

Syed, S. T., Gerber, B. S., & Sharp, L. K. (2013). Traveling towards disease: Transportation barriers to health care access. *Journal of Community Health, 38*(5), 976–993. https://doi.org/10.1007/s10900-013-9681-1

Tambalis, K. D., Panagiotakos, D. B., Psarra, G., & Sidossis, L. S. (2020). Screen time and its effect on dietary habits and lifestyle among schoolchildren. *Central European Journal of Public Health, 28*(4), 260–266. https://doi.org/10.21101/cejph.a6097

Tayal, U., Pompei, G., Wilkinson, I., Adamson, D., Sinha, A., Hildick-Smith, D., Cubbon, R., Garbi, M., Ingram, T. E., Colebourn, C. L., Camm, C. F., Guzik, T. J.,

Anderson, L., Page, S. P., Wicks, E., Jenkins, P., Rosen, S. D., Eftychiou, S., Roberts, E., Eftekhari, H., & Kunadian, V. (2024). Advancing the access to cardiovascular diagnosis and treatment among women with cardiovascular disease: A joint British Cardiovascular Societies' consensus document. *Heart, 110*(22), e4. https://doi.org/10.1136/heartjnl-2024-324625

Thurber, K. A., Banks, E., Joshy, G., Soga, K., Marmor, A., Benton, G., White, S. L., Eades, S., Maddox, R., Calma, T., & Lovett, R. (2021). Tobacco smoking and mortality among Aboriginal and Torres Strait Islander adults in Australia. *International Journal of Epidemiology, 50*(3), 942–954. https://doi.org/10.1093/ije/dyaa274

Tiedeman, C., Suthers, B., Julien, B., Hackett, A., & Oakley, P. (2019). Management of stroke in the Australian Indigenous population: From hospitals to communities. *Internal Medicine Journal, 49*(8), 962–968. https://doi.org/10.1111/imj.14303

Tobb, K., Kocher, M., & Bullock-Palmer, R. P. (2022). Underrepresentation of women in cardiovascular trials - It is time to shatter this glass ceiling. *Cardiology Research and Practice, 13,* 100109. https://doi.org/10.1016/j.ahjo.2022.100109

Tomiyama A. J. (2014). Weight stigma is stressful. A review of evidence for the Cyclic Obesity/Weight-Based Stigma model. *Appetite, 82,* 8–15. https://doi.org/10.1016/j.appet.2014.06.108

Trayhurn, P. (2007). Adipocyte biology. *Obesity, 8*(1), 41–44. https://doi.org/10.1111/j.1467-789X.2007.00316.x

Tsao, C. W., Aday, A. W., Almarzooq, Z. I., Anderson, C. A. M., Arora, P., Avery, C. L., Baker-Smith, C. M., Beaton, A. Z., Boehme, A. K., Buxton, A. E., Commodore-Mensah, Y., Elkind, M. S. V., Evenson, K. R., Eze-Nliam, C., Fugar, S., Generoso, G., Heard, D. G., Hiremath, S., Ho, J. E., Kalani, R. ... American Heart Association Council on Epidemiology and Prevention Statistics Committee and Stroke Statistics Subcommittee (2023). *Heart disease and stroke statistics-2023 update: A report from the American Heart Association. Circulation, 147*(8), e93–e621. https://doi.org/10.1161/CIR.0000000000001123

Tuffrey-Wijne, I., & Davies, J. (2007). This is my story: I've got cancer. *British Journal of Learning Disabilities, 35,* 7–11. https://doi.org/10.1111/j.1468-3156.2006.00421.x

Tuffrey-Wijne, I., Bernal, J., Hubert, J., Butler, G., & Hollins, S. (2009). People with learning disabilities who have cancer: An ethnographic study. *The British Journal of General Practice, 59*(564), 503–509. https://doi.org/10.3399/bjgp09X453413

US Bureau Labor Statistics (2023). *BLS Reports: Labor force statistics by race and ethnicity 2022.* Retrieved December 12, 2024, from https://www.bls.gov/opub/reports/race-and-ethnicity/2022/

U.S. Department of Health and Human Services, Office of Minority Health. (2021). *Heart disease and Hispanic Americans.* Retrieved September 27, 2025, from https://minorityhealth.hhs.gov/heart-disease-and-hispanic-americans/

Vaccarella, S., Lortet-Tieulent, J., Saracci, R., Conway, D. I., Straif, K., & Wild, C. P. (Eds.). (2019). *Reducing social inequalities in cancer: Evidence and priorities for research.* International Agency for Research on Cancer. Retrieved September 27, 2025, from https://publications.iarc.who.int/Book-And-Report-Series/Iarc-Scientific-Publications/Reducing-Social-Inequalities-In-Cancer-Evidence-And-Priorities-For-Research-2019

Valentelyte, G., Holman, N., James, S., Clarke, N., Bhatia, D., Bennett, K., Sorensen, J., & Gregg, E. W. (2025). Socioeconomic disparities in diabetes prevalence among the population in Ireland. *BMC Public Health, 25,* 2206. https://doi.org/10.1186/s12889-025-23022-6

Vancampfort, D., Schuch, F., Van Damme, T., Firth, J., Suetani, S., Stubbs, B., & Van Biesen, D. (2022). Prevalence of diabetes in people with intellectual disabilities and age- and gender-matched controls: A meta-analysis. *Journal of Applied Research in Intellectual Disabilities, 35*(2), 301–311. https://doi.org/10.1111/jar.12949

Victor, R. G., Lynch, K., Li, N., Blyler, C., Muhammad, E., Handler, J., Brettler, J., Rashid, M., Hsu, B., Foxx-Drew, D., Moy, N., Reid, A. E., & Elashoff, R. M. (2018).

A cluster-randomized trial of blood-pressure reduction in Black barbershops. *The New England Journal of Medicine, 378*(14), 1291–1301. https://doi.org/10.1056/NEJMoa1717250

Vogel, E. A., Humfleet, G. L., Meacham, M., Prochaska, J. J., & Ramo, D. E. (2019). Sexual and gender minority young adults' smoking characteristics: Assessing differences by sexual orientation and gender identity. *Addictive Behaviors, 95*, 98–102. https://doi.org/10.1016/j.addbeh.2019.03.005

Vogel, B., Acevedo, M., Appelman, Y., Bairey Merz, C. N., Chieffo, A., Figtree, G. A., Guerrero, M., Kunadian, V., Lam, C. S. P., Maas, A. H. E. M., Mihailidou, A. S., Olszanecka, A., Poole, J. E., Saldarriaga, C., Saw, J., Zühlke, L., & Mehran, R. (2021). The Lancet women and cardiovascular disease Commission: Reducing the global burden by 2030. *Lancet, 397*(10292), 2385–2438. https://doi.org/10.1016/S0140-6736(21)00684-X

Vögele, C., & Steptoe, A. (1993). Anger inhibition and family history as modulators of cardiovascular responses to mental stress in adolescent boys. *Journal of Psychosomatic Research, 37*(5), 503–514. https://doi.org/10.1016/0022-3999(93)90006-2

Volaco, A., Cavalcanti, A. M., Filho, R. P., & Précoma, D. B. (2018). Socioeconomic status: The missing link between obesity and diabetes mellitus? *Current Diabetes Reviews, 14*(4), 321–326. https://doi.org/10.2174/1573399813666170621123227

von Wagner, C., Baio, G., Raine, R., Snowball, J., Morris, S., Atkin, W., Obichere, A., Handley, G., Logan, R. F., Rainbow, S., Smith, S., Halloran, S., & Wardle, J. (2011). Inequalities in participation in an organized national colorectal cancer screening programme: Results from the first 2.6 million invitations in England. *International Journal of Epidemiology, 40*(3), 712–718. https://doi.org/10.1093/ije/dyr008

Waapihk Research (2024). *Indigenous Peoples and type 2 diabetes*. Retrieved September 28, 2025, from https://waapihk.com/2024/08/16/indigenous-peoples-and-type-2-diabetes/?utm_

Wang, H., Lee, P. M. Y., Zhang, J., Svendsen, K., Li, F., & Li, J. (2023). Association of intellectual disability with overall and type-specific cardiovascular diseases: A population-based cohort study in Denmark. *BMC Medicine, 21*(1), 41. https://doi.org/10.1186/s12916-023-02747-4

Warbrick, I., Came, H., & Dickson, A. (2019). The shame of fat shaming in public health: Moving past racism to embrace Indigenous solutions. *Public Health, 176*, 128–132. https://doi.org/10.1016/j.puhe.2018.08.013

Ward, L. M., Cooper, S. A., Sosenko, F., Morrison, D., Fleming, M., McCowan, C., Robb, K., Hanna, C. R., Hughes-McCormack, L., Dunn, K., Conway, D., Henderson, A., Smith, G., Truesdale, M., & Cairns, D. (2024). Population-based cancer incidence and mortality rates and ratios among adults with intellectual disabilities in Scotland: A retrospective cohort study with record linkage. *BMJ Open, 14*(8), e084421. https://doi.org/10.1136/bmjopen-2024-084421

Wardle, J. (2007). Eating behaviour and obesity. *Obesity Reviews, 8*(1), 73–75. https://doi.org/10.1111/j.1467-789X.2007.00322.x

Webber-Ritchey, K. J., Habtezgi, D., Wu, X., & Samek, A. (2023). Examining the association between parental factors and childhood obesity. *Journal of Community Health Nursing, 40*(2), 94–105. https://doi.org/10.1080/07370016.2022.2125809

Wen, M., Zhang, X., Harris, C. D., Holt, J. B., & Croft, J. B. (2013). Spatial disparities in the distribution of parks and green spaces in the USA. *Annals of Behavioral, 45*(1), S18–S27. https://doi.org/10.1007/s12160-012-9426-x

Witham, G., & Haigh, C. (2018). A narrative literature review examining cancer treatment issues for patients living with intellectual disabilities. *European Journal of Oncology Nursing, 36*, 9–15. https://doi.org/10.1016/j.ejon.2018.07.004

World Heart Federation (2023). *World heart report 2023: Confronting the world's number one killer.* https://world-heart-federation.org/resource/world-heart-report-2023/

World Health Organization (n.d.-a). *Social determinants of health.* Retrieved November 25, 2024, from https://www.who.int/health-topics/social-determinants-of-health#tab=tab_1

World Health Organization (n.d.-b) *Cancer.* Retrieved September 24, 2025, from https://www.who.int/health-topics/cancer#tab=tab_1

World Health Organization (2008). *Waist circumference and waste to hip ratio: A report of a WHO expert consultation.* Retrieved September 24, 2025, from https://www.who.int/publications/i/item/9789241501491

World Health Organization (2020). *Healthy diet.* Retrieved 24 September, 2025, from https://www.who.int/news-room/fact-sheets/detail/healthy-diet

World Health Organization (WHO) (2021a). *Tobacco responsible for 20% of deaths from coronary heart disease.* Retrieved September 24, 2025, from https://www.who.int/news/item/22-09-2020-tobacco-responsible-for-20-of-deaths-from-coronary-heart-disease

World Health Organization (WHO) (2021b). *MPOWER package of data-driven tobacco control measures helps protect up to 5 billion lives.* Retrieved November 20, 2024, from https://www.who.int/news-room/feature-stories/detail/mpower-package-of-data-driven-tobacco-control-measures-helps-protect-up-to-5-billion-lives

World Health Organization (WHO). (2021c). *Physical activity.* Retrieved June 6, 2025, from https://iris.who.int/server/api/core/bitstreams/a137d0b6-64ec-4e86-a69a-ae38ca7cef59/content

World Health Organization (2024a). *Noncommunicable diseases.* Retrieved February 18, 2025, from https://www.who.int/news-room/fact-sheets/detail/noncommunicable-diseases

World Health Organization (2024b). *The top 10 causes of death.* Retrieved September 24, 2025, from https://www.who.int/news-room/fact-sheets/detail/the-top-10-causes-of-death

World Health Organization (2024c). *World Health Statistics, monitoring health for SDG, sustainable Development Goals.* Retrieved October 30, 2024, from https://www.who.int/publications/i/item/9789240094703

World Health Organization (2024d). *Chronic obstructive pulmonary disease (COPD).* Retrieved September 26, 2025, from https://www.who.int/news-room/fact-sheets/detail/chronic-obstructive-pulmonary-disease-(copd)

World Health Organization (2025a). *Cardiovascular diseases.* Retrieved September 1, 2024, from https://www.who.int/news-room/fact-sheets/detail/cardiovascular-diseases-(cvds)

World Health Organization (2025b). *Obesity and overweight.* Retrieved June 6, 2025, from https://www.who.int/news-room/fact-sheets/detail/obesity-and-overweight

Wu, H., Wu, J., Zhang, Z., Zheng, Y., Niu, W., Zheng, L., & Li, J. (2021). Prevalence and associated risk factors of hypertension in adults with disabilities: A cross-sectional study in Shanghai, China. *Clinical Epidemiology, 13,* 769–777. https://doi.org/10.2147/CLEP.S322791

Wu, J., Huang, L., Wu, A., Xu, J., Wu, Z., Le, M., Jiang, C., & Wu, H. (2023). Risk factors and characteristics of new-onset coronary heart disease in adults with physical disabilities: A retrospective cohort study. *Heliyon, 9*(3), e13841. https://doi.org/10.1016/j.heliyon.2023.e13841

Wu, J., Wang, Y., Li, Y., Liu, H., Yang, S., Zhai, H., & Wu, H. (2024). Are physically disabled people at high risk of coronary heart disease among disabled population - Evidence from 7.5-year retrospective cohort study. *Annals of Epidemiology, 90,* 42–48. https://doi.org/10.1016/j.annepidem.2023.11.001

Wyszyńska, J., Podgórska-Bednarz, J., Dereń, K., Baran, J., Czenczek-Lewandowska, E., Leszczak, J., & Mazur, A. (2020). Associations between adiposity indicators and hypertension among children and adolescents with intellectual disability - A case-control study. *Journal of Applied Research in Intellectual Disabilities, 33*(5), 1133–1140. https://doi.org/10.1111/jar.12735

Xu, F., Earp, J. E., Adami, A., Lofgren, I. E., Delmonico, M. J., Greene, G. W., & Riebe, D. (2022). The sex and race/ethnicity-specific relationships of abdominal fat distribution and anthropometric indices in US adults. *International Journal of Environmental Research and Public Health, 19*(23), 15521. https://doi.org/10.3390/ijerph192315521

Xu, R., Huang, S., Shi, C., Wang, R., Liu, T., Li, Y., Zheng, Y., Lv, Z., Wei, J., Sun, H., & Liu, Y. (2023). Extreme temperature events, fine particulate matter, and myocardial Infarction mortality. *Circulation, 148*(4), 312–323. https://doi.org/10.1161/CIRCULATIONAHA.122.063504

Xue, Y. T., Tan, Q. W., Li, P., Mou, S. F., Liu, S. J., Bao, Y., Jiao, H. C., & Su, W. G. (2015). Investigating the role of acute mental stress on endothelial dysfunction: A systematic review and meta-analysis. *Clinical Research in Cardiology, 104*(4), 310–319. https://doi.org/10.1007/s00392-014-0782-3

Yang, H. S., Kim, S. Y., Jo, M. J., Kim, Y. Y., & Park, J. H. (2023). Early-onset stroke among people with disabilities: A national database study in South Korea from 2008 to 2017. *The Lancet Regional Health – Western Pacific, 38*, 100819. https://doi.org/10.1016/j.lanwpc.2023.100819Yang et al., 2023

Yang, Z., Liu, C., He, L., Zhao, H., Jian, J., Chen, H., Wei, H., Niu, J., & Luo, B. (2025). Social isolation and loneliness increase the risk of coronary heart disease: Insights from a prospective cohort study. *Social Science & Medicine, 366*, 117701. https://doi.org/10.1016/j.socscimed.2025.117701

Yoo, J. E., Lee, D., Kim, B., Chang, W. H., Jin, S. M., Han, K., & Shin, D. W. (2025). Increased risk of type 2 diabetes after traumatic amputation: A nationwide retrospective cohort study. *Frontiers in Endocrinology, 15*, 1437860. https://doi.org/10.3389/fendo.2024.1437860

Yusuf, S., Reddy, S., Ounpuu, S., & Anand, S. (2001). Global burden of cardiovascular diseases: Part II: variations in cardiovascular disease by specific ethnic groups and geographic regions and prevention strategies. *Circulation, 104*(23), 2855–2864. https://doi.org/10.1161/hc4701.099488

Yusuf, S., Hawken, S., Ounpuu, S., Dans, T., Avezum, A., Lanas, F., McQueen, M., Budaj, A., Pais, P., Varigos, J., Lisheng, L. & INTERHEART Study Investigators (2004). Effect of potentially modifiable risk factors associated with myocardial infarction in 52 countries (the INTERHEART study): Case-control study. *Lancet, 364*(9438), 937–952. https://doi.org/10.1016/S0140-6736(04)17018-9

Zorbas, H., & Elston, J. (2016). Sharing the challenge of cancer control for Indigenous Australians: A national agenda. *European Journal of Cancer Care, 25*, 222–224. https://doi.org/10.1111/ecc.12475

10 Pain

Chapter contents

- What is pain?
- Theories of pain.
- Pain in specific populations.
- Measuring pain.
- Pain management.

Chapter objectives

After reading this chapter, you should be able to answer the following questions:

- Discuss why the definition of pain is important.
- Explain the difference between acute and chronic pain and the impact of chronic pain on people's lives.
- Consider the role of gender identity in the experience and expression of chronic pain.
- Explore how discrimination and stigma may influence pain experiences across different groups.
- Discuss different ways of measuring pain, taking culture into account.
- Explain why culture is an important consideration when developing pain management strategies.

What is pain?

The International Association for the Study of Pain (IASP) defines pain as "An unpleasant sensory and emotional experience with, or resembling that associated with, actual or potential tissue damage" (Raja et al., 2020, p. 1976). Within this definition, it is important to note that pain is subjective and not always due to tissue damage, injury or disease. Psychological factors, such as learning from own or others' pain experiences, depression, anxiety and cultural factors, can influence perceptions of pain. Even though pain is unpleasant, it does have a survival function. Pain is a signal to tell the individual that something is wrong and it prompts action to protect the individual from greater harm or further injury. This may involve moving away from the thing that had caused the pain (e.g. pulling your hand away from something hot), taking action to protect an injury (by holding it), seeking medical treatment to deal with the pain or taking medication to control pain. Arthur and Rolan (2019) referred to pain as a 'near universal experience', meaning that it is something that almost everyone would have experienced, regardless of culture, ethnicity, sexual orientation, gender identity and disability. The meaning, expression of pain and degree of pain reported can be influenced by psychosocial factors and within Indigenous cultures, the concept

DOI: 10.4324/9781003423157-10

of pain is linked to experiences of colonisation, stolen land rights, the spirit world, emotions and mental wellbeing (Bailey et al., 2023).

Acute pain

Acute pain is relatively short lasting; it acts as a warning signal that something is wrong and typically results from a specific injury or disease process that causes tissue damage, e.g. a broken limb, the pain from an acute infection, chest pain due to lack of blood supply to the heart muscle, etc. Pain usually prompts a person to engage in pain reduction behaviours, which may involve some type of self-help, such as taking analgesic medication or seeking help and advice from family, friends and healthcare professionals. Usually when remedial action is taken, acute pain reduces and eventually goes away. Pain has survival value, but some people are born with the inability to feel pain, which is a genetic condition called congenital insensitivity to pain (see Box 10.1). It can cause repeated injuries, disease and inflammation that may go unnoticed, leading to permanent tissue and bone damage or even death.

BOX 10.1
CONGENITAL INSENSITIVITY TO PAIN

Al-Hroub et al. (2024) outlined the case study of a 13-year-old girl who presented at a clinic with a history of recurrent episodes of swelling in both ankles, the right knee, joint deformities, high temperatures, multiple falls, blisters, sores on the lower limbs, mouth ulcers, evidence of bite damage to the tongue and multiple bodily scars. Despite these injures, the girl never displayed any signs of being in pain. Medical staff were initially concerned that the girl was being physically abused, but genetic testing confirmed a diagnosis of congenital insensitivity to pain (CIP.)

A case study by Kosmidis et al. (2013) described a 33-year-old man with CIP, who had been unable to feel pain, temperature or hardly sweated since birth. From birth through to adulthood, the man suffered from unnoticed injuries that included multiple bone fractures, joint dislocations and infections. In addition, the consequences of being unable to sweat left the man at risk of developing heatstroke, as sweating is a bodily cooling mechanism. At 33 years old, the man had deformed, unstable joints and limited mobility, which contributed to obesity and poor quality of life.

Chronic pain

When pain lasts beyond the expected recovery time of three months, it is considered to be chronic in nature. It is estimated that around 31% of people across the world live with **chronic pain** (Steingrímsdóttir et al., 2017), which can interfere with mental and physical wellbeing, impact quality of life (QoL) and become a source of disability. Chronic pain is a feature of many diseases and it can be a condition on its own, without any injury or tissue damage. The lack of a validating diagnosis to legitimise chronic pain can result in stigma and discrimination, as the invisibility of chronic pain may cause others, including healthcare professionals, to doubt its existence (Perugino et al., 2022). People who are in chronic pain are at risk of developing anxiety and depression (Lerman et al., 2015). Pain can also have negative impacts on daily life, work and have financial and social consequences, which include emotional withdrawal from social situations and leisure activities (Rios & Zautra, 2011). The non-specific nature of chronic pain means it is more difficult to manage than acute pain.

Theories of pain

The specificity theory of pain

Descartes, a French philosopher in the 17th century, believed that a person felt pain when receptors were activated by a stimulus (e.g. injury), resulting in a signal being transmitted along a nerve pathway to specific areas in the brain. The specificity part of the theory referred to there being separate receptors and nerve pathways for different sensations, such as touch and pain, with the pain being sensed by nociceptors and touch by mechanoreceptors. Each receptor was thought to send signals along independent nerve pathways, terminating in separate brain areas for pain and touch. During the 1800s, **the Specificity Theory** was expanded, Von Frey (1894, as cited in Moayedi & Davis, 2013), agreed with the idea of there being specific nerve endings on the skin but suggested that these consisted of special receptors for different types of stimuli, e.g. cold, heat touch and pain.

The pattern theory of pain

Around the same time, Goldscheider (1886), as cited in Moayedi & Davis (2013), put forward **the pattern theory of pain**, which explained that distinct types of pain were due to the pattern of impulses from nerve endings, which were received and blended in a specialised part of the spinal cord (the dorsal horn) and then sent to the brain. This theory superseded the idea of there being a separate sensory system for pain, with the receptors for pain being shared with other senses and only perceived as pain when the sensations became intense. This biomedical view of pain emphasised that actual tissue damage and the degree of pain were related, more damage equalled more pain. However, Beecher (1956) who had been a doctor during World War 2 found that soldiers who had been injured in battle required 47% less pain-relieving medication than civilian patients who had sustained similar non-war injuries. This was a groundbreaking discovery, as it showed that the size of the injury or wound was not directly related to the degree of pain; moreover, the meaning that an individual attached to pain could influence how pain was experienced. For soldiers, the context of the injury was important, when they were injured, it meant that they were unfit for duty, they could go home and they were welcomed back as war heroes. In this context, pain was something positive for solders, whereas for civilians, injury often resulted in an unwelcome interruption of valued activities. This showed that the context in which an injury occurred and how the individual interpreted it could exert an influence on the amount of pain experienced. These findings were impossible to understand using a purely biomedical explanation of pain, as mental processes, such as attention, perception and emotion, have a role to play in the perception and sensation of pain.

The gate control theory of pain

In Melzack and Wall's (1965) **Gate Control Theory**, pain is influenced by multidimensional factors that interact with neural impulses going to (via afferent pathway) and coming from the brain (efferent pathway), via the spinal cord. When we sustain an injury, specialised pain receptors called nociceptors (see Box 10.2) initiate a pain signal that goes from the area of the injury to the **dorsal horn** of the spinal cord, which contains a hypothetical gate; the pain signal has to travel through this gate to get to the brain. The GCT agreed with previous ideas of there being different types of nerve fibres that relayed information about the type of damage or sensations, for example, a cut, burn, scrape, muscle pain, dull internal pain, etc. **A-delta nerve fibres** are myelinated, which means they are covered in a sheath, which helps to insulate the nerve signal and the signal is transmitting more quickly to the brain. These types of fibres are associated with pain that is well localised and sharp. Smaller diameter **C fibres** are not myelinated, they transmit pain more slowly, with pain typically characterised as being dull and diffuse. Non-painful sensations such as light touch and pressure are transmitted by larger diameter **A-beta nerve fibres**, which compete with pain signals at the gate and can help inhibit the sensation of pain. For example, when you hit your elbow, the sharp pain travels along the A-delta fibres to the gate, you might hold and rub your elbow, which can reduce the sensation of pain. This is due to the gate being blocked by the competing A-beta signal which prevents or reduces the pain signal from getting to the brain.

BOX 10.2
NOCICEPTION

We have specialised skin receptors (nociceptors) for pain related to cold, hot, pressure and chemical stimuli; the name given to the physiological activation of pain receptors and nerve fibres is nociception. When tissue is damaged, nociceptors are activated, whether or not we feel the pain immediately may be influenced by psychological factors, which can compete with pain signals received by brain, as explained by the Gate Control Theory of Pain.

Pain may also be mediated by descending signals coming down the spinal cord from the brain, which include attention, anxiety, fear, depression, excitement, happiness and concentration. A pain signal coming from an injury will have to compete with the descending neural impulses to get through the 'gate'. The GCT of pain brought psychology into the biomedical view of pain via perceptual processes involving interpretation, past experience, culture, environmental factors and psychosocial factors. Factors that help pain signal get through the gate to the brain include anxiety, stress, depression, helplessness, fatigue, fear associated with pain, beliefs about having little personal control over pain and past experience.

The neuromatrix model of pain

The neuromatrix model of pain proposed that the brain and spinal cord (central nervous system; CNS) are not just passive recipients of pain signals (Melzack

& Katz, 2014). For example, in order to explain the puzzle of **phantom limb pain**, which is characterised by the perception of pain in limb has been amputated, these authors postulated that pain must be generated somewhere within the CNS itself. In addition, we know that there is no correlation between the extent of an injury and the amount of pain experienced and there are many occasions when people go to their doctor complaining of being in pain, only to be told that examinations, X-rays and scans have shown no damage or disease to account for their pain experiences. This is a common finding in people who have **fibromyalgia**, a chronic condition that is characterised by pain and tender points throughout the body, fatigue and sleep problems. Melzack and Katz (2014) and Melzack (2001) explained that many structures within the CNS work together in the generation of pain, which include the spinal cord, brainstem, the limbic system and parts of the cerebral cortex. This helps explain how sensory information, thinking, emotions, personality, behavioural and physical activity can each exert an influence on pain experiences, especially in chronic pain. Melzack and Katz believed that the bodily response to stress could impact pain, with elevated stress resulting in greater sensitivity to pain.

BOX 10.1
CRITICAL THINKING

Think of a time when you experienced physical pain, did your thoughts, emotions and the social situation affect how you expressed and coped with the pain? For example, have you ever fallen down, got back up and pretended not to be hurt? What does this tell us about the interaction between biological, psychological and social factors and the pain experience?

Pain in specific populations

The ISAP designated their Global theme for 2025 as, "pain management, education, and research in low- and middle-income settings" (Calvo & Sharma, 2025, p. 1). Their focus also includes marginalised communities within high-income countries, such as Indigenous Peoples, culturally diverse groups, migrants and people of low socioeconomic status. In 2024, the ISAP also recognised the need for further research into gender differences in chronic pain. This included all gender identities, sexual orientations and intersections of ethnicity (Blyth et al., 2024).

Sex hormones and pain

Female sex hormones such as oestrogen and progesterone may make people more sensitive to pain (see Box 10.3), with the primarily male hormone testosterone, having the opposite effect (Craft et al., 2004). This led researchers to explore pain during the menstrual cycle with inconclusive findings (Bartley & Fillingim, 2013). Older adults tend to report greater pain than their younger counterparts, with women experiencing even more pain compared to men. de Kruijf et al. (2016) examined the association between sex hormones and musculoskeletal (bone, joint and muscle) chronic pain in people over the age of 45 and found that women who had lower levels of oestrogen had higher levels of chronic pain, but there was no relationship between chronic pain and testosterone levels in men. More promising evidence comes from brain imaging studies, which indicate that there are sex differences when the brain responds to chronic pain. Females show greater emotional processing of pain, whereas for men, greater activity is found in areas associated with sensing and localising pain, but these are also influenced emotions and stress (Gupta et al., 2017).

Gender and pain

The relationship between pain, gender and sex can be confounded by researchers excluding the full spectrum of gender and sexual identities and by conflating sex with gender, using the terms interchangeably within the same study. In a survey across 17 countries, Tsang et al. (2008, p. 889) reported that females reported more pain than males, attributing possible differences to "hormonal and/or psychosocial factors specific to the female gender". The title of this paper referred to the term 'gender'; however, researchers referred to both sex and gender, using the terms interchangeably, making interpretation and applicability of results unclear. Picking up on this point, Boerner et al. (2018) reviewed all papers published in the journal Pain in 2017. They found over 75% of authors used the descriptor of gender when they were in fact referring to biological sex and nearly 33% of authors alternated between the descriptors sex and gender within their publications. This is of importance, as gender can impact pain perceptions, experiences and behaviours due to socialisation and cultural expectations, while differences in biological sex and pain may be mediated by sex hormones (Fillingim et al., 2009). Furthermore, there is general agreement for the need to look beyond binary categories of sex and gender to better understand how chronic pain is experienced across diverse identities.

BOX 10.3
PAIN TERMINOLOGY

Sensation and perception are related, but they are different. Sensation involves receipt of sensory information (seeing, hearing, smell, touch and taste) from the external environment. This information is physiological in nature, to be meaningful, sensations need to be interpreted by the brain. Perception involves interpretation of sensations, these interpretations are influenced by past experiences, memories, emotions, culture and expectations.

You may read about pain threshold, pain tolerance and pain sensitivity and wonder how they differ. The point at which pain no longer feels just uncomfortable and starts to feel painful is known as the pain threshold. For example, if you put your hand into hot water, you may feel comfortable, but if the temperature is gradually increased, your pain threshold is the point at which the heat becomes painful. Pain tolerance is concerned with the amount of pain an individual can endure over time. Using the same example, once the heat of the water becomes hot enough to cause pain, tolerance is concerned with how long you can keep your hand in the water before removing it due to pain. Pain sensitivity is concerned with your reaction to pain. If you have higher pain sensitivity, it means you react to pain more easily or feel pain more intensely than others under the same conditions.

In 2008, Tsang et al. (2008) reported a gender gap in chronic pain prevalence, 13 years later not much had changed, with 63.3% of women and 55.5% of men in Europe reporting chronic pain, with back pain being the most commonly reported condition (Bimpong et al., 2022). It seems that women experience more pain than men (Keogh, 2022) and have greater sensitivity to experimentally induced pain, such as extremes of temperature and pressure; in addition, women are also more likely to admit to being in pain compared to men. The reasons for this are not clear, but women are more likely to have chronic conditions that have pain as the main symptom, e.g. low back pain, osteoarthritis, fibromyalgia, headaches and abdominal pain (Blyth et al., 2024). Explanations of gender differences in pain are thought to involve an interplay of biopsychosocial factors in how people experience and express pain.

Pain catastrophising (Sullivan et al., 1995) refers to thinking about pain in an overly exaggerated, negative way. It involves **rumination**, magnification, helplessness and a belief that nothing can be done to stop or reduce pain (see Box 10.4). People who exhibit high levels of pain catastrophising report greater intensity of pain, have increased emotionally distressed responses to pain and are less responsive to pain treatments. Sullivan et al. (2000) found that women reported a higher intensity of pain and displayed a longer duration of pain behaviours during experimentally induced pain (immersing an arm in ice water for one minute) compared to men. However, when catastrophising was statistically controlled for, the gender difference was no longer apparent. Similarly, when comparing levels of pain, pain behaviours and physical disability between men and women who had osteoarthritis (due to wear and tear) of the knee, women exhibited higher scores on all three pain variables, but gender differences were accounted for women having higher catastrophising scores (Keefe et al., 2000). Emotional factors such as depression can also have a negative impact on the experience of chronic pain. Keogh et al. (2006) found that women who had higher depression scores reported greater pain-related disability compared to men. Gender differences have also been noted in relation to anxiety and pain, with men tending to worry about intensity of the pain itself (Edwards et al., 2003), whereas women have greater anxiety sensitivity, that is, they worry more about the pain-related anxiety symptoms, such as increased heart rate and feeling dizzy, which is especially prevalent in chest pain (Keogh et al., 2004). However, findings are not entirely consistent, as some studies report conflicting results or no significant gender differences in pain experiences.

BOX 10.4 CATASTROPHIZING

This is a way of thinking which is very negative, the worst-case scenario or worst possible outcome. Quite often people who have chronic pain find themselves in a vicious circle whereby they wake up with pain and have a negative automatic thought of 'another day of agony'; this may be followed by 'I cannot stand another day of this' and it can lead to anger and increased muscular tension, which may cause the pain to get worse. It may be necessary for healthcare professional to gently challenge some of these types of thoughts, 'another day of agony' may not be truly representative of the whole day, but this must be done in a very sensitive manner. One way of approaching this is to ask, 'what is the worst-case scenario?' and 'what is the best-case scenario?', then lead onto 'what would be the most realistic outcome?'

Socialisation and culture have a role to play in learning about gender and can exert influences on pain experiences and behaviours. Keogh (2021) used the Gender Context Model of pain to explore the association between social norms, gender identity, gender expression and pain. This model suggests that gender can influence how an individual reacts to their own and other's pain; in addition, the experience of pain can also influence a person's own gender identity. For example, an individual's gender identity influences how they think about themselves in relation to the social labels of being masculine or feminine and the traits linked to them. Traditionally, masculinity has been associated with traits of toughness, independence and not showing emotion, femininity with being caring, expressive and social (Keogh & Boerner, 2020; Keogh & Denford, 2009). Men who identify with traditional masculine roles tend to have high pain tolerances and pain thresholds (Alabas et al., 2012) but often interpret chronic pain as a threat to their masculinity (Ahlsen et al., 2014; Conversano et al., 2021), which may make them try to 'push through' pain (Côté & Coutu, 2010; Flurey et al., 2016). Women may also feel that chronic pain has negative impacts on their traditionally viewed feminine roles of being able to care for others and provide emotional support. Hence, those who identify with traditional gender roles may adapt self-perceptions and behaviours to cope with the impact of chronic pain (Ahlsen et al., 2014; Côté & Coutu, 2010). Despite Keogh's Gender Context Model offering a more inclusive framework to consider gender identity, most studies still utilise binary conceptions of gender, overlooking non-binary and gender-neutral individuals. Similarly, the literature on chronic pain and sexual orientation tends to focus on biological sex ascribed at birth, negating the experiences of those who do not identify as heterosexual. This has resulted in the pain experiences and voices of people from across different gender identities and sexual orientations being under researched (Blyth et al., 2024).

LGBTQI+ individuals and pain

People from sexual and gender minority groups tend to experience more pain and limitations in ability to engage in everyday tasks compared to heterosexual and cisgender populations (Fredriksen-Goldsen et al., 2017). Such disparities have been correlated with stigma and discrimination, especially from healthcare professionals, which can result in underreporting, exacerbation and chronicity of pain. In a study assessing pain responses between transgender and cisgender adults who had HIV, Strath et al. (2020) found that gender was a an important factor in pain sensitivity. Compared to cisgender men, transgender women and cisgender women were more sensitive to experimental pain (heat and pressure) and transgender women tolerated less pressure-based pain. From this, the authors concluded that transgender women may be at greater risk for chronic pain. The stress of stigma and discrimination can have a negative impact on how pain is perceived and experienced. Moreover, transgender individuals experience multiple risk factors that predispose them to the development of chronic pain, such as higher levels of anxiety, depression, lack of or difficulty in accessing gender affirming care, housing and job insecurity (Stocking et al., 2025).

Zajacova et al. (2023) examined data from a large, nationally representative health survey in the US that measured chronic pain across different sexual identity groups, which included heterosexual, gay/lesbian, bisexual and people from other sexual minority groups (referred to as others by the authors). Pain prevalence was lowest in the heterosexual group at 11.5% compared to 21.5% in people who identified as bisexual or other. Zajacova et al. suggested that this higher pain prevalence could be explained by **double discrimination**, as individuals in the 'other' group faced rejection from the heterosexual population and gay/lesbian communities. This increased marginalisation can contribute to bisexual individuals and people of other sexual identities feeling unseen, misunderstood and unsupported. In addition, psychological stress was higher in these two sexual minority groups (bisexual = 12.2%; other = 14.1%) compared with heterosexual (3.5%) and gay/lesbian (6.2%) groups. Such findings are in keeping with the minority stress theory that stigma, discrimination and social exclusion can have negative impacts on health and more specifically chronic pain. In addition to being from an LGBTQI+ community, the intersections of poverty, being isolated from family and coming from an ethnic minority background can increase vulnerability to pain and increase barriers to healthcare (Craig et al., 2020). Bale and Epperson (2015) concluded that there may be biological sex and gender differences in how chronic pain signals are interpreted by the brain and how people behave in response to pain.

Ethnicity and pain

Research has indicated that there may be differences in sensitivity to pain across ethnic groups, with African Americans exhibiting more severe clinical (associated with disease or injury) and experimental (induced by cold water, heat, electrical stimulation or reduced blood flow to a limb) pain than non-Hispanic Whites (Rahim-Williams et al., 2012). However, these authors acknowledged that pain sensitivity can be influenced by beliefs, culture, perceived discrimination, environmental factors, social roles, language and gender.

In summarising the findings of 20 years of research into pain management in the US, Meghani et al. (2012) reported that ethnic minority patients had a lower likelihood of receiving opioid pain medication compared to White patients. This supported the findings of Staton et al. (2007) who reported that healthcare professionals were twice as likely to underestimate the extent of pain experienced by Black patients compared with other ethnicities. An interesting study by Mende-Siedlecki et al. (2021) assessed bias in pain recognition by asking participants to look at pictures of Black and White men's facial expressions of pain, anger, happiness, fearfulness and sadness. Participants identified pain more easily on White faces, they were less likely to recognise sadness on Black faces, but no differences were found for recognition of anger, fear and happiness. When participants were asked how much pain-relieving cream should be prescribed for people who had equal intensities of facial pain expression, less cream was recommended for pictures showing Black faces. The inability to perceive pain in the faces of Black people may help explain why healthcare professionals may unconsciously perceive Black patients as being in less pain. This can have adverse treatment outcomes in terms of Black patients receiving less effective painkillers, a reduced dose of medication or their verbalisations of pain being dismissed.

Healthcare professionals may exhibit bias towards ethnic minority groups that can result in less-than-optimal treatment outcomes. Across the UK and US, a common misperception still prevails in healthcare professional thinking that patients of African or Caribbean descent have less sensitivity to pain. To some extent, this may also help explain disparities in pain assessment, treatment and the provision of pain-relieving medications for these groups (Hoffman et al., 2016). Ethnic disparities in pain assessment and management are due to historical biases embedded within the medical system and action is still required to address these inequities in care (Hood (2025).

Pain within Indigenous populations

Across the world, Indigenous people are more likely to experience chronic pain compared to their non-Indigenous counterparts. In New Zealand, 24.2% of Māori (over 15 years old) have chronic pain, compared to 21.3% for the rest of the population. Within Australia, there is no governmental information on the prevalence of pain in Aboriginal and Torres Strait Islanders. A small survey of those living in remote areas of Western Australia found that Indigenous Australians had levels of chronic pain that were comparable to those of their non-Indigenous counterparts (Wong et al., 2021); Bernardes et al. (2022) reported that the Indigenous population had 1.4 times more **musculoskeletal pain** compared to non-Indigenous people. The prevalence of chronic pain within Native American and Alaskan Natives is around 5% higher than the average for the rest of the US population (Zajacova et al., 2022).

Indigenous Peoples hold a conception of pain that is different to Western views, with the latter mainly focusing on the physical nature of pain. For Indigenous People, pain is not just physical, it has emotional, mental and spiritual aspects, it is associated with the community, land, culture and ancestors. The history of colonisation, intergenerational trauma and loss are all facets of pain for Indigenous People, and this helps to explain why Indigenous people often report that their pain is minimised or disregarded by healthcare professionals (Bailey et al., 2023).

According to Fenwick (2006), the way in which people express pain can be influenced by their culture, which can have direct consequences for measuring and treating pain. Often culture and ethnic origin are thought of as one entity, but the former is much more than just nationality, it includes beliefs, customs, societal organisation, the environment and historical injustices. Thus, healthcare professions must address the concept of pain, assessment and management within the holistic cultural context of Indigenous populations (Fenwick & Stevens, 2004). Within Indigenous settings, the traditional healer engaged in observation, **palpation** and told the person what to do to get better. The Indigenous healer knew what was wrong, without the need for asking questions. This contrasts with Western healthcare interactions in which the patient is asked a variety of questions, and the responses are often used to inform subsequent questioning to collect all relevant information to come to a diagnosis, necessary investigations and treatment. When Western healthcare professionals question Indigenous people about their pain, their questions may be met with silence; this is due to the type of questioning not being congruent with Indigenous healing practices. Additionally, some questions may seem nonsensical to Indigenous People, for example, asking if the person is in pain, when the extent of a serious injury is evident. Usually when someone is in pain, they display pain behaviours, but due to past injustices and previously negative interactions with the healthcare system, Indigenous people can be hesitant to report pain to healthcare professionals (Strong et al., 2015). This contributes to health disparities, as Western trained healthcare professionals may think that the patient has a high pain tolerance, which can result in undertreatment of pain.

Incorporating Indigenous lived experiences into research and practice is crucial for developing culturally appropriate pain assessment and management strategies that promote health equity. In a review of qualitative studies that focused on chronic pain in Indigenous adults, Gaspar Fernandes et al. (2025) found that pain is not viewed as being an isolated symptom that requires a medical fix. Pain is seen as something that influences and is influenced by the whole body, it is linked with the natural cycles of the seasons, the moon and climatic temperature, which humans have little control over. Indigenous people view pain as something that is closely connected to their identity and something to be endured. Pain helps to build inner strength and associations have been made with ancestors who also endured pain and developed wisdom from it. A salient aspect of chronic pain within Indigenous communities is acknowledgement of the impact of colonisation and intergenerational trauma. Pain is not just physical but is symptomatic of cultural loss and oppression. Current use of Western-only methods to assess and treat chronic pain only helps reinforce colonial dominance within healthcare systems, meaning that Indigenous people not only experience chronic pain within their bodies, but also within society through continued oppression. This makes Indigenous people reluctant to seek help for chronic pain, as the experience of discrimination and stigma just helps to perpetuate their pain and suffering. Participating in community life can help Indigenous people cope with chronic pain. However, as in Western societies, chronic pain may be a barrier to full participation in community activities, as physical limitations can impact cultural roles, identity and spiritual power, leading to feelings of shame and embarrassment.

Western treatments to alleviate chronic pain for Indigenous populations often ignores traditional health practices and knowledge, which can have negative consequences for treatment adherence. To counter this, Bartlett et al. (2012) suggested the use of the 'Two Eyed Seeing' approach (see Chapter 7), in which traditional Indigenous knowledge and Western medicine are viewed as being of equal standing. This mutual respect of Indigenous and Western healthcare knowledge working together can be extremely beneficial for Indigenous patients.

Intersectionality and pain

A paucity of studies has explored pain through an intersectional lens. Brady et al. (2019) conducted focus groups with a sample of refugees and migrants who were from a range of different cultural backgrounds. They shared a common experience of having recently arrived in Australia, were from the non-dominant culture and had chronic pain. Previous research with culturally and linguistic diverse communities and consultation with community leaders representing the different cultures and ethnicities were used to inform focus group questions. Findings showed that being a woman, who was a refugee, on a low income and being visibly different from the culturally dominant group, made managing pain more difficult. Participants could not afford private specialist care or avail of preferred therapies and they had to endure long waiting times for treatment, which had poor outcomes. In addition, some participants felt their migrant or refugee status and the support already received from Australia led the dominant culture to expect them not to complain about delayed medical treatments. This made it even more difficult for participants to speak up about their pain and contributed to feelings of isolation.

The cause of fibromyalgia remains illusive, but it is more commonly diagnosed in women, who due to gendered stereotypes may struggle to have their symptoms validated by others and health professionals. Women have often been portrayed as overly emotional, irrational, prone to exaggeration and more likely to complain about pain more than men (Hoffmann & Tarzian, 2001). Due to the lack of an objective test to confirm diagnosis, some healthcare professionals and people within the general population question the legitimacy of fibromyalgia as a real entity (Häuser & Fitzcharles, 2018). Pryma (2017) explored women's experiences of living with chronic pain due to fibromyalgia. Most Black women had faced gendered stigma and had been dismissed as being **hypochondriacal**, as they did not look unwell. Regardless of ethnicity, women from lower socioeconomic backgrounds felt they were perceived by others as exaggerating their pain and were blamed for not working hard enough to get better or to support themselves financially. The intersection of ethnicity and gender was experienced differently by Black women who explained how they faced both ethnic and gender-based judgemental attitudes about the legitimacy of their pain and disability, they felt doubted or dismissed. Pryma suggested this may be perpetuated by the way in which fibromyalgia is portrayed in the media as mainly affecting White people, making it more of a struggle for women of colour to be seen and heard and leaving them to prove they were deserving of care. Some Black women reported that healthcare professionals had dismissed their pain and felt they had been denied treatment due to the stereotypic notions of, Black people feel less pain or Black people are more likely to misuse medication. These intersectional biases of socioeconomic status, ethnicity and gender made Black women's struggles with the invisibility of chronic pain even harder.

BOX 10.2
CRITICAL THINKING

How can personal biases or cultural assumptions influence your perception of someone else's pain?

Measuring pain

Scales and questionnaires to measure pain

There are a range of ways to measure pain, one simple method is to use a visual analogue scale (VAS), which is displayed as a 100-millimetre line, one end states, 'no pain' and the opposite end, has 'worst pain'. The individual is asked to place an X or mark where they think their pain intensity is along this line (see Figure 10.1). The distance from the left side (no pain) to where the point where the X is placed is measured with a ruler and can be expressed in millimetres. This

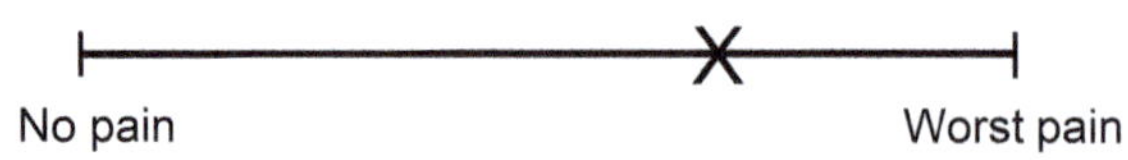

Figure 10.1
Visual analogue scale to rate pain

Source: Author

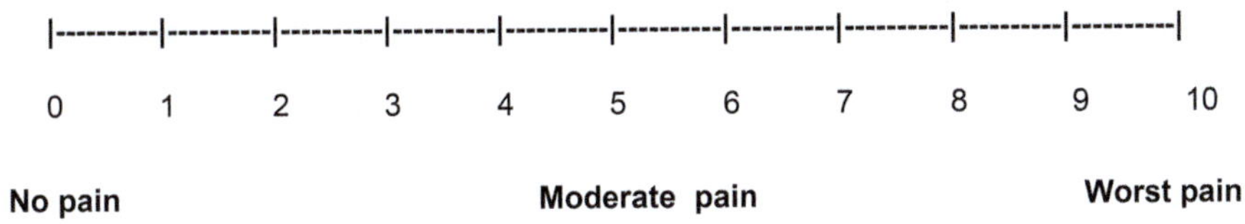

Figure 10.2
Numerical rating scale for pain

Source: Author

type of pain assessment can be completed at multiple time points to assess if pain is diminishing or increasing.

Another simple method of pain measurement is the numerical rating scale ([NRS]; see Figure 10.2). This permits the individual to represent their pain on a line from no pain to worst pain possible using numbers.

Facial expressions may be used to measure pain, one such example is the Wong-Baker FACES® Pain Rating Scale (referred to from here as FACES scale). This self-report measure is commonly used with children three years and older, Unlike the VAS and NRS, the FACES scale is copyrighted, thus permission is required from the owners before use. In addition to facial expressions, the FACES contains numbers and words to describe pain severity, which ranges from 'no hurt' to 'hurts worst' (see Figure 10.3). The scale may also be used by adults, with the word 'hurt' replaced with 'pain'. Users are asked to select the face that that is the best describes the pain they are feeling.

The McGill pain questionnaire

One of the best-known **multidimensional pain scales** used to measure pain is the McGill Pain Questionnaire (MPQ) (Melzack, 1975). This provides an assessment of various types and duration of pain, the overall intensity of pain (mild, moderate and severe), emotional effects (e.g. sickening, tiring, punishing) and the sensory aspects (throbbing, dull, piercing). There is a VAS to indicate the extent

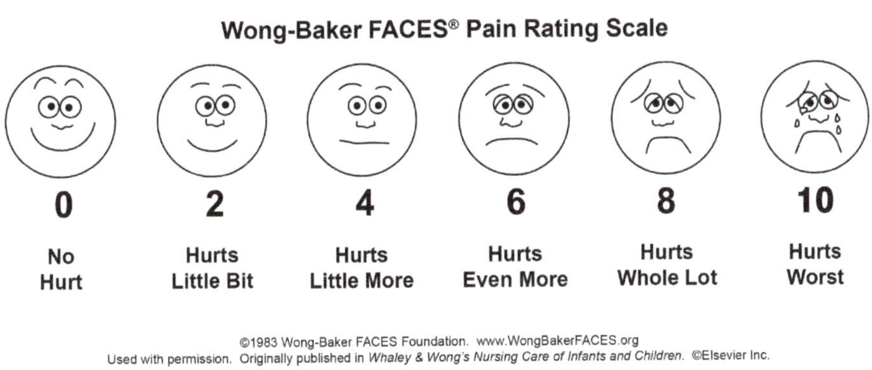

Figure 10.3
Wong-Baker FACES® Pain Rating Scale

Source: Reproduced with kind permission from the Wong-Baker FACES Foundation. https://wongbakerfaces.org/

of pain and a body chart to indicate the site of the pain and whether it feels internal or external. Another commonly used measure is the Brief Pain Inventory (Cleeland & Ryan, 1994), which asks about the location of pain, impact on daily activities, use of pain medication and degree of pain relief. While the Brief Pain Inventory (BPI) was initially developed for assessing cancer-related pain, it has been used extensively in a range of other chronic conditions. There are also disease-specific measures of pain and disability, for example, the Arthritis Impact Measurement Scale (Meenan et al., 1980), the Oswestry Disability Index for low back pain (Fairbank & Pynsent, 2000) and the Roland-Morris Disability Index (Roland & Fairbank, 2000). These scales also measure the multidimensional aspects of pain, along with functional limitations in specific disease populations.

Verbal and nonverbal aspects of pain measurement

Within most Western societies, pain behaviours are often associated with various facial expressions, which may be accompanied by verbalisations. This includes complaining about pain and verbal utterances such as moaning and groaning, behaviours such as changes in posture, rest and activity. However, verbal and nonverbal communication about pain can vary across cultures. Fenwick (2006) explained that Aboriginal and Torres Strait Islanders may use nonverbal behaviours, such as head and eye movements, to indicate they are in pain; these methods of communication may be imperceptible to Western trained healthcare practitioners, who lack cultural sensitivity to such cues. Even though many Indigenous people are multilingual and can communicate effectively in English, when in a healthcare setting, they tend to initiate conversations that centre around social interactions rather than pain, which may be perceived by Western-trained healthcare practitioners as wasting time and irrelevant to the assessment and management of pain.

Cultural sensitivity of pain measures

When assessing a patient's subjective pain intensity, healthcare professionals tend use a specific range tools across all patients, but this can be problematic, as the chosen tool may not be validated for the culture in which it is used. For example, using a VAS of 1–10 can produce inaccurate findings for some Indigenous populations, such as those in central Australia, as they have their own complex 'number systems' that do not specifically accord with Western numerical representations (Fenwick, 2006). Similarly, the use of facial expression tools, such as that in Figure 10.3, presupposes a universality in facial pain expressions. This perpetuates the Westernisation of pain symbolism and may negate culturally appropriate pain assessment in Indigenous populations. An example of this is the FACES® scale in which 'no hurt' (pain) is depicted by eyes being wide open and eyebrows raised; this type of eye and eyebrow expression among the Canadian Inuit people is an indication of agreement, rather than a pain status. While Ellis et al. (2011) attempted to adapt the FACES® scale among Inuit communities, this adapted scale (Northern Pain Scale) has not been widely used in clinical settings and it is unclear if it is a culturally valid measure of pain expression for Indigenous people. Moreover, a recent scoping review that focused on measuring physical pain in Canadian Indigenous Peoples found scant research into the validity of Western pain measurement scales for use with these populations Bailey et al. (2023). This has implications for underrecognition of pain and may contribute to a stereotypic notion that Indigenous People feel less pain compared to their non-Indigenous counterparts. Such practices can lead to Indigenous pain going unnoticed, disregarded or underestimated (Bailey et al., 2023). In a mixed methods study, Zhang et al. (2024) developed a culturally responsive pain scale by working with an Elder and a Knowledge Keeper from Indigenous Cree Peoples in Northern Saskatchewan. This involved adaptation to the FACES® to add descriptors in the local language, four facial expressions, including a closed mouth indicating silence, which is a common Cree pain behaviour meaning the worst pain. In addition, in Cree culture, colour has meaning, hence different colours were used for each face, with yellow indicating no pain and blue the worst pain. This Community Directed Pain Scale (CDPS) was developed for use in chronic musculoskeletal pain and tested with Indigenous People undergoing physiotherapy treatment for chronic low back pain. Findings indicated that providing a variety of ways to denote pain in one brief scale, which used local language descriptors, a horizontal scale, faces that were culturally representative of Cree pain experiences and colour was meaningful to patients and the healthcare professionals who were treating them. However, as previously noted, when measuring pain within Indigenous populations there may be a need to consider other facets of the pain experience that are culturally appropriate. In a scoping review, Bailey et al. (2023) highlighted that Indigenous storytelling was a salient part of pain expression for Indigenous Peoples and suggested that incorporating this into routine healthcare practices may be a more culturally respectful and appropriate way to assess pain. The concept of chronic pain is much broader for Indigenous People than how it has been defined by Western science. As a result, studies that compare the extent of pain between Indigenous and non-Indigenous populations may not be comparing like with like, which can lead to miscommunication and underdiagnosis of chronic pain.

Pain management

Culture can influence how people interpret the meaning of pain and pain behaviours (Callister, 2003). Preferred pain management strategies may also be influenced by ethnicity, for example, some groups such as African Americans favour passive coping methods such as prayer and hope (Campbell & Edwards, 2012). This may relate to beliefs about pain being a punishment from God; a test of an individual's religious belief and that endurance of pain can lead to spiritual growth. In addition, some patients may be reluctant to take **opioid-based medications** due to concerns about possible addiction (Unruh, 2007) and in some countries prescribing and use of opioids are prohibited (see Chapter 11).

Pain management programmes

Knowledge about the management of pain is mainly based on Western White Eurocentric research that has been conducted in high-income countries (Morais et al., 2022). In the UK, **cognitive behaviour therapy** (CBT) has been advocated as an effective part of pain management programmes (PMPs), as it can lead to improvements in mood, reductions in disability and reduce pain catastrophising in people with chronic pain (Williams et al., 2012). However, the majority of PMPs within the UK have been developed for White English-speaking patients and seen as universally suited to all, without considering cultural and ethnic applicability (Burton & Shaw, 2015).

People in the UK and US who identify as Black or Asian are more likely to report chronic pain but face more problems in getting treatment than their White majority counterparts (Zajacova et al., 2021) and access to chronic pain management services differs across ethnic groups. Added to this, people from ethnic minorities may also experience intersectional healthcare system disparities (Brady et al., 2017) due to difficulties relating to language, health literacy, cultural insensitivity from healthcare systems and bias from healthcare staff. Within the UK, people who have chronic pain may be referred to PMPs that utilise structured group interventions based on education about and coping with pain, exercise, relaxation and discussions about beliefs relating to pain. Little attention has been given to assessing whether PMPs developed for White English UK populations meet the needs of people from other ethnic minority backgrounds. In a service evaluation of pain rehabilitation services within the North of England, Bull et al. (2023) found that education about chronic pain was only discussed from a Western perspective. This contrasted with first-generation immigrants' understanding of pain and coping, which was based on their culture and faith. Ethnic minority patients stressed the importance of the role that faith played in accepting that their pain was God's will and they were optimistic about the role of prayer to help pain, which was at odds with the more secular discussions in PMPs. The latter centred on coming to terms with pain and learning to cope with it (Bull et al., 2023).

Davies et al. (2025) used the Te Whare Tapa Whā (see Chapter 2) in designing a culturally appropriate six-week PMP for Māori communities. This was co-designed with a local Māori healthcare provider, patients and their families. Participants highlighted the need to include traditional Māori methods, such as herbs, prayer and spiritual healing. In keeping with the collective nature of health, patients emphasised the importance of family members being included within the PMP. Delivery needed to happen within community venues rather than hospitals due to the latter being associated with discrimination, stigma and lack of cultural safety. To ensure cultural relevance, visual and written materials used within the programme were assessed for suitability by an expert in Māori health literacy, Māori metaphors and illustrations used to describe pain were co-designed with a Māori illustrator and the PMP was delivered by Māori community partners. This culturally tailored, co-designed PMP was highly valued and culturally acceptable to participants. It improved confidence and skills to manage pain and improved relationships between families and healthcare providers. These two examples highlight the need for pain management approaches that are culturally sensitive and recognise diverse beliefs and treatment strategies.

Psychological interventions for chronic pain

Psychological interventions have a lot to offer people who have chronic pain. They can be used to educate the patient about the negative cycle of pain, how it occurs and the factors that help perpetuate it. In the early stages after an injury, it is often necessary for the patient to avoid movements or behaviours that cause pain; however, these 'pain behaviours' may persist long past the acutely painful stage. These avoidance behaviours can have negative consequences both physically (loss of mobility and muscular strength) and psychologically (loss of confidence and self-esteem). There is also some evidence to suggest that avoidance behaviours are linked to catastrophic thinking about pain, which may be amenable to cognitive behaviour therapy (CBT).

Cognitive behaviour therapy

Cognitive behaviour therapy (CBT) is a structured brief therapeutic intervention that involves core beliefs and automatic thoughts. It is necessary to assess each patient's needs to include their specific difficulties and to determine treatment goals. Establishing a good therapeutic relationship with the patient is necessary, along with an emphasis on the collaborative nature of CBT to ensure the patient understands what is happening to them and why. CBT will only be of use to a patient who is willing to engage with it and agree to complete homework activities linked to their pain. To use CBT in chronic pain, patient assessment usually includes self-report questionnaires (e.g. MPQ, a depression inventory and perhaps an anxiety inventory), along with a patient diary and clinical interview. Completion of the pain diary is essential as it will include information on the activities that the patient is engaging in, their pain severity, their irritability (or mood) and any coping strategies that have had some success in reducing pain. The pain diary also provides a baseline measurement of pain and shows associations between activity, pain, emotions and coping.

Cognitive and behavioural elements that can maintain pain chronicity can include situations or factors that make the pain worse, but it is also important to explore those that help reduce pain. This can be facilitated using the ABC formulation. A refers to the antecedents or triggers that make the pain worse, B corresponds to the beliefs attached to the problem and C refers to the emotional and behavioural consequences of pain chronicity. Sometimes patients are not totally aware of the feelings associated with their pain, so it will be necessary to ask them to describe a recent activity that made their pain worse. This will define not only the context, but also their associated beliefs and emotions. For example, a single event may help explain how pain catastrophising developed (see Figure 10.4).

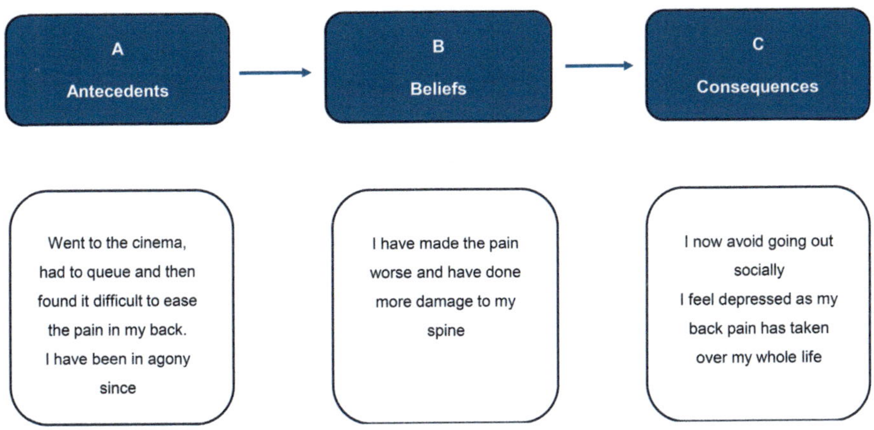

Figure 10.4
Behavioural and cognitive antecedents, beliefs and consequences associated with pain chronicity

Source: Author

Patients may be unaware that they engage in biased thinking about their pain always being unbearable. It is unlikely that a patient really has a pain score of 10 out of 10 (worst pain imaginable) for 24 hours per day, but they may say this. The patient's biased thinking about pain should not be dismissed, rather it is appropriate to discuss the rating of pain, while empathising and helping them identify any time during the day when their pain feels worse or slightly better. CBT includes helping the patient to become aware of their **negative automatic thoughts** (NATs), such as 'my pain will never get better'; 'I have pain 24 hours a day'; my pain is worse, so there must be something seriously wrong'. The NATs are challenged by asking 'what is the evidence for this' and helping the patients to consider if they really have pain 24 hours per day, by querying if they are always in pain when resting. The patient may say that at certain times of the day rest can be helpful, this permits discussion of the NAT, 'always being in pain'.

Some patients rate pain in terms of the overall feeling, that is, feelings of helplessness and lack of control rather than just the intensity of the pain itself. Due to this, it will be necessary to seek clarification regarding the meaning of pain in terms of emotions and physical abilities. Pain diaries can also give information on activities or emotions that precipitate the pain getting worse and this information may be used in treatment strategies. Other types of information may be elicited from the patient, for example, beliefs about pain control and health locus of control. Pain beliefs are quite important because they may be related to illness representations in terms of controllability or cure (see Chapter 5). Questions may probe what the patient thinks has caused the pain and makes it continue and what they have been told about their pain. Relationships can be affected by chronic pain and chronic pain behaviours, so information about these and home life, along with any work-related issues, may also need to be explored.

Other interventions

Relaxation, imagery, biofeedback and hypnosis can help divert a patient's focus away from pain. Pain that is made worse by muscular tension may be helped by a relaxation programme that encourages muscular relaxation and visualisation. Biofeedback may be used to provide an individual with a visual or an auditory indication of how tense a muscle is, whereas relaxation can be used to help the individual to consciously reduce muscular tension. Feelings of anxiety and helplessness can make pain feel worse and reduce an individual's ability to cope with pain. Interventions such as mindfulness or relaxation can help reduce anxiety and make pain more manageable. Being able to exert some control over chronic pain through the use of specific activities, such as taking pain medication before doing prescribed exercises or planning activities so that an individual can sit down and rest when required can help reduce helplessness and provide some sense of control over the pain.

Chronic pain has negative effects on individuals, families, communities and health services. It can have psychosocial and economic consequences. Sources and consequences of pain need to be considered in a holistic sense, as it is not just the nociceptive component that needs attention, but also the patient's pain behaviours and psychological distress. Moreover, there needs to be recognition that how we define pain goes beyond the narrow Western biomedical conceptualisation to consider the impact of stigma and discrimination faced by minority groups along with the disruption to relationships, lives and culture caused by colonisation. To ignore these social and cultural determinants of pain just serves to perpetuate health inequities.

Chapter summary

Discuss why the definition of pain is important?

A clear definition recognises that pain is more than just nociception. It includes cognitive and emotional factors and acknowledges that it is possible to experience pain in the absence of tissue damage. This helps shape the types of therapeutic interventions that can be used to treat pain, moving away from sole reliance on medication and addressing the role of psychosocial processes and culture on the experience and treatment of pain.

Explain the difference between acute and chronic pain and the impact of chronic pain on people's lives

Acute pain is short lasting and has survival value as it tells the individual that something is wrong and can prevent the person from doing further damage. Chronic pain persists longer than the expected recovery time (more than three months) and is not always associated with tissue damage. Chronic pain can be disabling, can impact quality of life and have implications for other family members and the community.

Consider the role of gender identity in the experience and expression of chronic pain

There are variations in how people with different gender identities experience and respond to pain, which is influenced by socialisation and social expectations. This suggests women have a higher sensitivity to pain and are more likely to express pain, whereas men may view pain expression as a threat to masculinity. Most research into pain and gender still uses binary terminology, often conflating gender with biological sex. Further research is required into the pain experience of minority gender groups, as they often experience stigma and discrimination, which are risk factors for the development and maintenance of chronic pain.

Explore how discrimination and stigma may influence pain experiences across different groups

People from gender, sexual, ethnic, Indigenous and lower socioeconomic groups may be at higher risk of the development of chronic pain due to greater exposure to poverty, discrimination and stigma. The effects of chronic pain may be perpetrated by lack of cultural sensitivity from healthcare professionals and the public.

Taking culture into account, discuss different ways of measuring pain?

Pain is subjective and culture may determine a patient's pain behaviours. Various measurement scales have been used to assess pain, which range from simple visual analogue scales to multidimensional scales, which are based on Western conceptualisations of pain. When assessing pain, it is essential that the scale or method being used is suited to the culture and situation it will be used in. Adapting measures designed and validated in other cultures may miss important nuances of pain that are culturally specific.

Explain why culture is an important consideration when developing pain management strategies

Pain management strategies, such as pain management programmes (PMPs), need to be culturally relevant to the population they serve as culture shapes people's perceptions of the cause of pain and how it can be managed. Patient beliefs are shaped by culture and/or religion, which can influence an individual's engagement with a PMP and acceptability of treatments.

Keywords

Acute pain: Short-term pain related to injury, tissue damage or illness; it has survival value in that it is a warning something is wrong.
Chronic pain: Pain that lasts beyond the expected recovery time and it can be a condition on its own.
Specificity theory of pain: Separate receptors and nerve pathways for different sensations.
Pattern theory of pain: Distinct types of pain are due to the pattern of impulses from nerve endings.
Gate control theory of pain: Pain signals can be modulated by a hypothetical gate within the dorsal horn of the spinal cord.
Dorsal horn: The location of the gate within the spinal cord that can block or permit pain signals getting to the brain.
A-delta fibres: Myelinated nerve fibres involved in fast transmission of well-localised sharp pain signals.
C-fibres: Unmyelinated nerve signals that transmit pain more slowly than A-delta fibres, pain is characteristically dull and diffuse.
A-beta fibres: Large diameter nerve fibres that transmit nonpainful signals, such as touch and pressure.
Neuromatrix model of pain: Pain is not just received by the central nervous system (CNS) but can be generated within the CNS itself.
Phantom limb pain: Pain that is experienced in a limb, even though it has been amputated.
Fibromyalgia: A chronic condition that is characterised by widespread pain, bodily tender points and fatigue.
Pain catastrophising: Thinking about pain in an overly exaggerated negative way.
Rumination: Repetitive thinking about the same negative thoughts or problems.
Double discrimination: Simultaneous discrimination from two sources, e.g. the general population and from within the LGBTQI+ community.
Musculoskeletal pain: Pain that originates from the muscles, bones, joints, ligaments and/or tendons.
Palpation: Using the hands to feel the body to detect areas of tension and imbalances which are interpreted by an Indigenous healer.
Hypochondriacal: Having excessive worry or fear of having a serious illness, which may be due to interpretation of bodily symptoms.

Opioid-based medication: A strong analgesic drug used to treat severe pain, which carries the risk of addiction.
Cognitive behaviour therapy: A psychotherapeutic treatment that helps people to identify and change negative thought patterns and behaviours.
Negative automatic thoughts: These are spontaneous thoughts that may focus on negative outcomes related to pessimism, self-criticism or fear.

Key Readings

Boerner, K. E., Chambers, C. T., Gahagan, J., Keogh, E., Fillingim, R. B., & Mogil, J. (2018). Conceptual complexity of gender and its relevance to pain. *Pain, 159*(11), 2137–2141, https://doi.org/10.1097/j.pain.0000000000001275
Craig, K. D., Holmes, C., Hudspith, M., Moor, G., Moosa-Mitha, M., Varcoe, C., & Wallace, B. (2020). Pain in persons who are marginalized by social conditions. *Pain, 161*(2), 261–265. https://doi.org/10.1097/j.pain.0000000000001719
Gaspar Fernandes, L., Davies, C., Jaye, C., Hay-Smith, J., & Devan, H. (2025). "We do not stop being Indigenous when we are in pain": An integrative review of the lived experiences of chronic pain among Indigenous peoples. *Social Science & Medicine, 373*, 117991. https://doi.org/10.1016/j.socscimed.2025.117991
Moayedi, M., & Davis, K. D. (2013). Theories of pain: From specificity to gate control. *Journal of Neurophysiology, 109*(1), 5–12. https://doi.org/10.1152/jn.00457.2012

These reflective questions are designed to encourage you to think about the material presented in this chapter

1 Outline the differences between acute and chronic pain, how might chronic pain affect an individual's daily life.
2 How do factors, such as gender and ethnicity, influence an individual's experience or expression of pain?
3 How have various models of pain influenced our understanding of the multidimensional nature of pain?

References

Ahlsen, B., Bondevik, H., Mengshoel, A. M., & Solbrække, K. N. (2014). (Un)doing gender in A rehabilitation context: A narrative analysis of gender and self in stories of chronic muscle pain. *Disability and Rehabilitation, 36*(5), 359–366. https://doi.org/10.3109/09638288.2013.793750
Alabas, O. A., Tashani, O. A., Tabasam, G., & Johnson, M. I. (2012). Gender role affects experimental pain responses: A systematic review with meta-analysis. *European Journal of Pain, 16*(9), 1211–1223. https://doi.org/10.1002/j.1532-2149.2012.00121.x
Al-Hroub, N. N., Al-Salahat, A. A., Taamreh, M. A., Abunejma, F. M., & Dukmak, O. N. (2024). Congenital insensitivity to pain: A case study of a rare genetic disorder. *Cureus, 16*(9), e69414. https://doi.org/10.7759/cureus.69414
Arthur, L., & Rolan, P. (2019). A systematic review of Western medicine's understanding of pain experience, expression, assessment and management for Australian Aboriginal and Torries Strait Islander Peoples. *Pain Reports, 4*(6), e764. https://doi.org/10.1097/PR9.0000000000000764

Bailey, N. G. N., Knott, R., Grenier, G., Craig, K. D., & Kramer, J. L. K. (2023). Physical pain among Indigenous Peoples in Canada: A scoping review. *Canadian Journal of Anaesthesia, 70*(6), 1047–1063. https://doi.org/10.1007/s12630-023-02461-y

Bale, T. L., & Epperson, C. N. (2015). Sex differences and stress across the lifespan. *Nature Neuroscience, 18*(10), 1413–1420. https://doi.org/10.1038/nn.4112

Bartlett, C., Marshall, M., & Marshall, A. (2012). Two-eyed seeing and other lessons learned within a co-learning journey of bringing together indigenous and mainstream knowledges and ways of knowing. *Journal of Environmental Studies and Sciences, 2*, 331–340. https://doi.org/10.1007/s13412-012-0086-8

Bartley, E. J., & Fillingim, R. B. (2013). Sex differences in pain: A brief review of clinical and experimental findings. *British Journal of Anaesthesia, 111*(1), 52–58. https://doi.org/10.1093/bja/aet127

Beecher, H. K. (1956). Relationship of significance of wound to the pain experienced. *The Journal of the American Medical Association, 161*(17), 1609–1613. https://doi.org/10.1001/jama.1956.02970170005002

Bernardes, C. M., Houkamau, K., Lin, I., Taylor, M., Birch, S., Claus, A., Bryant, M., Meuter, R., Isua, J., Gray, P., Kluver, J. P., Jones, C., Ekberg, S., & Pratt, G. (2022). *Communication and access to healthcare*: Experiences of Aboriginal and Torres Strait Islander people managing pain in Queensland, Australia. *Frontiers in Pain Research, 3*, 1041968. https://doi.org/10.3389/fpain.2022.1041968

Bimpong, K., Thomson, K., Mcnamara, C. L., Balaj, M., Akhter, N., Bambra, C., & Todd, A. (2022). The gender pain gap: Gender inequalities in pain across 19 European countries. *Scandinavian Journal of Public Health, 50*(2), 287–294. https://doi.org/10.1177/1403494820987466

Blyth, F., Parker, R., Strath, L., & Wesselmann, U. (2024). *ISAP Global year 2024: Gender differences in chronic pain conditions, Fact Sheet.* Retrieved August 13, 2025, from https://www.iasp-pain.org/wp-content/uploads/2024/06/gender-differences-chronic-pain-fact-sheet_R1.pdf

Boerner, K. E., Chambers, C. T., Gahagan, J., Keogh, E., Fillingim, R. B., & Mogil, J. (2018). Conceptual complexity of gender and its relevance to pain. *Pain 159*(11), 2137–2141, https://doi.org/10.1097/j.pain.0000000000001275

Brady, B., Veljanova, I., & Chipchase, L. (2017). An exploration of the experience of pain among culturally diverse migrant communities. *Rheumatology Advances in Practice, 1*(1), 1–14. https://doi.org/10.1093/rap/rkx002

Brady, B., Veljanova, I., & Chipchase, L. (2019). The intersections of chronic noncancer pain: Culturally diverse perspectives on disease burden. *Pain Medicine, 20*(3), 434–445. https://doi.org/10.1093/pm/pny088

Bull, E., Young, D., Etchebarne, A., & Malpus, Z. (2023). Understanding ethnic minority service user experiences of being invited to and attending group pain programmes: A qualitative service evaluation. *British Journal of Pain, 17*(1), 58–70. https://doi.org/10.1177/20494637221129196

Burton, A. E., & Shaw, R. L. (2015). Pain management programmes for non-English-speaking Black and minority ethnic groups with long-term or chronic pain. *Musculoskeletal Care, 13*(4), 187–203. https://doi.org/10.1002/msc.1099

Callister, L. C. (2003). Cultural influences on pain perceptions and behaviors. *Home Health Care Management & Practice, 15*(3), 207–211. https://doi.org/10.1177/1084822302250687

Calvo, M., & Sharma, S. (2025). ISAP Global year 2025: *Introduction to the IASP 2025 global year: Pain management, research, and education in low- and middle-income settings, fact sheet.* Retrieved August 10, 2025, from https://www.iasp-pain.org/wp-content/uploads/2025/05/intro-to-global-year-2025-fact-sheet_R1.pdf

Campbell, C. M., & Edwards, R. R. (2012). Ethnic differences in pain and pain management. *Pain Management, 2*(3), 219–230. https://doi.org/10.2217/pmt.12.7

Cleeland, C. S., & Ryan, K. M. (1994). Pain assessment: Global use of the Brief Pain Inventory. *Annals of the Academy of Medicine, 23*(2), 129–138.

Conversano, C., Ciacchini, R., Orrù, G., Bazzichi, M. L., Gemignani, A., & Miniati, M. (2021). Gender differences on psychological factors in fibromyalgia: A systematic review on the male experience. *Clinical and Experimental Rheumatology, 39*(3), 174–185. https://doi.org/10.55563/clinexprheumatol/73g6np

Côté, D., & Coutu, M. F. (2010). A critical review of gender issues in understanding prolonged disability related to musculoskeletal pain: How are they relevant to rehabilitation? *Disability and Rehabilitation, 32*(2), 87–102. https://doi.org/10.3109/09638280903026572

Craft, R. M., Mogil, J. S., & Aloisi, A. M. (2004). Sex differences in pain and analgesia: The role of gonadal hormones. *European Journal of Pain, 8*(5), 397–411. https://doi.org/10.1016/j.ejpain.2004.01.003

Craig, K. D., Holmes, C., Hudspith, M., Moor, G., Moosa-Mitha, M., Varcoe, C., & Wallace, B. (2020). Pain in persons who are marginalized by social conditions. *Pain, 161*(2), 261–265. https://doi.org/10.1097/j.pain.0000000000001719

Davies, C., Devan, H., Reid, S., Haribhai-Thompson, J., Hempel, D., Aho-White, I. J. T., & Te Morenga, L. (2025). "When you're in pain you do go into your shell": A community-based pain management programme co-designed with Māori whānau to address inequities to pain management - A qualitative case study. *The Journal of Pain, 37S*, 104760. Advance online publication. https://doi.org/10.1016/j.jpain.2024.104760

de Kruijf, M., Stolk, L., Zillikens, M. C., de Rijke, Y. B., Bierma-Zeinstra, S. M. A., Hofman, A., Huygen, F. J. P. M., Uitterlinden, A. G., & van Meurs, J. B. J. (2016). Lower sex hormone levels are associated with more chronic musculoskeletal pain in community-dwelling elderly women. *Pain, 157*(7), 1425–1431. https://doi.org/10.1097/j.pain.0000000000000535

Edwards, R., Augustson, E., & Fillingim, R. (2003). Differential relationships between anxiety and treatment-associated pain reduction among male and female chronic pain patients. *The Clinical Journal of Pain, 19*(4), 208–216. https://doi.org/10.1097/00002508-200307000-00003

Ellis, J. A., Ootoova, A., Blouin, R., Rowley, B., Taylor, M., Decourtney, C., Joyce, M., Greenley, W., & Gaboury, I. (2011). Establishing the psychometric properties and preferences for the Northern Pain Scale. *International Journal of Circumpolar Health, 70*(3), 274–285. https://doi.org/10.3402/ijch.v70i3.17823

Fairbank, J. C., & Pynsent, P. B. (2000). The Oswestry Disability Index. *Spine, 25*(22), 2940–2952. https://doi.org/10.1097/00007632-200011150-00017

Fenwick, C., & Stevens, J. (2004). Post operative pain experiences of Central Australian Aboriginal women. What do we understand? *Australian Journal of Rural Health, 12*, 22–27. https://doi.org/10.1111/j.1440-1584.2004.00541.x

Fenwick, C. (2006). Assessing pain across the cultural gap: Central Australian Indigenous Peoples' pain assessment. *Contemporary Nurse, 22*(2), 218–227. https://doi.org/10.5172/conu.2006.22.2.218

Fillingim, R. B., King, C. D., Ribeiro-Dasilva, M. C., Rahim-Williams, B., & Riley, J. L., 3rd (2009). Sex, gender, and pain: A review of recent clinical and experimental findings. *The Journal of Pain, 10*(5), 447–485. https://doi.org/10.1016/j.jpain.2008.12.001

Flurey, C. A., Hewlett, S., Rodham, K., White, A., Noddings, R., & Kirwan, J. (2016). Men, rheumatoid arthritis, psychosocial impact and self-management: A narrative review. *Journal of Health Psychology, 21*(10), 2168–2182. https://doi.org/10.1177/1359105315572452

Fredriksen-Goldsen, K. I., Kim, H. J., Shui, C., & Bryan, A. E. B. (2017). Chronic health conditions and key health indicators among lesbian, gay, and bisexual older US adults, 2013-2014. *American Journal of Public Health, 107*(8), 1332–1338. https://doi.org/10.2105/AJPH.2017.303922

Gaspar Fernandes, L., Davies, C., Jaye, C., Hay-Smith, J., & Devan, H. (2025). "We do not stop being Indigenous when we are in pain": An integrative review of the lived experiences of chronic pain among Indigenous peoples. *Social Science & Medicine, 373*, 117991. https://doi.org/10.1016/j.socscimed.2025.117991

Gupta, A., Mayer, E. A., Fling, C., Labus, J. S., Naliboff, B. D., Hong, J. Y., & Kilpatrick, L. A. (2017). Sex-based differences in brain alterations across chronic pain conditions. *Journal of Neuroscience Research, 95*(1–2), 604–616. https://doi.org/10.1002/jnr.23856

Häuser, W., & Fitzcharles, M. A. (2018). Facts and myths pertaining to fibromyalgia. *Dialogues in Clinical Neuroscience, 20*(1), 53–62. https://doi.org/10.31887/DCNS.2018.20.1/whauser

Hoffman, K. M., Trawalter, S., Axt, J. R., & Oliver, M. N. (2016). Racial bias in pain assessment and treatment recommendations, and false beliefs about biological differences between Blacks and Whites. *Proceedings of the National Academy of Sciences, 113*(16), 4296–4301. https://doi.org/10.1073/pnas.1516047113

Hoffmann, D. E., & Tarzian, A. J. (2001). The girl who cried pain: A bias against women in the treatment of pain. *The Journal of Law, Medicine & Ethics, 29*(1), 13–27. https://doi.org/10.1111/j.1748-720x.2001.tb00037.x

Hood, A. M. (2025). Racism in pain management causes needless suffering. *British Medical Journal, 389*, r848. https://doi.org/10.1136/bmj.r848

Keefe, F. J., Lefebvre, J. C., Egert, J. R., Affleck, G., Sullivan, M. J., & Caldwell, D. S. (2000). The relationship of gender to pain, pain behavior, and disability in osteoarthritis patients: The role of catastrophizing. *Pain, 87*(3), 325–334. https://doi.org/10.1016/S0304-3959(00)00296-7

Keogh, E. (2021). The gender context of pain. *Health Psychology Review, 15*(3), 454–481. https://doi.org/10.1080/17437199.2020.1813602

Keogh, E. (2022). Sex and gender differences in pain: Past, present, and future. *Pain, 163*(1), S108–S116. https://doi.org/10.1097/j.pain.0000000000002738

Keogh, E., & Boerner, K. E. (2020). Exploring the relationship between male norm beliefs, pain-related beliefs and behaviours: An online questionnaire study. *European Journal of Pain, 24*(2), 423–434. https://doi.org/10.1002/ejp.1499

Keogh, E., & Denford, S. (2009). Sex differences in perceptions of pain coping strategy usage. *European Journal of Pain, 13*(6), 629–634. https://doi.org/10.1016/j.ejpain.2008.07.002

Keogh, E., Hamid, R., Hamid, S., & Ellery, D. (2004). Investigating the effect of anxiety sensitivity, gender and negative interpretative bias on the perception of chest pain. *Pain, 111*(1–2), 209–217. https://doi.org/10.1016/j.pain.2004.06.017

Keogh, E., McCracken, L. M., & Eccleston, C. (2006). Gender moderates the association between depression and disability in chronic pain patients. *European Journal of Pain, 10*(5), 413–422. https://doi.org/10.1016/j.ejpain.2005.05.007

Kosmidis, I., Krallis, P., Tsiamasfirou, D., & Filiopoulos, K. (2013). Congenital insensitivity to pain with anhidrosis: A case report of a 33-year-old patient. *Journal of Pediatric Orthopedics. Part B, 22*(1), 70–75. https://doi.org/10.1097/BPB.0b013e3283524c52

Lerman, S. F., Rudich, Z., Brill, S., Shalev, H., & Shahar, G. (2015). Longitudinal associations between depression, anxiety, pain, and pain-related disability in chronic pain patients. *Psychosomatic Medicine, 77*(3), 333–341. https://doi.org/10.1097/PSY.0000000000000158

Meenan, R. F., Gertman, P. M., & Mason, J. H. (1980). Measuring health status in arthritis. The arthritis impact measurement scales. *Arthritis and Rheumatism, 23*(2), 146–152. https://doi.org/10.1002/art.1780230203

Meghani, S. H., Byun, E., & Gallagher, R. M. (2012). Time to take stock: A meta-analysis and systematic review of analgesic treatment disparities for pain in the United States. *Pain Medicine, 13*(2), 150–174. https://doi.org/10.1111/j.1526-4637.2011.01310.x

Melzack, R. (1975). The McGill Pain Questionnaire: Major properties and scoring methods. *Pain, 1*(3), 277–299. https://doi.org/10.1016/0304-3959(75)90044-5

Melzack, R. (2001). Pain and the neuromatrix in the brain. *Journal of Dental Education, 65*(12), 1378–1382. https://doi.org/10.1002/j.0022-0337.2001.65.12.tb03497.x

Melzack, R., & Katz, J. (2014). The neuromatrix in behavioral medicine. In D. I. Mostofsky (ed), *The handbook of behavioral medicine* (pp. 759–774). Wiley Blackwell. https://doi.org/10.1002/9781118453940.ch35

Melzack, R., & Wall, P. D. (1965). Pain mechanisms: A new theory. *Science, 150*(3699), 971–979. https://doi.org/10.1126/science.150.3699.971

Mende-Siedlecki, P., Lin, J., Ferron, S., Gibbons, C., Drain, A., & Goharzad, A. (2021). Seeing no pain: Assessing the generalizability of racial bias in pain perception. *Emotion, 21*(5), 932–950. https://doi.org/10.1037/emo0000953

Moayedi, M., & Davis, K. D. (2013). Theories of pain: From specificity to gate control. *Journal of Neurophysiology, 109*(1), 5–12. https://doi.org/10.1152/jn.00457.2012

Morais, C. A., Aroke, E. N., Letzen, J. E., Campbell, C. M., Hood, A. M., Janevic, M. R., Mathur, V. A., Merriwether, E. N., Goodin, B. R., Booker, S. Q., & Campbell, L. C. (2022). Confronting racism in pain research: A call to action. *The Journal of Pain, 23*(6), 878–892. https://doi.org/10.1016/j.jpain.2022.01.009

New Zealand Government (2022). *Health and independence report 2022*. Ministry of Health. Retrieved August 15, 2025, from https://www.health.govt.nz/system/files/2023-07/health_and_independence_report_2022_online_version.pdf

Perugino, F., De Angelis, V., Pompili, M., & Martelletti, P. (2022). Stigma and chronic pain. *Pain and Therapy, 11*(4), 1085–1094. https://doi.org/10.1007/s40122-022-00418-5

Pryma, J. (2017). "Even my sister says I'm acting like a crazy to get a check": Race, gender, and moral boundary-work in women's claims of disabling chronic pain. *Social Science & Medicine, 181*, 66–73. https://doi.org/10.1016/j.socscimed.2017.03.048

Rahim-Williams, B., Riley, J. L., Williams, A. K., & Fillingim, R. B. (2012). A quantitative review of ethnic group differences in experimental pain response: Do biology, psychology, and culture matter? *Pain Medicine, 13*(4), 522–540. https://doi.org/10.1111/j.1526-4637.2012.01336.x

Raja, S. N., Carr, D. B., Cohen, M., Finnerup, N. B., Flor, H., Gibson, S., Keefe, F. J., Mogil, J. S., Ringkamp, M., Sluka, K. A., Song, X., Stevens, B., Sullivan, M. D., Tutelman, P. R., Ushida, T., & Vader, K. (2020). The revised international association for the study of pain definition of pain: Concepts, challenges, and compromises. *Pain, 161*(9), 1976–1982. https://doi.org/10.1097/j.pain.0000000000001939

Rios, R., & Zautra, A. J. (2011). Socioeconomic disparities in pain: The role of economic hardship and daily financial worry. *Health Psychology, 30*(1), 58–66. https://doi.org/10.1037/a0022025

Roland, M., & Fairbank, J. (2000). The Roland-Morris Disability Questionnaire and the Oswestry Disability Questionnaire. *Spine, 25*(24), 3115–3124. https://doi.org/10.1097/00007632-200012150-00006

Staton, L. J., Panda, M., Chen, I., Genao, I., Kurz, J., Pasanen, M., Mechaber, A. J., Menon, M., O'Rorke, J., Wood, J., Rosenberg, E., Faeslis, C., Carey, T., Calleson, D., & Cykert, S. (2007). When race matters: Disagreement in pain perception between patients and their physicians in primary care. *Journal of the National Medical Association, 99*(5), 532–538.

Steingrímsdóttir, ÓA., Landmark, T., Macfarlane, G. T., & Nielsen, C. S. (2017). Defining chronic pain in epidemiological studies: A systematic review and meta-analysis. *Pain, 158*(11), 2092–2107. https://doi.org/10.1097/j.pain.0000000000001009

Strath, L. J., Sorge, R. E., Owens, M. A., Gonzalez, C. E., Okunbor, J. I., White, D. M., Merlin, J. S., & Goodin, B. R. (2020). Sex and gender are not the same: Why identity is important for people living with HIV and chronic pain. *Journal of Pain Research, 13*, 829–835. https://doi.org/10.2147/JPR.S248424

Stocking, S. Q., Webb, C. K., Miller, G. H., Thomeer, M. B., Goodin, B. R., & Sorge, R. E. (2025). Understanding risk of chronic pain development and related mental health disparities among transgender people: A review of current literature and future directions. *The Journal of Pain, 37S*, 104681. https://doi.org/10.1016/j.jpain.2024.104681

Strong, J., Nielsen, M., Williams, M., Huggins, J., & Sussex, R. (2015). Quiet about pain: Experiences of Aboriginal people in two rural communities. *The Australian Journal of Rural Health, 23*(3), 181–184. https://doi.org/10.1111/ajr.12185

Sullivan, M. J. L., Bishop, S. R., & Pivik, J. (1995). The Pain Catastrophizing Scale: Development and validation. *Psychological Assessment, 7*(4), 524–532. https://doi.org/10.1037/1040-3590.7.4.524

Sullivan, M. J. L., Tripp, D. A., & Santor, D. (2000). Gender differences in pain and pain behavior: The role of catastrophizing. *Cognitive Therapy and Research, 24*, 121–134. https://doi.org/10.1023/A:1005459110063

Tsang, A., Von Korff, M., Lee, S., Alonso, J., Karam, E., Angermeyer, M. C., Borges, G. L., Bromet, E. J., Demytteneare, K., de Girolamo, G., de Graaf, R., Gureje, O., Lepine, J. P., Haro, J. M., Levinson, D., Oakley Browne, M. A., Posada-Villa, J., Seedat, S., & Watanabe, M. (2008). Common chronic pain conditions in developed and developing countries: Gender and age differences and comorbidity with depression-anxiety disorders. *The Journal of Pain, 9*(10), 883–891. https://doi.org/10.1016/j.jpain.2008.05.005

Unruh, A. M. (2007). Spirituality, religion, and pain. *The Canadian Journal of Nursing, 39*(2), 66–86.

Williams, A. C., Eccleston, C., & Morley, S. (2012). Psychological therapies for the management of chronic pain (excluding headache) in adults. *The Cochrane Database of Systematic Reviews, 11*(11), CD007407. https://doi.org/10.1002/14651858.CD007407.pub3

Wong, A., Hyde, Z., Smith, K., Flicker, L., Atkinson, D., Skeaf, L., Malay, R., & LoGiudice, D. (2021). Prevalence and sites of pain in remote-living older Aboriginal Australians, and associations with depressive symptoms and disability. *Internal Medicine Journal, 51*(7), 1092–1100. https://doi.org/10.1111/imj.14870

Wong-Baker FACES Foundation (2018). *Wong-Baker FACES® Pain Rating Scale*. Retrieved May 2, 2025, from http://www.WongBakerFACES.org.

Zajacova, A., Grol-Prokopczyk, H., & Fillingim, R. (2022). Beyond Black vs White: Racial/ethnic disparities in chronic pain including Hispanic, Asian, Native American, and multiracial US adults. *Pain, 163*(9), 1688–1699. https://doi.org/10.1097/j.pain.0000000000002574

Zajacova, A., Grol-Prokopczyk, H., Liu, H., Reczek, R., & Nahin, R. L. (2023). Chronic pain among U.S. sexual minority adults who identify as gay, lesbian, bisexual, or "something else". *Pain, 164*(9), 1942–1953. https://doi.org/10.1097/j.pain.0000000000002891

Zajacova, A., Grol-Prokopczyk, H., & Zimmer, Z. (2021). Sociology of chronic pain. *Journal of Health and Social Behavior, 62*(3), 302–317. https://doi.org/10.1177/00221465211025962

Zhang, T., Bath, B., McKinney, V., Swidrovich, J., Johnson, R., Foulds, H., Makar, N., Montgrand, M., & Lovo, S. (2024). Understanding needs for chronic musculoskeletal pain management in a Northern Dene and Métis community: A community-based needs assessment. *Canadian Journal of Pain, 8*(2), 2412560. https://doi.org/10.1080/24740527.2024.2412560

1 Palliative and end-of-life care

Chapter contents

- Palliative care.
- Culture and palliative care.
- Palliative care and hospice care.
- Advanced care planning.
- Pain relief in palliative and end-of-life care.

Chapter objectives

After reading this chapter you should be able to answer the following questions:

- Discuss what is meant by palliative care.
- Explain key factors that influence access to palliative care across various populations.
- Differentiate between palliative care and hospice care.
- Describe what is meant by advanced care planning and outline its role in supporting choice and dignity in dying.
- Identify common barriers to accessing effective pain relief and symptom management at end-of-life care.

Palliative care

Due to medical advances, not only are people living longer, but they are also managing a multiplicity of chronic conditions, some of which will be life-limiting. When people have a disease that is life limiting, **palliative care** may be provided; however, the public has limited knowledge about this type of care. Most people associate palliative care with relief of pain when close to death due to cancer (Li et al., 2025; McIlfatrick et al., 2021a) and it is commonly perceived as only being available in hospitals or hospices (Flieger et al., 2020). While this was its initial focus, modern palliative care aims to reduce suffering and improve quality of life (QoL) for people of all ages and at all stages of serious and **progressive disease** (Flieger et al., 2020). Across the globe, the Worldwide Hospice Palliative Care Alliance (WHPCA) (2020) reported that around 70% of palliative care is provided for people with diseases other than cancer. This includes chronic respiratory diseases, cardiovascular disease (CVD), stroke, end-stage kidney disease, Alzheimer's disease, neurological diseases, congenital abnormalities, diabetes and acquired immunodeficiency syndrome (AIDS), to name but a few. Rather than taking a biomedical approach, palliative care is holistically orientated, it includes delivery of care in hospital, **hospices** and the community. Palliative care uses a

DOI: 10.4324/9781003423157-11

patient-centred approach to help manage physical, emotional, social and spiritual aspects of wellbeing and can also assist patients and their families to make informed decisions about treatment and care options.

Palliative care involves the assessment of physical, psychological and spiritual wellbeing, along with interventions to provide symptom management, including pain relief. A range of treatments and interventions may be put in place to support the individual who is in receipt of care, along with their family and/or carers, this also includes bereavement support. Patients, families and carers can be involved in a partnership of shared decision-making, involving a range of healthcare professionals. This includes doctors, nurses, physiotherapists, occupational therapists, dieticians, psychologists, social workers, religious and spiritual leaders, who may be collectively referred to as a **multidisciplinary team**. Care may also involve volunteers, complementary and alternative therapists.

Depending on patient preference, palliative care can be introduced as early as desired in the disease trajectory, but quite often palliative care does not feature until an individual becomes quite unwell and, in some cases, it is not initiated at all (Collins et al., 2018). Two main reasons for this include lack of knowledge on the part of patients and families that they can avail of palliative care at any time in the course of the disease and that they can request initiation of this type of care (Collins et al., 2020). While not everyone with a life-limiting disease may think about the need for palliative care, healthcare professionals can help individuals, families and in some cases close friends, think about preferences regarding the type of care and desired interventions that they want when they near end of life. Such discussions can be documented to ensure that health professionals and other people are aware of an individual's wishes (Rietjens et al., 2017).

Knowledge about palliative care

In a cross-sectional survey, Collins et al. (2020) found that having positive views and good health literacy about palliative care was linked to previously having cared for someone with a serious illness. These researchers found that most people lacked awareness about palliative care, a finding that was confirmed by McIlfatrick et al. (2021a). The public often view palliative care as synonymous with passively waiting to die and do not consider it to be a model of high-quality care. While many people may express a desire to find out more about palliative care, there is a reluctance to introduce the topic due to concerns about causing upset to others. However, lack of knowledge and understanding about palliative care can create a vicious circle of palliative care invisibility and silence (Black et al., 2024).

Availability of palliative care

According to the World Health Organization (WHO) (2020), palliative care is a basic universal human right, income, age, type and stage of disease should not be barriers to receipt. However, across the globe in 2013, up to one-third of counties lacked any type of palliative care services (Lynch et al., 2013) and in 2020, only around 14% of people who needed palliative care received it (WHO, 2020). A range of factors have contributed to this, which include insufficient knowledge on the part of policymakers about the need for palliative care and limited healthcare provision in some low- and middle-income countries, which leaves little or no resources for palliative care provision. Within Africa, only 37 out of 54 countries have palliative or hospice care services (Hospice Africa Uganda, n.d.) and this despite having the greatest need for palliative care across all world regions (Worldwide Hospice Palliative Care Alliance, 2020). Barriers to the provision of palliative care in many countries include lack of financial support and healthcare personnel, limited or no training for healthcare professionals, along with continued misconceptions about who palliative care should be offered to (Akiyama et al., 2016).

A systematic review that examined access to hospice care in high-income countries across Australia, Canada, New Zealand and the UK found that some sections of society, such as ethnic minorities, Indigenous Peoples, the very elderly, those living in deprived areas and people with a non-cancer diagnosis, had a lower likelihood of receiving care provided by hospice services (Tobin et al., 2022). The authors of this review were unable to identify any literature pertaining to hospice access for LGBTQI+ (lesbian, gay, bisexual, transgender, queer plus) groups. However, previous research shows that people from Indigenous (Waran et al., 2016), ethnic (Bassah et al., 2024; Jawed & Comer, 2024), gender and sexual minority groups (Wakefield et al., 2021) may avoid hospice or palliative care because of previous life exposure to discriminatory healthcare treatment, stigma, cultural and religious barriers. In addition, the almost ubiquitous Eurocentric approach to palliative and **end-of-life care** may not be compatible with the beliefs and spiritual aspects of being ill and dying within some countries and cultures.

Culture and palliative care

Death is universal, but the experience of receiving a palliative prognosis, along with the experience of death and dying, is very much influenced by culture. Patients and family members may have differing beliefs about disease, disease progression, the amount and extent of information and or treatments they wish to receive and engagement with advanced care planning. A person's culture, age, ethnicity, gender identity, sexual orientation, socioeconomic status, where they live, disability and type of disease may influence their attitudes to death and dying and the nature of the palliative and end-of-life care that is acceptable to them. In some societies and cultures, discussions about death and dying are avoided and healthcare professional discussions of the topic are viewed as culturally insensitive (Givler et al., 2023). Not all individuals want to know their prognosis, whereas others request as much information as possible to make plans, be they financial, social, family related or for their end-of-life care, which may include **advanced plans** and **directives**.

In previous chapters, we learned that people from LGBTQI+ communities often experience discrimination in healthcare settings. These experiences may create anticipatory discrimination, which includes how they and their partner will be perceived or discriminated against by healthcare professionals. Due to fear of rejection by other patients, healthcare professionals and visitors, showing affection for a same-sex partner, along with gender identity and sexual orientation may need to remain hidden when receiving palliative care. Unconscious bias from healthcare professionals may be exhibited in presumptions about partners being cisgender and heterosexual (Wakefield et al., 2021). Furthermore, healthcare professionals may not always acknowledge the role of same-sex partners in key decision-making, which can lead to the patient and their partner feeling isolated and rejected (Bristowe et al., 2018). This can culminate in avoidance of palliative care services, which may mean that informal carers (family and friends) need to care for loved ones who have more advanced disease and for longer.

Palliative care and hospice care

The terms palliative care and hospice care have been used interchangeably, which has caused confusion and concern among patients and families. Added to this confusion is the differential use of the term '**hospice care**' by country. The word hospice can be used to refer to a place or a type of care that has similar aims to palliative care in reducing suffering and improving quality of life (QoL). In the United Kingdom (UK), palliative and hospice care does not necessarily equate with end-of-life care, as patients may receive palliative care alongside curative treatments and supportive hospice care to help symptom control for months (Hui & Bruera, 2016). In the US, hospice care is typically provided for patients who have advanced disease that is not capable of curative treatment and end of life is six months or less. Hospice care is more commonly associated with end-of-life care, which means that treatment is focused on ensuring that the individual does not suffer in terms of symptom burden (e.g. pain, respiratory problems, nausea) or other psychosocial symptoms (e.g. anxiety). However, not everyone who is in receipt of end-of-life care needs to be in a hospital or hospice, as this type of care can be provided in the community, which permits patients, if they wish, to die at home in the presence of family and friends.

Advanced care planning

In terms of death and dying, Western medicine has a focus on patient autonomy. If a patient is unable to communicate for themselves or unconscious, healthcare professionals ask family members if the patient had any advanced care plans or views about death and dying, thus emphasising the rights and autonomy of the patient. Palliative care was developed through a Western lens and applied within developing countries and in non-Western cultures (Ntizimira et al., 2022), such an approach negates consideration of colonialised people, whose culture, traditions and beliefs differ to those of Western countries. While the World Health Organization (WHO, 2020) stated that there should be universal palliative care around the globe, they also recognised the need to consider diversity of communities, cultures and countries.

As a disease progresses or treatment side effects become more problematic, a patient's wishes and goals about treatment and care may need to change accordingly. Initially a patient may want to be as active and cognitively aware as possible, but the encroachment of pain and disability or treatment-related burdens may result in a renegotiation of goals and stronger pain relief can affect levels of consciousness. It can be helpful for patients, family members and healthcare professionals to understand a patient's wishes and goals in relation to treatment. Advanced care planning gives patients the autonomy to detail their preferences regarding future care. It can include where the individual would like to be cared for and means the patient's wishes can be respected, especially if they are no longer capable of communicating. Patients in conjunction with family members may decide to stop all active forms of treatment in favour of being made comfortable and pain free, with a desire to die at home instead of in a healthcare setting. McIlfatrick et al. (2021b) found that only around 29% of people had heard about advanced care planning and most people linked it with having a terminal diagnosis and being near end of life (Li et al., 2025). However, a consensus statement by the European Association for Palliative Care (EAPC) highlighted that advanced care plans can be put in place at any time during an adult's life and not just when they are seriously or terminally ill (Sudore et al., 2017). While McIlfatrick et al. (2021b) found there was an acknowledgement that advanced care planning was beneficial for patients and families, most survey participants (68%) were not in favour of receiving information about it. Advanced care planning is flexible, voluntary and an ongoing process that can change over time, unlike advanced directives, which involves formal decision making. In certain jurisdictions advanced directives are legally binding (see Box 11.1).

BOX 11.1
ADVANCED DIRECTIVES AND CAPACITY

An advanced directive is also known as an advanced decision to refuse treatment (ADRT). It is a legal document that permits an individual to state in advance which medical treatments they wish to refuse, enabling their decisions to be known and respected. An individual must have the mental capacity to make an ADRT, they must be quite specific about the types of treatment being refused, under what circumstances this will happen and in the UK, they need to be aged 18 and over. An ARDT is a written document that is signed by the patient and witnessed by another person.

Within England and Wales, the **Mental Capacity Act** (MCA; 2005) was put in place to protect people who may lack the mental capacity, to make decisions and includes anyone aged 16 and over. It applies to health and medical treatments, social care and living arrangements and covers five main points.

1. Presumed capacity: It is assumed everyone has capacity, unless it is proven otherwise. If there is any doubt about an individual's capacity, then that capacity must be assessed.
2. Support to make decisions: Before determining if someone does not have capacity, every opportunity must be afforded to the individual to make their own decisions. This may include presenting information in a more simplistic way and/or using pictures to explain things.
3. Right to make unwise decisions: If an individual makes a decision, just because someone else sees that decision as being unwise, it does not mean that the individual lacks capacity.
4. Best interests: If a decision is made on behalf of an individual, that decision must be in the best interests of the individual.
5. Least restrictive option: Any decisions taken in the best interests of the individual must limit their freedom and rights as little as possible.

An example of the application of the MCA.

A patient with advanced incurable cancer has decided that in the situation that they are close to death and become unconscious or confused, they do not want their life to be prolonged by receiving **cardiopulmonary resuscitation** (CPR), their breathing to be taken over or assisted by **artificial ventilation** and they do not want to receive nutrition through **tube feeding**.

The patient goes to their general practitioner (GP), who assesses the patient's capacity to make this decision by ensuring that the patient understands what treatment is being refused, that the patient can weigh up the consequences of refusal, that they can retain this information long enough to make the decision and they are able to communicate their decision to the GP. If the GP decides that the patient has capacity to make an ADRT and is over 18 years old, the ADRT can be signed and dated by the patient, signed and witnessed by the GP and placed on the patient's medical record.

A few months later, the patient is admitted to hospital, not fully conscious and has difficulty communicating. The patient's notes contain the ADRT, under the MCA, the medical team must check that the document is valid (that the patient had capacity when it was made, that it was signed and witnessed and there is no other updated document that overrides the initial ADRT). The medical team tries talking to the patient about their ADRT, but the patient is not responsive; the team have to ensure that the ADRT is valid under the current circumstances i.e. the circumstances under which treatment was to be refused and the types of treatment refused. Even if the medical team feels that they can prolong the patient's life with CPR, ventilation or tube feeding, they must not provide the refused treatments. This is a very simple explanation and real life can be much more complex.

Culture and advanced care planning

In the US, White non-Hispanic patients are more likely to have formal advanced care plans and advanced directives in place compared to minority ethnic groups (Carr, 2011; Crooks et al., 2023), likewise within the UK (McAdoo et al., 2012). The exact reasons for this are unclear but may be linked with ethnic differences regarding decisions about death, dying and the role of the wider family in decision-making. African American and Hispanic patients prefer informal end-of-life planning through trusted relationships with leaders from their communities. It has been suggested that this preference has been shaped by a combination of distrust from past discriminatory treatment, unsatisfactory communication with healthcare professionals in the past and historical injustices such as slavery and racism (Cain et al., 2018).

Cultural and religious beliefs may influence how individuals and their families approach the end of life, which includes withholding information about disease prognosis from the patient, as not all countries subscribe to Western views of patient autonomy. In China, there is a reluctance to tell a patient that they have a life-limiting disease for fear that such information will have a detrimental impact on the patient, making their disease worse and accelerating death (Li et al., 2025). In addition, withholding information from the patient is based on the belief that any discussion would cause the patient unnecessary emotional suffering (Lunn, 2003). In Taiwan, the doctor informs a patient's family about life-limiting disease and the family is responsible for conveying the diagnosis to the patient. This contrasts with Western medicine in which patients do have the right to know about their disease status, but they also have a choice to request that they are not told everything. For example, an individual may want to know if they have cancer but may request not to be informed of their prognosis. In some cultures, discussion and engaging in advance care planning and putting ADRTs in place are seen as going against God's will and a challenge to one's faith (Cervantes et al., 2017; Li et al., 2021; Periyakoil et al., 2015).

LGBTQI+ and advanced care planning

Family estrangement is common within LGBTQI+ communities and social support may be limited compared to those experienced by cisgender and heterosexual individuals. Thus, it is essential that healthcare professionals ascertain from the patient, who should be included in their care and decision-making (Harding et al., 2012). While there have been positive legal changes in Europe, the UK and the US to protect and legitimise the relationship rights of LGBTQI+ people, many counties still criminalise these relationships. There may be barriers to a partner's participation in a patient's end-of-life care decisions and ensuring that the patient's gender identity is respected. Legislation can also change, for example, on January 20, 2025, President Donald Trump signed Executive Order that has affected LGBTQI+ rights in the US, along with access to healthcare (Warbelow, 2025).

Indigenous Peoples and advanced care planning

In Chapter 6, we learned about the importance of health literacy in helping patients to follow healthcare instructions and advice. Similarly, within palliative and end-of-life care, the terminology used by healthcare professionals needs to be matched with the needs of patients, family members and culture. When healthcare professionals lack cultural sensitivity, patients and their families may struggle to understand the nature of and reasons for the care or treatment that is being provided. This can lead to negative experiences, feelings of discrimination and have consequences for future communication and healthcare interactions. For example, according to Waran et al. (2016), Indigenous Peoples of Australia do not refer to end of life, dying or death, the culturally respectful term to use in interactions is 'finishing up'. It is essential that healthcare professionals who often deliver healthcare within a biomedical context, understand, respect and take into account the cultural aspects of the communities in which they work. Research within Indigenous communities indicates that receipt of palliative and/or end-of-life care in urban-based medical facilities can lead to a sense of isolation for patients and families. Additionally, fear, mistrust and racism, as a consequence of colonialisation, have contributed to Indigenous Peoples across the globe being apprehensive of accepting palliative and end-of-life care (Anderson & Woticky, 2018). They fear that their choices and voices will go unheard, that they will be separated from their family, community, way of life and culture. Indigenous patients located within an urban hospital or hospice, in receipt of end-of-life care, may experience barriers to traditional grieving processes, which can impact on families and communities. Barriers can include refusal to permit traditional Indigenous ceremonial practices within healthcare facilities, the patient being placed long distances from family and restrictions on the number of visitors, culminating in feelings of isolation (Kelly et al., 2009). These researchers explored the experiences of family members whose relatives had died at a health centre that had been designated as providing culturally sensitive and competent care for Indigenous Peoples. While the centre did permit multiple visitors, restrictions on the timing of visits and the size of patients' bedrooms, limited how many people could be with patients at any given time. These barriers had negative implications for supporting and fulfilling the spiritual needs of Indigenous people who were dying (Duggleby et al., 2015) and highlighted the need for collaborative working between health professionals, healthcare organisations and Indigenous People (Racine et al., 2022). Peters and Andersen (2013) reported that within Canada, many Indigenous people who live in urban areas are second and third generation, hence their links to ancestral lands may not be as strong as those living in rural areas, but their cultural identity and heritage are still highly important (Anderson & Woticky, 2018). Indigenous people who live in urban areas may have family, community members and Elders who live far away. When a death occurs, it can take time for extended family to reach the bedside. After death, healthcare providers are often reluctant to permit the patient's body to remain in the room until the extended family arrives, which can prevent the completion of ceremonial tasks that are in keeping with Indigenous ceremonial procedures of 'finishing up'.

For Indigenous People, the end of life is a natural aspect of the life cycle and a social celebratory event that marks the person's transition to the spirit world (Canadian Partnership Against Cancer, 2022). The land, family, community and spirit world all hold particular relevance to Indigenous People. Even though a family member may be in discomfort, distress or can avail of treatments that may prolong life, they often prioritise returning to their community over dying in what they perceive to be 'alien' hospitals or hospices (McGrath, 2007) and this is especially the case for older people. Dying at home means the person's animal spirit is 'tied' to the land and provides the opportunity for sacred knowledge to be passed on to another family member prior to death. Most Indigenous People prefer to receive end-of-life care at home, especially those who live in rural communities (Canadian Society of Palliative Care Physicians, 2016). This may not always be possible due to unavailability of appropriate palliative and end-of-life care services. In addition, dying at home may mean that Indigenous People have less access to equipment that will help them to feel more comfortable (e.g. moving and handling equipment to help transfer the individual from bed, airflow mattresses and seating to prevent pressure sores, etc.) and limited access to medications for symptom control (Waran et al., 2016). To Western healthcare professions, the choice to die at home with reduced support may be viewed as falling short of 'clinical standards' associated with their perceptions of a 'good death'. However, such a view shows a lack of insight into the cultural and spiritual importance of the land, ancestors and community within Indigenous belief systems and that death is part of the natural four-stage cycle of life (birth, youth, adulthood, elder), as noted in Chapter 5.

Within Western healthcare settings, when no advanced care plans are in place, it is usually the close family (next of kin) who are asked to make important decisions about ongoing treatment options. This contrasts with Indigenous decision-making that involves both the family and the wider community who discuss stories about the patient. Anderson and Woticky (2018) provided information about a fatally injured Indigenous individual who was unlikely to survive. Rather than the immediate family making decisions, those who knew the patient the best articulated what treatment and extent of intervention they thought the patient would have wanted. While health professional staff were sympathetic to this decision-making, they rejected it and following Western procedures by seeking decisions and permission only from the patient's immediate next of kin. Rejecting these Indigenous ways of living undermined collective values and decision-making traditions, perpetuating colonialist perspectives, the medicalisation of death and culturally inappropriate care.

BOX 11.1
CRITICAL THINKING

Do you think that more health education is needed about palliative care and advanced care planning? If so, where should this information be available and how should it be delivered? For example, leaflets, posters, within schools and workplaces?

Pain relief in palliative and end-of-life care

Many people with advanced diseases, such as cancer, end-stage kidney disease and lung disease, experience significant pain and other symptoms that have major consequences for quality of life. A central aspect of Western biomedical end-of-life care is the management of physical pain, usually by the administration of powerful opioid drugs (Middleton-Green, 2008). Patients and their families may have beliefs regarding opioid medications being linked with **euthanasia**, imminent death and concerns about addiction (Givler et al., 2023). Across the globe the Worldwide Hospice Palliative Care Alliance (2020) reported that just over 84% of people who needed opioid medications for pain control were unable to access them and this was a pressing issue for patients in low- and middle-income countries. The limited or non-availability of opioid medications is of concern, as the two most frequent and serious symptoms at the end of life that can be reduced by these medications are moderate to severe pain (63%) and respiratory problems (Saphire et al., 2020). In low- and middle-income countries, rather than cost being the barrier to opioid prescribing, restrictions or total bans are due to concerns about substance misuse (Frau et al., 2021), such governmental substance control leads to undue suffering (Sallnow et al., 2022). The WHO (2020) viewed this as a challenge for palliative care in developing countries, but Kunonga et al. (2025) pointed out that even within high-income countries, disparities in prescribing opioid drugs for palliative symptom control are a pressing concern for some sections of the population.

Ethnicity can be a barrier to receipt of appropriate pain relief when people are near end of life. Black and White-Hispanic patients with a diagnosis of cancer were more likely to receive lower doses and more short-acting opioid medications to control their pain over the final month of life compared to their non-Hispanic White counterparts. Furthermore, Black patients received less medication than Hispanic patients (Enzinger et al., 2023). These researchers suggested that such disparities may have been due to healthcare professionals' conscious and unconscious biases in relation to societal beliefs about Black patients being 'at risk' for substance abuse and an inability of healthcare professionals to read the facial pain expressions on Black faces (Mende-Siedlecki et al., 2021). Access to pain relief is also influenced by the intersections of gender and age, with men and older patients being less likely to receive medications (Saphire et al., 2020).

Ascertaining the extent of pain that a patient is experiencing can be fraught with difficulty, especially if the patient and healthcare professional do not share a common language. In Chapter 10, we learned about potential issues in using standardised pain scales that are not suited to a patient's language or culture. While family members may be of use as informal translators, this can cause miscommunication about the extent of pain the patient is experiencing and be influenced by the family member's own beliefs about pain, which can result in under- or overestimations of a patient's pain (Givler et al., 2023). This may be especially true in cultures where pain is considered as part of accepting God's will and that pain must be endured (Anandarajah et al., 2016). We learned in Chapter 10 that Indigenous Peoples' conception of pain is somewhat different to that of Western medicine, as the former also includes hurt and pain associated with colonisation. Palliative care promotes a patient-centred approach, recognising emotional, physical, social and spiritual connections (Gone, 2009). To manage pain, palliative and end-of-life care from an Indigenous viewpoint, healthcare professionals need to utilise a Two-Eyed Seeing approach (Bartlett et al., 2012), by including traditional healing practices, alongside Western healthcare practices.

Palliative care needs to be responsive to the physical, emotional, social, spiritual and cultural needs of people of all ages, all stages and types of disease. We need to educate the public about palliative care not being synonymous with end-of-life care. Likewise with advanced care planning and advanced directives, which can give people the autonomy to choose the care that is consistent with their own values and beliefs.

Chapter summary

Discuss what is meant by palliative care

Modern palliative care aims to improve quality of life and reduce suffering in people who have serious, progressive or life-limiting disease. It is holistically orientated, helping to manage physical, emotional, social and spiritual aspects of care for patients and their families. Palliative care can be provided at any stage of disease and in conjunction with other treatments aimed at curing or controlling disease.

Explain key factors that influence access to palliative care across various populations

Access to palliative care is a basic human right, but not everyone can avail of it due to limited healthcare resources in low- and middle-income countries, financial barriers, lack of trained staff and misconceptions about who palliative care is for. People from minority ethnic backgrounds, LGBTQI+ communities and Indigenous Peoples may avoid palliative care due to previous experiences of discrimination, stigma, cultural and religious barriers. In addition, a reluctance to discuss palliative care can act as a barrier to receipt of this type of treatment.

Differentiate between palliative care and hospice care

Palliative care is appropriate at any stage of a disease and can be provided alongside treatments that prolong life. In the UK, hospice care may be provided to manage symptoms for many months, but in the US, hospice care is usually provided for patients whose end of life is six months or less. Both palliative and end-of-life care are typically delivered by multidisciplinary teams.

Describe what is meant by an advanced directive and outline its role in supporting choice in dignity and dying

In Western healthcare settings, patient autonomy is respected and an advanced directive planning permits individuals to discuss and legally record (in writing) their preferences for future healthcare. This means that if an individual becomes unconscious or is unable to communicate, their wishes are known and can be respected. Advanced directives must be quite specific, detailing the circumstances under which treatment can be refused and the exact types of treatments that are refused. The aim of an advanced directive is to support patient autonomy, but there are cross-cultural differences that need to be respected.

Identify common barriers to accessing effective pain relief and symptom management at end-of-life care

In many Western societies, end-of-life care often involves the use of opioid drugs to help manage symptom burden associated with respiratory distress and pain. However, some people view opioids as a mechanism for hastening death, have concerns about addiction and fear that they will not be able to communicate with family members at end of life. In low- and middle-income countries, access to opioids for use in end-of-life care is often prohibited by governments, due to concerns about substance misuse and addiction. Bias on the part of healthcare professionals can also limit the amount and type of opioid prescribed for certain ethnic groups.

Keywords

Palliative care: A holistic type of care that includes physical, emotion, social and spiritual needs that can be introduced at any stage of progressive or serious life-limiting disease.

Progressive disease: A disease that gets worse over time, leading to increased symptom burden and eventual loss of life.

Patient-centred approach: An approach to care that responds to individual patient needs, preferences and values.

Hospice care: A type of care that may be provided alongside palliative care for symptom control. It can also refer to a place where end-of-life care is provided.

Multidisciplinary team: A group of healthcare professionals from different disciplines (e.g. doctors, nurses, physiotherapists, occupational therapists, social workers, etc.), who work together to provide the best care for a patient.

End-of-life care: Medical care and support that help with symptom management, comfort and dignity when a person is dying.

Advanced care planning: A way in which an individual can make decisions about future healthcare, in case they are unable to communicate their wishes. It may include types of treatments and where they would like to receive that care.

Advanced decision to refuse treatment (advanced directive): A written, witnessed, legal document that details the specific treatments that an individual does not want to receive should they become unable to communicate.

Capacity: The ability of an individual to understand and retain information in order that they can make informed decisions about their healthcare and communicate these decisions.

Cardiopulmonary resuscitation: An emergency technique that involves chest compressions to pump blood to the brain and often combined with rescue breaths to provide oxygen for someone who has stopped breathing.

Artificial ventilation: A machine such as a ventilator that assists in or completely takes over an individual's breathing.

Tube feeding: Delivery of nutrition through a tube into the stomach or intestines, usually used when a person cannot eat.

Finishing up: A term used by some Indigenous People to describe death and traditional ceremonial practices that take place after death that honours the person and their transition into the spirit world.

Euthanasia: The consensual, intentional and painless ending of an individual's life in order to relieve suffering.

Key Readings

Cain, C. L., Surbone, A., Elk, R., & Kagawa-Singer, M. (2018). Culture and palliative care: Preferences, communication, meaning, and mutual decision making. *Journal of Pain and Symptom Management, 55*(5), 1408–1419. https://doi.org/10.1016/j.jpainsymman.2018.01.007

Wakefield, D., Kane, C. E., Chidiac, C., Braybrook, D., Harding, R. (2021). Why does palliative care need to consider access and care for LGBTQ people? *Palliative Medicine*, 35(10), 1730–1732. https://doi.org/10.1177/02692163211055011

Waran, E., O'Connor, N., Zubair, M. Y., & May, P. (2016). 'Finishing up' on country: Challenges and compromises. *Internal Medicine Journal, 46*(9), 1108–1111. https://doi.org/10.1111/imj.13186

Worldwide Hospice Palliative Care Alliance. (2020). *Global atlas of palliative care* (2nd edn.). Worldwide Hospice Palliative Care Alliance. https://www.palliativecare.in/wp-content/uploads/2020/10/Global-Atlas-2nd-Edition-2020.pdf

Reflective questions

These reflective questions are designed to encourage you to think about the material presented in this chapter

1 Why is it important to understand a person's culture, background or identity (such as being LGBTQI+ or Indigenous) when providing palliative care?

2 Of what benefit is an advanced decision to refuse treatment (advanced directive)?

3 How has palliative care changed from its initial focus on pain relief and cancer?

References

Akiyama, M., Hirai, K., Takebayashi, T., Morita, T., Miyashita, M., Takeuchi, A., Yamagishi, A., Kinoshita, H., Shirahige, Y., & Eguchi, K. (2016). The effects of community-wide dissemination of information on perceptions of palliative care, knowledge about opioids, and sense of security among cancer patients, their families, and the general public. *Supportive Care in Cancer, 24*(1), 347–356. https://doi.org/10.1007/s00520-015-2788-4

Anandarajah, G., Roseman, J., Lee, D., & Dhandhania, N. (2016). A 10-year longitudinal study of effects of a multifaceted residency spiritual care curriculum: Clinical ability, professional formation, end of life, and culture. *Journal of Pain and Symptom Management, 52*(6), 859–872.e1. https://doi.org/10.1016/j.jpainsymman.2016.06.006

Anderson, M., & Woticky, G. (2018). The end of life is an auspicious opportunity for healing: Decolonizing death and dying for urban Indigenous People. *International Journal of Indigenous Health, 13*(2), 48–60. https://doi.org/10.32799/ijih.v13i2.32062

Bartlett, C., Marshall, M., & Marshall, A. (2012). Two-Eyed Seeing and other lessons learned within a co-learning journey of bringing together indigenous and mainstream knowledges and ways of knowing. *Journal of Environmental Studies and Sciences, 2*, 331–340. https://doi.org/10.1007/s13412-012-0086-8

Bassah, N., Beranek, J., Kennedy, M., Onabadejo, J., & Santos Salas, A. (2024). Inequities in access to palliative and end-of-life care in the black population in Canada: A scoping review. *International Journal for Equity in Health, 23*(1), 81. https://doi.org/10.1186/s12939-024-02173-9

Black, R., Hasson, F., Slater, P., Beck, E., & McIlfatrick, S. (2024). Building public engagement and access to palliative care and advance care planning: A qualitative study. *BMC Palliative Care, 23*(1), 98. https://doi.org/10.1186/s12904-024-01420-8

Bristowe, K., Hodson, M., Wee, B., Almack, K., Johnson, K., Daveson, B. A., Koffman, J., McEnhill, L., & Harding, R. (2018). Recommendations to reduce inequalities for LGBT people facing advanced illness: ACCESSCare national qualitative interview study. *Palliative Medicine, 32*(1), 23–35. https://doi.org/10.1177/0269216317705102

Cain, C. L., Surbone, A., Elk, R., & Kagawa-Singer, M. (2018). Culture and palliative care: Preferences, communication, meaning, and mutual decision making. *Journal of Pain and Symptom Management, 55*(5), 1408–1419. https://doi.org/10.1016/j.jpainsymman.2018.01.007

Canadian Partnership Against Cancer (2022). Beginning the journey into the spirit world: First Nations, Inuit and Métis approaches to palliative and end-of-life care in Canada. Retrieved August 28, 2025, from https://s22457.pcdn.co/wp-content/uploads/2023/02/Beginning-the-journey-into-the-spirit-world_2022.pdf

Canadian Society of Palliative Care Physicians. (2016). *How to improve palliative care in Canada*. Retrieved February 2, 2025, from https://pallmed.ca/wp-content/uploads/2023/02/Full-Report-How-to-Improve-Palliative-Care-in-Canada-FINAL-Nov-2016.pdf

Carr, D. (2011). Racial differences in end-of-life planning: Why don't Blacks and Latinos prepare for the inevitable? *Omega, 63*(1), 1–20. https://doi.org/10.2190/OM.63.1.a

Cervantes, L., Jones, J., Linas, S., & Fischer, S. (2017). Qualitative interviews exploring palliative care perspectives of Latinos on dialysis. *Clinical Journal of the American Society of Nephrology, 12*(5), 788–798. https://doi.org/10.2215/CJN.10260916

Collins, A., Sundararajan, V., Burchell, J., Millar, J., McLachlan, S. A., Krishnasamy, M., Le, B. H., Mileshkin, L., Hudson, P., & Philip, J. (2018). Transition points for the routine integration of palliative care in patients with advanced cancer. *Journal of Pain and Symptom Management, 56*(2), 185–194. https://doi.org/10.1016/j.jpainsymman.2018.03.022

Collins, A., McLachlan, S. A., & Philip, J. (2020). Community knowledge of and attitudes to palliative care: A descriptive study. *Palliative Medicine, 34*(2), 245–252. https://doi.org/10.1177/0269216319888371

Crooks, J., Trotter, S., Patient Public Involvement Consortium, & Clarke, G. (2023). How does ethnicity affect presence of advance care planning in care records for individuals with advanced disease? A mixed-methods systematic review. *BMC Palliative Care, 22*(1), 43. https://doi.org/10.1186/s12904-023-01168-7

Duggleby, W., Kuchera, S., MacLeod, R., Holyoke, P., Scott, T., Holtslander, L., Letendre, A., Moeke-Maxwell, T., Burhansstipanov, L., & Chambers, T. (2015). Indigenous people's experiences at the end of life. *Palliative & Supportive Care, 13*(6), 1721–1733. https://doi.org/10.1017/S147895151500070X

Enzinger, A. C., Ghosh, K., Keating, N. L., Cutler, D. M., Clark, C. R., Florez, N., Landrum, M. B., & Wright, A. A. (2023). Racial and ethnic disparities in opioid access and urine drug screening among older patients with poor-prognosis cancer near the end of life. *Journal of Clinical Oncology, 41*(14), 2511–2522. https://doi.org/10.1200/JCO.22.01413

Flieger, S. P., Chui, K., & Koch-Weser, S. (2020). Lack of awareness and common misconceptions about palliative care among adults: Insights from a national survey. *Journal of General Internal Medicine, 35*(7), 2059–2064. https://doi.org/10.1007/s11606-020-05730-4

Frau, S., Kananga, A. M., Kingolo, J. N., Kanyunyu, G. M., Zongwe, A. K. H., Tshilengi, A. N., & Ravinetto, R. (2021). Training on adequate use of opioid analgesics in West and Central Africa: A neglected step on the way to access to essential medicines? *Journal of Pharmaceutical Policy and Practice, 14*(1), 104. https://doi.org/10.1186/s40545-021-00388-7

Givler, A., Bhatt, H., & Maani-Fogelman, P. A. (2023, May 22). *The importance of cultural competence in pain and palliative care.* In StatPearls. StatPearls Publishing. https://www.ncbi.nlm.nih.gov/books/NBK493154/

Gone, J. P. (2009). A community-based treatment for Native American historical trauma: Prospects for evidence-based practice. *Journal of Consulting and Clinical Psychology, 77*(4), 751–762. https://doi.org/10.1037/a0015390

Harding, R., Epiphaniou, E., & Chidgey-Clark, J. (2012). Needs, experiences, and preferences of sexual minorities for end-of-life care and palliative care: A systematic review. *Journal of Palliative Medicine, 15*(5), 602–611. https://doi.org/10.1089/jpm.2011.0279

Hospice Africa Uganda (n.d.) *Our history: Spreading the vision through education and training*. Retrieved September 1, 2025, from https://www.hospice-africa.org/history

Hui, D., & Bruera, E. (2016). Integrating palliative care into the trajectory of cancer care. *Nature Reviews Clinical Oncology, 13*(3), 159–171. https://doi.org/10.1038/nrclinonc.2015.201

Jawed, A., & Comer, A. R. (2024). Disparities in end-of-life care for racial minorities: A narrative review. *Annals of Palliative Medicine, 13*(2), 309–321. https://doi.org/10.21037/apm-23-459

Kelly, L., Linkewich, B., Cromarty, H., St Pierre-Hansen, N., Antone, I., & Giles, C. (2009). Palliative care of First Nations people: A qualitative study of bereaved family members. *Canadian Family Physician, 55*(4), 394–395.e7.

Kunonga, T. P., Johnson, E. E., Din, U., Westhead, E., Dewhurst, F., & Hanratty, B. (2025). Ethnic inequalities in palliative care prescribing in high income countries - A rapid systematic review. *BMC Palliative Care, 24*(1), 119. https://doi.org/10.1186/s12904-025-01742-1

Li, Z., Beck, E., McIlfatrick, S., & Hasson, F. (2025). A qualitative study exploring overseas Chinese understanding and experiences of advance care planning. *International Journal of Palliative Nursing, 31*(7), 326–336. https://doi.org/10.12968/ijpn.2024.0018

Li, I. F., Huang, S. M., Lee, C. F., Chen, Y. H., & Hsiung, Y. (2021). Perceptions of behavioral awareness, intention, and readiness for advance care planning: A mixed-method study among older Indigenous patients with late-stage cancers in remote areas of eastern Taiwan. *International Journal of Environmental Research and Public health, 18*(16), 8665. https://doi.org/10.3390/ijerph18168665

Lunn, J. S. (2003). Spiritual care in a multi-religious context. *Journal of Pain & Palliative care Pharmacotherapy, 17*(3-4), 153–169.

Lynch, T., Connor, S., & Clark, D. (2013). Mapping levels of palliative care development: A global update. *Journal of Pain and Symptom Management, 45*(6), 1094–1106. https://doi.org/10.1016/j.jpainsymman.2012.05.011

Mende-Siedlecki, P., Lin, J., Ferron, S., Gibbons, C., Drain, A., & Goharzad, A. (2021). Seeing no pain: Assessing the generalizability of racial bias in pain perception. *Emotion, 21*(5), 932–950. https://doi.org/10.1037/emo0000953

McAdoo, S. P., Brown, E. A., Chesser, A. M., Farrington, K., & Salisbury, E. M.; Pan-Thames Renal Audit Group (2012). Measuring the quality of end of life management in patients with advanced kidney disease: Results from the pan-Thames renal audit group. *Nephrology, Dialysis, Transplantation, 27*(4), 1548–1554. https://doi.org/10.1093/ndt/gfr514

McGrath, P. (2007). 'I don't want to be in that big city; this is my country here': Research findings on Aboriginal peoples' preference to die at home. *The Australian Journal of Rural Health, 15*(4), 264–268. https://doi.org/10.1111/j.1440-1584.2007.00904.x

McIlfatrick, S., Slater, P., Beck, E., Bamidele, O., McCloskey, S., Carr, K., Muldrew, D., Hanna-Trainor, L., & Hasson, F. (2021a). Examining public knowledge, attitudes and perceptions towards palliative care: A mixed method sequential study. *BMC Palliative Care, 20*(1), 44. https://doi.org/10.1186/s12904-021-00730-5

McIlfatrick, S., Slater, P., Bamidele, O., Muldrew, D., Beck, E., & Hasson, F. (2021b). *'It's almost superstition: If I don't think about it, it won't happen'*. Public knowledge and attitudes towards advance care planning: A sequential mixed methods study. *Palliative Medicine, 35*(7), 1356–1365. https://doi.org/10.1177/02692163211015838

Middleton-Green, L. (2008). Managing total pain at the end of life: A case study analysis. *Nursing Standard, 23*(6), 41–46. https://doi.org/10.7748/ns2008.10.23.6.41.c6708

Ntizimira, C., Deo, M. S., Dunne, M., & Krakauer, E. (2022). Decolonizing end-of-life care: Lessons and opportunities. *Ecancer, 16*, ed121. https://doi.org/10.3332/ecancer.2022.ed121

Periyakoil, V. S., Neri, E., & Kraemer, H. (2015). No easy talk: A mixed methods study of doctor reported barriers to conducting effective end-of-life conversations with diverse patients. *PloS One, 10*(4), e0122321. https://doi.org/10.1371/journal.pone.0122321

Peters, E. J., & Andersen, C. (2013*). Indigenous in the city: Contemporary identities and cultural innovation*. UBC Press.

Racine, L., Fowler-Kerry, S., & Aiyer, H. (2022). Integrative review of the needs and challenges of indigenous palliative care in rural and remote settings. *Journal of Advanced Nursing, 78*, 2693–2712. https://doi.org/10.1111/jan.15287

Rietjens, J. A. C., Sudore, R. L., Connolly, M., van Delden, J. J., Drickamer, M. A., Droger, M., van der Heide, A., Heyland, D. K., Houttekier, D., Janssen, D. J. A., Orsi, L., Payne, S., Seymour, J., Jox, R. J., Korfage, I. J.; European Association for Palliative Care (2017). Definition and recommendations for advance care planning: An international consensus supported by the European Association for Palliative Care. *The Lancet. Oncology, 18*(9), e543–e551. https://doi.org/10.1016/S1470-2045(17)30582-X

Sallnow, L., Smith, R., Ahmedzai, S. H., Bhadelia, A., Chamberlain, C., Cong, Y., Doble, B., Dullie, L., Durie, R., Finkelstein, E. A., Guglani, S., Hodson, M., Husebø, B. S., Kellehear, A., Kitzinger, C., Knaul, F. M., Murray, S. A., Neuberger, J., O'Mahony, S., & Rajagopal, M. R.... Lancet Commission on the value of death (2022). Report of the Lancet Commission on the Value of Death: Bringing death back into life. *Lancet, 399*(10327), 837–884. https://doi.org/10.1016/S0140-6736(21)02314-X

Saphire, M. L., Prsic, E. H., Canavan, M. E., Wang, S. J., Presley, C. J., & Davidoff, A. J. (2020). Patterns of symptom management medication receipt at end-of-life among Medicare beneficiaries with lung cancer. *Journal of Pain and Symptom Management, 59*(4), 767–777.e1. https://doi.org/10.1016/j.jpainsymman.2019.11.015

Sudore, R. L., Lum, H. D., You, J. J., Hanson, L. C., Meier, D. E., Pantilat, S. Z., Matlock, D. D., Rietjens, J. A. C., Korfage, I. J., Ritchie, C. S., Kutner, J. S., Teno, J. M., Thomas, J., McMahan, R. D., & Heyland, D. K. (2017). Defining advance care planning for adults: A consensus definition from a multidisciplinary Delphi panel. *Journal of Pain and Symptom Management, 53*(5), 821–832.e1. https://doi.org/10.1016/j.jpainsymman.2016.12.331

Tobin, J., Rogers, A., Winterburn, I., Tullie, S., Kalyanasundaram, A., Kuhn, I., & Barclay, S. (2022). Hospice care access inequalities: A systematic review and narrative synthesis. *BMJ Supportive & Palliative Care, 12*(2), 142–151. https://doi.org/10.1136/bmjspcare-2020-002719

Wakefield, D., Kane, C. E., Chidiac, C., Braybrook, D., & Harding, R.. (2021). Why does palliative care need to consider access and care for LGBTQ people? *Palliative Medicine*, 35(10), 1730–1732. https://doi.org/10.1177/02692163211055011

Waran, E., O'Connor, N., Zubair, M. Y., & May, P. (2016). 'Finishing up' on country: Challenges and compromises. *Internal Medicine Journal, 46*(9), 1108–1111. https://doi.org/10.1111/imj.13186

Warbelow, S. (2025). *Understanding executive orders and what they mean for the LGBTQ+ community*. Human Rights Campaign. Retrieved September 1, 2025, from https://www.hrc.org/news/understanding-executive-orders-and-what-they-mean-for-the-lgbtq-community

World Health Organization (2020). *Palliative care: Key facts*. Retrieved August 28, 2025, from https://www.who.int/news-room/fact-sheets/detail/palliative-care

Worldwide Hospice Palliative Care Alliance. (2020). *Global atlas of palliative care* (2nd edn.). Worldwide Hospice Palliative Care Alliance. https://www.palliativecare.in/wp-content/uploads/2020/10/Global-Atlas-2nd-Edition-2020.pdf

Index

Note: Page references in *italics* refer to figures and **bold** refer to tables.